Gastrointestinal System

D1333854

Short Term Book Loan

ONE WEEK

First and second edition authors:

Elizabeth Cheshire

Melanie Sarah Long

Third edition author:

Rusheng Chew

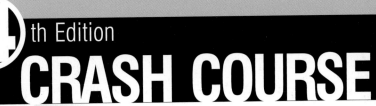

4th Edition
CRASH COURSE

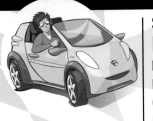

SERIES EDITOR:
Dan Horton-Szar
BSc(Hons) MBBS(Hons) MRCGP
Northgate Medical Practice
Canterbury
Kent, UK

FACULTY ADVISOR:
Martin Lombard
MD MSc FRCPI FRCP(Lond)
Consultant Gastroenterologist and Hepatologist
Royal Liverpool University Hospital
Liverpool, UK

Gastrointestinal System

Megan Griffiths
MBChB(Hons) Foundation Doctor
Wirral University Teaching Hospital
Merseyside, UK

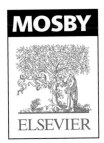

MOSBY

ELSEVIER

Edinburgh London New York Oxford Philadelphia St Louis Sydney Toronto 2012

MOSBY
ELSEVIER

Commissioning Editor: Jeremy Bowes
Development Editor: Sheila Black
Project Manager: Andrew Riley
Designer: Stewart Larking
Icon Illustrations: Geo Parkin
Illustrator: Cactus

First edition 1998

Second edition 2002

Reprinted 2003 (twice), 2005

Third edition 2008

Fourth edition 2012

ISBN: 978-0-7234-3620-1

British Library Cataloguing in Publication Data
A catalogue record for this book is available from the British Library

Library of Congress Cataloging in Publication Data
A catalog record for this book is available from the Library of Congress

ELSEVIER your source for books,
journals and multimedia
in the health sciences

www.elsevierhealth.com

Working together to grow
libraries in developing countries

www.elsevier.com | www.bookaid.org | www.sabre.org

ELSEVIER   **BOOK AID**
International   Sabre Foundation

The
Publisher's
policy is to use
**paper manufactured
from sustainable forests**

Printed in China

Series editor foreword

The *Crash Course* series first published in 1997 and now, 15 years on, we are still going strong. Medicine never stands still, and the work of keeping this series relevant for today's students is an ongoing process. These fourth editions build on the success of the previous titles and incorporate new and revised material, to keep the series up to date with current guidelines for best practice, and recent developments in medical research and pharmacology.

We always listen to feedback from our readers, through focus groups and student reviews of the *Crash Course* titles. For the fourth editions we have completely re-written our self-assessment material to keep up with today's 'single-best answer' and 'extended matching question' formats. The artwork and layout of the titles has also been largely re-worked to make it easier on the eye during long sessions of revision.

Despite fully revising the books with each edition, we hold fast to the principles on which we first developed the series. *Crash Course* will always bring you all the information you need to revise in compact, manageable volumes that integrate basic medical science and clinical practice. The books still maintain the balance between clarity and conciseness, and provide sufficient depth for those aiming at distinction. The authors are medical students and junior doctors who have recent experience of the exams you are now facing, and the accuracy of the material is checked by a team of faculty advisors from across the UK.

I wish you all the best for your future careers!

Dr Dan Horton-Szar

Series Editor

Author

Medical exams can be a daunting experience. This textbook aims to help prepare students by providing a comprehensive overview of the gastrointestinal system, presented in a clear and concise manner. It takes readers through a logical thought process starting with basic anatomy and physiology and culminating with clinical disorders. This provides a strong foundation which allows students to understand the basic sciences, and then apply this to a clinical scenario.

As well as aiding revision, hopefully this book will also prove a useful resource when making the transition from student to house officer. It provides a detailed overview of the common gastrointestinal problems that you will certainly face on the wards.

I hope that you enjoy reading this book and find it a useful resource.

Megan Griffiths

Liverpool
2012

Faculty advisor

Despite their best intentions and notice of timetables, all students find that exams come too soon. *Crash Course* is written by people who've been there for people who are getting there! The series is largely written by students in their final year or just after qualifying as doctors who have recently passed their exams and who know what you need to know to pass and excel in your exam. This book on the *Gastrointestinal System* tells you that, but I hope is comprehensive enough to give you even more – a good grounding in clinical gastroenterology and hepatology. It is an exciting subject area and *Crash Course* is designed to bring it alive with information. The illustrations in this book pack in a thousand more words than we could in the text and I hope you will enjoy learning from them.

Martin Lombard

Liverpool
2012

Acknowledgements

There are two people who deserve a special mention for their role in the production of the 4th edition of this book. The first is Martin Lombard, faculty advisor, whose knowledge of the gastrointestinal system and general medicine has ensured that this book has kept up to date with all the recent changes in clinical medicine. The second is Sheila Black, content development specialist, for all her guidance and patience in ensuring that this book would be completed on time.

To Rusheng Chew and the authors of previous editions, thank you for providing such a great format and starting base, upon which I have been able to build.

I would also like to take this opportunity to thank my family and friends for all their love and support.

Contents

Contents

Introduction to the gastrointestinal system ① 1

● Objectives

After reading this chapter you should be able to:
- Outline and reproduce the basic structure of the gastrointestinal system
- Describe the functions of the gastrointestinal system
- Name the major food groups and their roles
- Describe the embryological development of the gastrointestinal tract

ANATOMICAL OVERVIEW

The gastrointestinal (GI) system is comprised of several organs (Fig. 1.1). Anatomically, it is essentially a muscular tube which maintains the same basic structure throughout its length (Fig. 1.2). From the innermost to the outermost, the layers which comprise the basic structure are the mucosa (composed of the epithelial layer, lamina propria and muscularis mucosae), submucosa, two smooth layers (the inner is circular, and the outer longitudinal) and finally the serosa.

There are also intrinsic submucosal (Meissner's) and mucosal (Auerbach's) nerve plexuses, the activity of which is moderated by extrinsic innervations and hormones.

HINTS AND TIPS

It is essential to know the basic structure of the GI tract and the order of the layers; MCQs often test this.

Food moves through the GI tract by gravity, voluntary muscle action (from the oral cavity to the oesophagus) and peristalisis (a wavelike movement involving the co-ordinated contraction of muscle in one area followed by relaxation in the next area; see Chapter 4). A series of sphincters prevent any reflux or backflow of food (Fig. 1.3).

Clinical Note

Among other factors, the integrity of the lower oesophageal sphincter protects against reflux of acid contents from the stomach (gastro-oesophageal reflux disease, or GORD).

FUNCTIONS OF THE GASTROINTESTINAL TRACT

We need a gut because our body needs to extract small molecules from the large molecules which are bound up in food for metabolism. A complete list of functions is in Fig. 1.4, with the main ones being motility, secretion, digestion and absorption.

Motility refers to the muscular contractions which cause the propulsion and mixing of gut contents. The tone of the smooth muscle layers maintains a constant pressure on the contents of the GI tract, allowing peristalsis (propulsive movements) and mixing to occur. In addition, sympathetic and parasympathetic reflexes occurring in different parts of the tract act through hormonal and neuronal mechanisms to modify the speed of food movement through the tract. The contents move through the tract at a rate at which they can be processed.

The other three principal functions are closely related. Secretory glands release digestive juices into the gut lumen. These juices contain enzymes which break up complex food structures into smaller absorbable units by hydrolysis, i.e. digestion. Following this, the products of digestion are absorbed into the blood or lymph from the gut lumen, mainly in the small intestine.

Other functions related to the digestive process include:

- Storage of waste material in the sigmoid colon and rectum
- Exocrine, endocrine and paracrine secretions are all involved in active digestion and the control of digestion and motility in the gut
- Some GI peptide hormones have local and systemic effects
- Excretion of waste products.

Fig. 1.1 Anatomy of the gastrointestinal tract, showing its surface markings. The transpyloric plane (of Addison) passes midway between the jugular notch and the symphysis pubis, and midway between the xiphisternum and the umbilicus. Surface regions: A = right hypochondriac; B = epigastric; C = left hypochondriac; D = right lumbar; E = umbilical; F = left lumbar; G = right iliac fossa; H = hypogastric; I = left iliac fossa.

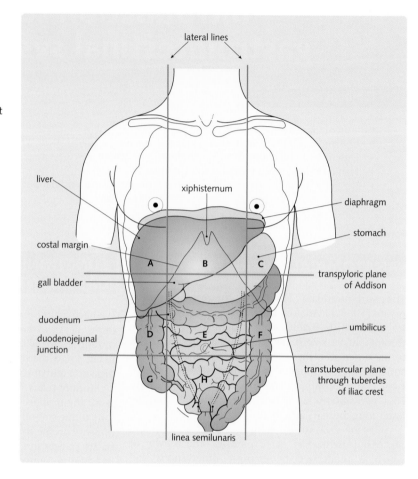

The GI tract is not sterile as it is open to the external environment. It is thus presented with a number of challenges on a daily basis, from harmful bacteria to toxic substances and so requires good defence mechanisms:

- *Sight, smell and taste* often alert us to the fact that food is contaminated. The vomit reflex exists to eject harmful material
- *The acid in the stomach* kills most of the bacteria ingested with food
- *The natural bacterial flora* of the gut prevent colonization by potentially harmful bacteria
- *Aggregations of lymphoid tissue* (part of the immune system) are present in the walls of the gut, known as Peyer's patches. These can mount an immune response to antigens found in the diet.

FOOD GROUPS

Food is a source of energy, minerals and vitamins which are required by the body for growth, maintenance and repair. The key food groups are carbohydrates, fat and protein, which are summarized in Fig. 1.5.

An average 70-kg male may survive for 5–6 weeks on body fat stores when deprived of food, provided he is able to drink water. Blood glucose levels drop during the initial few days, then rise and stabilize. During prolonged fasting, the body will also break down muscle, including heart muscle, to provide energy. This may lead to death from cardiac failure. However, most food-deprived people do not die from starvation directly, but from the inability to fight off infectious diseases.

Conversely, overeating is a major cause of morbidity. This is because excess food, which is stored as fat, leads to obesity and associated diseases such as ischaemic heart disease and type 2 diabetes.

A description of the major food groups follows. For a more comprehensive account of the food groups and the metabolic processes involved in starvation and overeating, see *Crash Course: Metabolism and Nutrition.*

Carbohydrate

Carbohydrates are the main energy source of most diets. They provide 17 kJ (4 kcal) of energy per gram. Most dietary carbohydrate is in the form of polysaccharides,

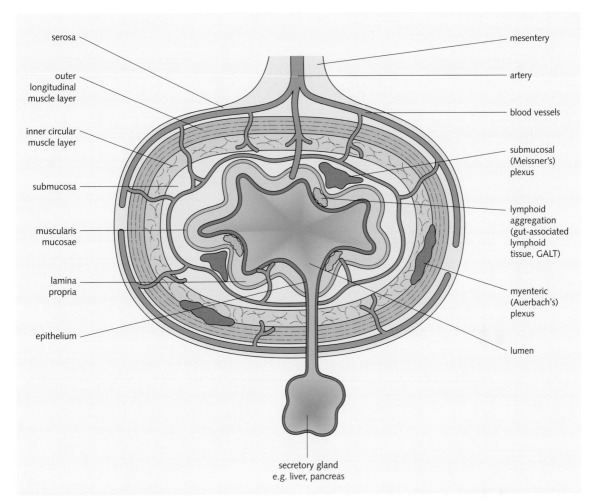

serosa

outer longitudinal muscle layer

inner circular muscle layer

submucosa

muscularis mucosae

lamina propria

epithelium

mesentery

artery

blood vessels

submucosal (Meissner's) plexus

lymphoid aggregation (gut-associated lymphoid tissue, GALT)

myenteric (Auerbach's) plexus

lumen

secretory gland e.g. liver, pancreas

Fig. 1.2   The basic structure of the gastrointestinal tract.

which consist of chains of glucose molecules. The principal ingested polysaccharides are starch, which is derived from plant sources, and glycogen from animal sources.

Other sources of carbohydrate are monosaccharides (glucose, fructose and galactose) and disaccharides (sucrose and lactose). Cellulose is an indigestible polysaccharide and is considered in the section on dietary fibre.

Carbohydrates are cheap forms of food, and so are easily taken in excess, often limiting the intake of other food constituents.

Protein

Protein is composed of amino acids linked by peptide bonds. Nine amino acids are essential for protein synthesis and nitrogen balance; the other necessary amino acids can be manufactured de novo in the body. Protein is required for tissue growth and repair. Meat is the principal source of protein, especially in the developed world.

We need 0.75 g of protein per kilogram of body weight per day, but in developed countries most people exceed this. In developing countries, combinations of certain foods can provide enough of the essential amino acids even though those foods, on their own, are low in some amino acids. A good example of a non-animal protein source which is high in essential amino acids is soybeans.

Proteins provide about the same amount of energy per gram as carbohydrates, but are not as easily utilized under normal circumstances.

Fat

Dietary fat is chiefly composed of triglycerides (esters of free fatty acids and glycerol, which may be saturated, monounsaturated or polyunsaturated). The essential fatty acids are linoleic acid and α-linoleic acid, which cannot be manufactured and so must be obtained from our diet.

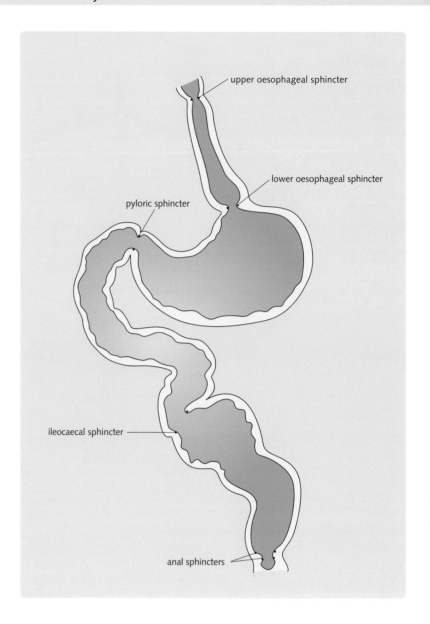

Fig. 1.3 Sphincters of the gastrointestinal tract.

upper oesophageal sphincter

lower oesophageal sphincter

pyloric sphincter

ileocaecal sphincter

anal sphincters

The body is efficient at manufacturing fats (triglycerides, sterols and phospholipids) and will lay down subcutaneous fat stores even on low-fat diets.

Dietary fat provides 37 kJ (9 kcal) of energy per gram. Nevertheless, due to its ill-effects when taken in excess, fats should comprise less than 35% of the total energy intake.

Water

Fluid intake and oxidation of food provides water for the body. About 1 litre of water is needed per day to balance insensible losses such as sweating, metabolism and exhalation of water vapour (more water is required in hot climates). Excess water is excreted in the urine by the kidneys; inadequate intake leads to dehydration.

Water is also needed for digestion, as digestion involves enzymatic hydrolysis of the bonds linking the smaller units which make up complex food structures.

Minerals

These are chemicals that must be present in the diet to maintain good health. Over 20 have so far been identified, e.g. iron and calcium.

Fig. 1.4 A summary of the functions of the gastrointestinal tract. (UOS = upper oesophageal sphincter.)

Function	Mechanism/process involved	Where it occurs
Digestion of food	(i) Mastication	Mouth: with teeth and tongue
	(ii) Swallowing	Oropharynx: relaxation of UOS
	(iii) Mixing	Stomach and small intestine
	(iv) Enzymatic digestion	Stomach and small intestine
	(v) Absorption	Stomach, small intestine and large intestine
Motility	(i) Peristalsis	Throughout gut
	(ii) Mass movement	Throughout gut
Storage of food waste		Stomach, sigmoid colon and rectum
Excretion	Defecation	Rectum and anus
Exocrine secretion	(i) Mucus/saliva secretion	Salivary gland
	(ii) HCl/pepsin/mucus secretion	Gastric glands of stomach
	(iii) HCO_3/amylase/lipase secretion	Pancreas
	(iv) Bile salt secretion	Liver
Endocrine secretion	(i) Gastrin secretion	Stomach
	(ii) Secretin secretion	Duodenal mucosa
	(iii) Insulin secretion	Pancreas
Paracrine secretions	Somatostatin secretion	Mucosa
Defence	(i) Smell, sight, taste	Oral cavity, cephalic region
	(ii) Gastric acid secretion	Stomach
	(iii) Vomit reflex	Stomach up to mouth
	(iv) Gut flora	Throughout gut
	(v) Mucus secretion	Throughout gut
	(vi) Immune response	Peyer's patches, macrophages in mucosa
	(vii) Secretion of IgA	Mucosal secretions

Trace elements (e.g. zinc, copper and iodine) are substances that, by definition, are present in the body in low concentrations (less than 100 parts per million) and include some minerals. It is not yet known whether all trace elements are essential for health.

Vitamins

Vitamins are classified as fat soluble or water soluble; vitamins A, D, E and K are fat soluble, the other vitamins are water soluble.

Fat-soluble vitamins are stored in fatty tissue in the body (mainly in the liver) and are not usually excreted in the urine. It is thus possible to have an excess of these vitamins, which may be toxic, e.g. vitamin A poisoning. On the other hand, absorption of fat-soluble vitamins is dependent upon the absorption of dietary fat: deficiency can occur in cases of fat malabsorption (see Chapter 4).

Body stores of water-soluble vitamins (other than vitamin B_{12}) are smaller than stores of fat-soluble vitamins. They are excreted in the urine and deficiencies of water-soluble vitamins are more common.

Dietary fibre

Dietary fibre consists of indigestible carbohydrates, primarily cellulose but also lignin and pectin. Cellulose cannot be digested as we do not have the enzymes

Fig. 1.5 A summary of the dietary food groups.

Food group		Source	Site of digestion	Function
Carbohydrates		Sugary foods, potatoes, pasta etc.	Mouth and small intestine	Energy source
Fats		Meats, oil, butter etc.	Small intestine	Energy source
Protein		Meat, pulses etc.	Stomach and small intestine	Synthesis and repair of tissues
Vitamins	Fat-soluble (A, D, E, K)	Meat, fish and vegetable oils	Not digested	Maintenance of general health
Vitamins	Water-soluble (B, C)	Milk, meat, fruit and vegetables	Not digested	
Minerals		Meat, milk, vegetables, cereals	Not digested	Maintenance of general health
Fibre		Plant foods	Not digested	Bulking agent, aids gut motility

necessary to hydrolyse the b-glycosidic bonds linking its glucose molecules, unlike starch where the glucose residues are linked by α-glycosidic bonds.

Although it does not provide energy, fibre adds bulk to the bowel contents and increases gut motility, thus preventing constipation. It also decreases absorption of toxic compounds, e.g. some carcinogens, due to its binding properties.

DEVELOPMENT

The gastrointestinal (GI) system (Fig. 1.1) develops entirely from the endoderm in the embryo. The formation of the tube is largely passive; it depends on the cephalo-caudal and lateral folding of the embryo.

The yolk sac produces blood cells and vessels, and is the site of haematopoiesis for the first 2 months from conception. Later, it becomes inverted and incorporated into the body cavity. The folding of the embryo constricts the initial communication between the embryo and the yolk sac.

The remnant of this communication is the vitelline duct, which normally disappears in utero. Where it persists, it is known as a Meckel's diverticulum.

The gut tube divides into foregut, midgut and hindgut. Their blood supply is from the coeliac trunk, superior mesenteric artery and inferior mesenteric artery respectively (Fig. 1.6). All derivatives from each division of the gut tube will thus have the same principal blood supply. The superior mesenteric artery is in the umbilicus.

The nerve supply of the foregut and midgut is from the vagus nerve (Xth cranial nerve), while the hindgut gets its nerve supply from the pelvic splanchnic nerves.

HINTS AND TIPS

The embryological development of the GI tract is a common question in exams – make sure you know the key stages, as well as the blood supply to the gut divisions and the developments during the herniation of the midgut.

The gut tube starts straight but twists during development and the midgut grows rapidly, with the developing liver occupying most of the space. As development progresses, there is not enough room in the fetal abdomen to accommodate the rapidly developing gut because of the large size of the liver and the two sets of kidneys. The midgut therefore herniates into the umbilical cord between weeks 7 and 11 of gestation, continuing its development outside the abdominal cavity.

The midgut, which forms an umbilical loop outside the abdominal cavity, undergoes a clockwise rotation of 180° around the axis of the superior mesenteric artery and what was the inferior limb becomes the superior limb (and vice versa). At the same time, it elongates to form the loops of the jejunum and ileum.

During the 11th week, the midgut returns into the abdomen, the process being known as the reduction of the physiological midgut hernia. The reason for this

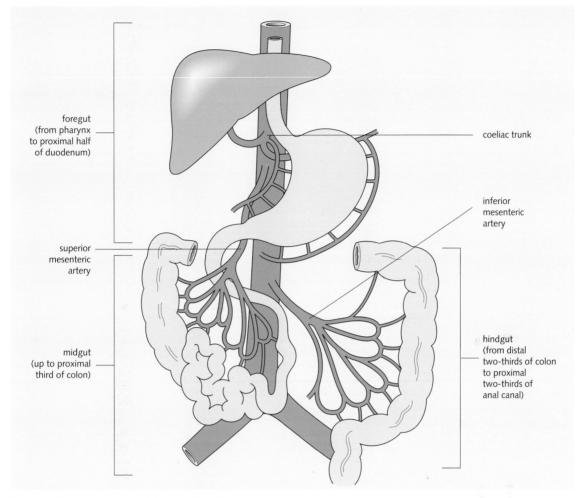

foregut
(from pharynx
to proximal half
of duodenum)

coeliac trunk

inferior
mesenteric
artery

superior
mesenteric
artery

midgut
(up to proximal
third of colon)

hindgut
(from distal
two-thirds of colon
to proximal
two-thirds of
anal canal)

Fig. 1.6 The arterial supply of the gastrointestinal tract.

is not well-explained, but is possibly due to the reduction in size of the liver and kidneys as well as the enlargement of the abdomen. The part forming the small intestine returns first to occupy the central part of the abdomen. The part forming the large intestine undergoes a 270° anticlockwise rotation as it returns so that the caecum lies under the liver. The tube then elongates again so that the caecum points downwards. The falciform ligament lies in front of the liver and the lesser omentum lies behind the liver. These developmental stages are shown in Fig. 1.7, while other organs and structures develop as described below:

- The liver and pancreas develop from endodermal diverticula that bud off the duodenum in weeks 4–6 (see Fig. 6.5)
- Much of the mouth (including the muscles of mastication and tongue) and the oesophagus develop from the branchial arches, of which there are six,

the first four being well-defined while the fifth and sixth are rudimentary

- The muscles of mastication, mylohyoid and anterior belly of digastric develop from the first (mandibular) arch, supplied by the trigeminal nerve (Vth cranial nerve)
- The anterior two-thirds of the tongue develop from three mesenchymal buds from the first pair of branchial arches. The posterior belly of digastric develops from the second arch, supplied by the facial nerve (VIIth cranial nerve)
- Stylopharyngeus develops from the third arch, supplied by the glossopharyngeal nerve (IXth cranial nerve)
- Cricothyroid, the constrictors of the pharynx and the striated muscles of oesophagus develop from the fourth and sixth arches, supplied by branches of the vagus nerve. The fifth arch is often absent.

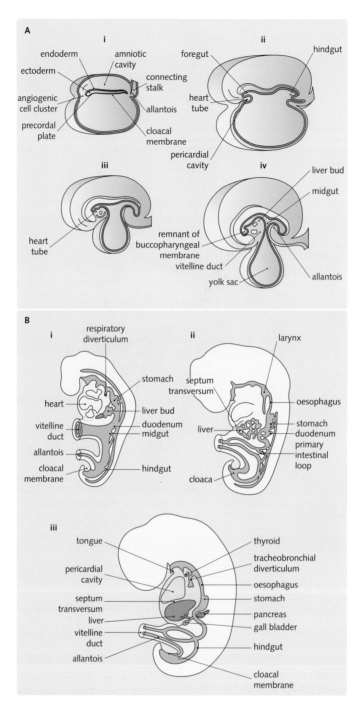

Fig. 1.7 (A) Stages of embryonic development of the gastrointestinal tract. Schematic drawings of sagittal sections through embryos at various stages of development, showing the development of the foregut, midgut and hindgut. (i) Presomite embryo. (ii) 7-somite embryo. (iii) 14-somite embryo. (iv) Embryo at 1 month. (B) Schematic drawings showing the primitive gastrointestinal tract and formation of the liver. (i) Diagram showing a 3-mm embryo (approx. 25 days). (ii) Embryo at 32 days (5 mm). (iii) Diagram of a 9-mm embryo (36 days) showing caudal expansion of the liver.

After reading this chapter you should be able to:
- List the components of the upper gastrointestinal tract
- Outline the embryological development of the structures making up the upper gastrointestinal tract
- Describe the anatomy and histological structure of the different components: tongue, oesophagus, salivary glands
- List the factors which affect appetite
- List the functions of saliva
- Describe the mechanism of swallowing
- Outline the factors which cause vomiting
- Outline the following types of disorders in the upper gastrointestinal tract: congenital abnormalities, infections and inflammatory disease, vascular disease and neoplastic disease

OVERVIEW

The upper gastrointestinal tract starts at the mouth and ends at the ligament of Trietze which separates the third and fourth parts of the duodenum. Associated structures include the tongue and salivary glands. Ingestion and the initial breaking up of food occur in the mouth, after which the food boluses are swallowed and enter the oesophagus. This is helped by the action of the tongue and pharyngeal muscles, as well as saliva secreted by the salivary glands.

FUNCTIONS AND PHYSIOLOGY

Food intake and its control

The control of food intake is complex and the hypothalamus plays an important role. Young people burn off excess intake as heat and through physical activity. They maintain a relatively constant weight, but this ability reduces with age.

Genetics have a huge influence on feeding and can account for up to 70% of the difference in body mass index in later life.

Signals which affect appetite

There are a number of factors which regulate appetite:

- *Blood glucose concentration* activates glucoreceptors in the hypothalamus, which act to up-regulate hunger when blood glucose levels fall, or up-regulate satiety when blood glucose concentrations rise
- *Fat ingestion* releases cholecystokinin (CCK), which slows stomach emptying, making us feel full
- *Calcitonin*, a peptide hormone secreted by the thyroid gland, acts to reduce appetite
- *Insulin* acts to up-regulate appetite, but glucagon down-regulates it
- Deposition of fat may lead to control of appetite by neuronal and hormonal signals. *Leptin*, a protein secreted by white fat cells, acts on the leptin receptors in the hypothalamus. This is thought to be part of the main satiety centre in the brain. Leptin produces a feedback mechanism between adipose tissue and the brain, acting as a 'lipostat', thus controlling fat stores. Leptin inhibits neuropeptide Y, which is the most potent peptide to stimulate feeding
- *Cold environments stimulate appetite*, whereas hot environments inhibit it
- *Distension of a full stomach inhibits appetite*, but contraction of an empty stomach stimulates it.

Central controls

The satiety centre is found in the ventromedial wall and the paraventricular nucleus of the hypothalamus. Stimulation of this inhibits food intake (aphagia), but lesions in this area may result in hyperphagia.

Glucostats in the brain measure the utilization of glucose. Diabetic patients feel hungry despite high blood glucose concentrations, because they lack insulin and, therefore, the cellular ability to take up glucose.

A feeding centre (not specific for hunger) is found in the lateral hypothalamus. Stimulation of this area increases eating and lesions here result in aphagia.

Other important central nervous system controls include opioids, somatostatin and growth-hormone-releasing hormone, all of which increase appetite. 5-Hydroxytryptamine (5-HT, serotonin), dopamine and γ-aminobutyric acid (GABA) all decrease appetite.

Diurnal variation

Carbohydrates are generally metabolized during the day, and fats at night. The hypothalamus is responsible for the switch between the two.

Mastication

Mastication breaks up large food particles, mixing them with salivary secretions and aiding subsequent digestion. Molecules dissolve in salivary secretions and stimulate taste buds. Odours are released that activate the olfactory system, leading to the initiation of reflex salivation and gastric acid secretions.

The muscles of mastication cause movement of the mandible at the temporomandibular joint. The digastric and mylohyoid muscles open the mouth, while the infrahyoid muscles stabilize the hyoid bone during mastication.

The teeth, gums, palate and tongue also play an important role, manipulating food and immobilizing it between the crushing surfaces of the teeth. The tongue then propels the bolus of food along the palate towards the pharynx, initiating the swallowing reflex.

Salivation

The average rate of salivary secretion is 1–2 L per day. Saliva composition varies according to the rate and site of production, but the main components are water, proteins and electrolytes. Primary secretion from the acini produces an isotonic fluid that is modified in the ducts (Fig. 2.1).

Control of salivary secretion

Secretion of saliva is under the control of the salivary centre in the medulla. Parasympathetic innervation causes an up-regulation in secretion and sympathetic innervation causes a downregulation. Parasympathetic cholinergic stimulation produces a watery secretion, which is blocked by atropine. This is given before surgery to reduce the risk of aspiration of saliva.

Sympathetic adrenergic and noradrenergic stimulation produce thick mucoid secretions, which add to the dry mouth sensation during the fright–fight–flight response.

There is a baseline level of salivary secretion, which is about 0.5 mL/min and is due to ongoing low-level parasympathetic stimulation. This baseline secretion prevents the mouth and pharynx from drying out.

On top of the baseline, increases in salivary secretion occur reflexively. There are two types of salivary

Fig. 2.1 Secretion of saliva. The primary secretion is released into the blind-ending acini and the fluid then flows through a series of converging ducts for secondary modification, before entering the oral cavity. The parotid glands produce the most serous secretions.

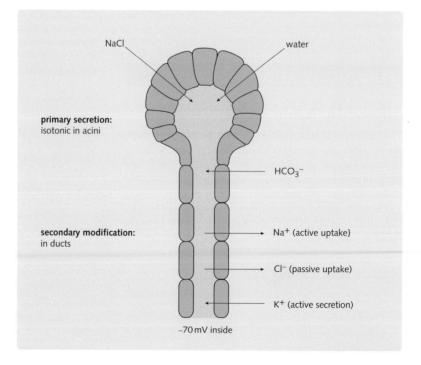

NaCl

water

primary secretion:
isotonic in acini

HCO_3^-

secondary modification:
in ducts

Na^+ (active uptake)

Cl^- (passive uptake)

K^+ (active secretion)

−70 mV inside

reflex: the simple reflex and the conditioned, or acquired, reflex. In the simple reflex, chemoreceptors in the mouth and oropharynx are activated by the taste of food; for example, amyl nitrate and citric acid produce copious secretion, hence sucking on a lemon wedge increases the rate of secretion about tenfold.

In the conditioned reflex, no oral stimulation is needed. Thinking, smelling and seeing food causes salivation by activating the salivary centre via the cerebral cortex. The conditioned reflex is acquired in response to previous experience.

Chewing produces saliva secretion by stimulating receptors in the masticatory muscles and joints. Paradontal mechanoreceptors around the teeth can also stimulate saliva.

However salivation is initiated, the impulses to the salivary glands travel via the autonomic nerves (Fig. 2.2).

Denervation causes dribbling. This is known as Canon's law of denervation hypersensitivity. Normally receptors are localized at neuroeffector junctions, but, if nerves are cut, receptors spread all over the gland and it becomes excessively sensitive to circulating acetylcholine, producing copious amounts of saliva.

There are four main sites at which the sympathetic and parasympathetic nerves can act to modify saliva secretion:

- The acini producing the primary secretion
- The ducts, which modify the secretions
- The blood vessels providing substances required for secretion and energy-containing nutrients, and removal of waste
- The myoepithelial cells surrounding the ducts and acini.

Salivary electrolytes

The major electrolytes found in saliva are Na^+, K^+, Cl^- and HCO_3^-. The concentrations vary according to the rate of flow (Fig. 2.3). Levels of Na^+ and Cl^- in saliva are hypotonic, but levels of HCO_3^- and K^+ are hypertonic at higher rates of flow. Saliva is hypotonic overall (about 200 mmol/L) and alkaline.

Salivary proteins

Salivary proteins include amylase, ribonuclease, R protein (which protects vitamin B_{12} as it passes through the duodenum, jejunum and ileum), lipase (important in cystic fibrosis when pancreatic lipase is lost), lysozyme, secretory IgA (immunoglobulin A), IgG and IgM.

Epidermal growth factor (EGF) is also secreted in saliva. This has a protective role at the gastroduodenal mucosa, by preventing the development of ulcers and promoting healing.

Functions of saliva and the salivary glands

The functions of saliva and the salivary glands include:

- General cleansing and protection of the buccal cavity, by washing away food particles which attract bacteria
- Moistening of the buccal cavity for speech (by aiding movements of the lips and tongue) and breastfeeding (saliva forms a seal around the mother's nipple)
- Secretion of digestive enzymes, especially salivary amylase, which hydrolyses linkages in starch
- Dissolving many food components, thus contributing to the taste of food
- Lubrication of the buccal cavity by mucus-secreting units of glands (under sympathetic and parasympathetic control), which helps swallowing
- Secretion of the antibacterial enzyme lysozyme, which protects teeth
- Secretion of IgA by plasma cells in connective tissue, which act to protect the body from invasion of microorganisms. The secretory component of IgA is synthesized by striated duct cells
- Neutralizing acid produced by bacteria as well as acids in food by the presence of bicarbonate; this helps to prevent dental caries.

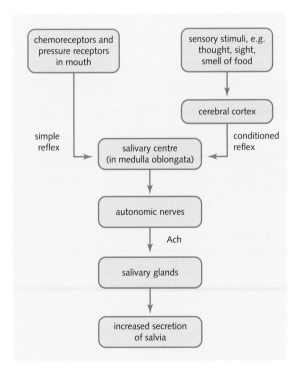

Fig. 2.2 Control of salivation. Two reflexes, the simple reflex and the conditioned (acquired) reflex, increase salivation above the baseline level of around 0.5 mL/min.

Fig. 2.3 Salivary composition against flow rate. (Redrawn with permission from Thaysen JH et al. Secretion control in salivation. Am J Physiol 1954; 178:155.)

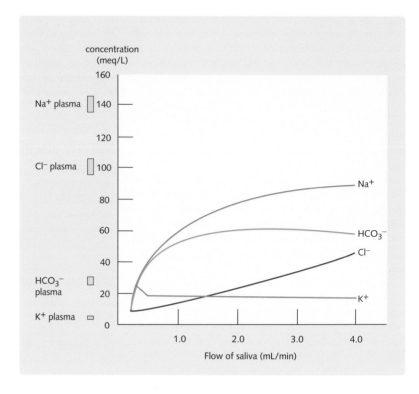

Oral mucosal absorption

The sublingual mucosa has an absorptive surface which, though unimportant for nutrition, can be exploited for the administration of some drugs. Most drugs are administered orally but this exposes drugs to first-pass metabolism in the liver. Drugs given orally must dissolve in the gastrointestinal fluids and penetrate the epithelial cell lining of the gastrointestinal tract by passive diffusion or active transport. Some drugs are poorly absorbed orally or are unstable in the tract.

Sublingual administration allows diffusion into the systemic circulation through the capillary network of the oral cavity, bypassing the liver and avoiding first-pass metabolism. Lower doses can, therefore, be given. Glyceryl trinitrate used in angina treatment is commonly given this way.

Oral defences

The alkaline pH of saliva neutralizes acid in food or in gastric contents following vomiting. Calcium and phosphate in saliva protect teeth by mineralizing newly erupted teeth and repairing pre-carious white spots in enamel.

Salivary proteins cover teeth with a protective coat called an acquired pedicle. Antibodies and antibacterial agents retard bacterial growth and tooth decay. The mucosa-associated lymphoid tissue (MALT) also plays an important role in protecting against microbial invasion at the mucosal membranes of the oral cavity.

Swallowing

We swallow about 600 times a day: 200 times while eating and drinking, 350 times while awake (when not eating or drinking) and 50 times while asleep.

Swallowing is the controlled transport of a food bolus from mouth to stomach, involving a sequential swallowing motor programme, which is generated in the medullary swallowing centre and consists of three phases: buccal, pharyngeal and oesophageal (Fig. 2.4). It is an 'all-or-nothing' reflex; it is initiated voluntarily, but once it is started, it cannot be stopped.

The buccal phase

The voluntary buccal phase occurs when the mouth is closed. The bolus of food is pushed upwards and backwards against the hard palate, forcing it into the pharynx. This phase initiates the subsequent phases, which are involuntary.

The pharyngeal phase

The pharyngeal phase lasts about 1 second, and is initiated by the bolus stimulating mechanoreceptors in the pharynx and firing impulses in the trigeminal

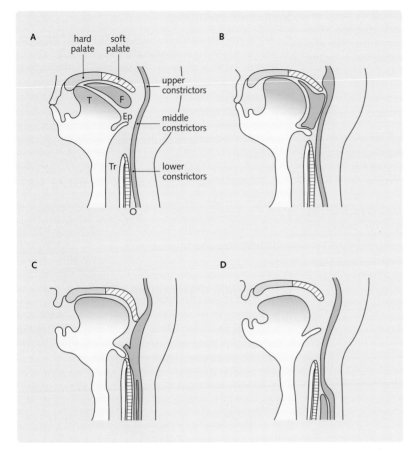

Fig. 2.4 The stages of swallowing. (A) The bolus of food, F is pushed into the pharynx by the tongue, T. (B) The bolus is propelled further back and the soft palate shuts off the nasopharynx. (C) The epiglottis, Ep, closes the opening to the trachea, Tr, and the bolus moves through the upper oesophageal sphincter. (D) Peristalsis now propels the bolus towards the lower oesophageal sphincter and stomach. (O = oesophagus.)

(Vth cranial nerve), glossopharyngeal (IXth cranial nerve) and vagus (Xth cranial nerve) nerves. Efferent fibres pass to the tongue and the pharyngeal muscles through the trigeminal, facial and hypoglossal nerves. This results in:

- The tongue being positioned against the hard palate, thus preventing the bolus re-entering the oral cavity
- The nasopharynx being closed off by the soft palate, in particular the uvula
- The larynx is elevated and its opening sealed off by the vocal folds
- The epiglottis closing the larynx
- The relaxation and opening of the upper oesophageal sphincter (UOS) for 0.5–1 s (once the bolus has passed through the upper oesophageal sphincter, it contracts tightly.

Clinical Note

Note also that respiration, which would be futile as the airway is closed, is temporarily stopped because the swallowing centre inhibits the respiratory centre, which is also located in the medulla.

The oesophageal phase

The oesophageal phase involves transport of the bolus along the oesophagus and takes between 6 and 10 seconds. Both primary and secondary peristaltic contractions are required.

The primary peristaltic wave is initiated by swallowing and sweeps down the entire length of the oesophagus. It involves sequential activation of the vagal efferents, which supply the striated muscle in the upper oesophagus directly. The smooth muscle is supplied by the enteric nerve plexus.

The bolus of food begins to move towards the stomach with the aid of gravity. The secondary peristaltic wave is triggered in response to local distension of the oesophagus and begins on the orad (mouth) side of the bolus and runs to the lower oesophageal sphincter (LOS). This occurs by an enteric reflex and helps clear food residues. Tertiary waves are common in the elderly, but they are not peristaltic or propulsive.

The LOS relaxes when the peristaltic wave meets it. It opens, allowing the bolus to pass into the stomach. Precision of tone is given by the vagal excitatory fibres (cholinergic) and the vagal inhibitory fibres (non-adrenergic non-cholinergic; NANC). These act reciprocally.

To tighten the LOS, an up-regulation in vagal excitatory fibre stimulation is required, coupled with a down-regulation in vagal inhibitory fibre stimulation. The opposite is true in relaxing or opening the LOS.

Vomiting

Vomiting (emesis) is one of the most common symptoms of illness, especially in children (where it is associated with almost any physical or emotional illness), pregnancy, alcohol dependency and some metabolic disorder.

The vomiting centre (Fig. 2.5) in the lateral reticular formation of the medulla 'coordinates' the process of vomiting. It is stimulated by:

- The chemoreceptor zone (CTZ) in the area postrema, which may itself be stimulated by circulating chemicals, drugs, motion sickness (induced by prolonged stimulation of the vestibular apparatus) and metabolic causes
- Vagal and sympathetic afferent neurons from the gut, which are stimulated by mucosal irritation
- The limbic system – less is known about these circuits, but sights, smells and emotional circumstances can induce vomiting.

Lesions of the chemoreceptor zones abolish vomiting induced by some emetic drugs, uraemia and radiation sickness, but not by gastrointestinal irritation.

Vomiting involves a retrograde giant contraction from the intestines, which expels some intestinal contents as well as gastric contents.

Stages of vomiting

- A feeling of nausea is often accompanied by autonomic symptoms of sweating, pallor and hypersalivation (which protects the mucosa of the mouth from the acid contents of the stomach)
- A deep breath is taken and the epiglottis closes, protecting the trachea and lungs
- At the same time, the retrograde giant contraction moves the contents of the upper intestine into the stomach
- The breath is held, fixing the chest. The muscles of the abdominal wall contract, increasing intra-abdominal pressure
- The oesophageal sphincters relax allowing expulsion of gastric contents through the mouth by reverse peristalsis.

Pharmacology of vomiting

It is important to understand the neural control of vomiting as most of the anti-emetic drugs act on the receptors of the neurotransmitters involved, i.e. 5-HT, dopamine, histamine and acetylcholine.

Anti-emetic drugs are used to prevent motion sickness; to prevent vomiting caused by other pharmacological agents, such as opioids; as well as vomiting due to other diseases, such as gastroenteritis or uraemia. Also, as prevention of vomiting is easier than stopping it once it has started, anti-emetics should be given before an emetic stimulus.

A description of the major classes of anti-emetics and how they work follows.

Fig. 2.5 The mechanisms controlling vomiting and the sites of action of anti-emetic drugs.

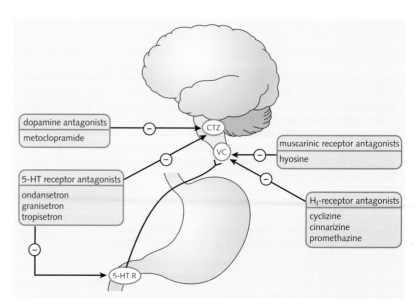

5-HT receptor antagonists (e.g. ondansetron)

5-HT is an important neurotransmitter in the vomiting reflex. As such, selective 5-HT receptor antagonists, for example ondansetron which blocks 5-HT3 receptors, are used to treat and prevent vomiting caused by cytotoxic drugs. These drugs act on the CTZ and visceral afferent nerves, as 5-HT3 receptors are found there.

Dopamime receptor blocker (e.g. metoclopramide)

Metoclopramide acts by blocking dopamine receptors in the CTZ. Dopamine, like 5-HT, is a neurotransmitter in the vomiting pathway. Metoclopramide also has a stimulant effect on gastrointestinal motility, which adds to its anti-emetic function.

H1-receptor antagonists (e.g. cyclizine)

H1-receptor antagonists are effective against motion sickness, as these receptors are found in the vestibular nuclei, and against vomiting caused by substances acting in the stomach. However, they are of no use against vomiting produced by substances acting on the CTZ.

Muscarinic-receptor antagonists (e.g. hyoscine)

Acetylcholine receptors are found in the vomiting centre and in the nucleus tractus solitarius. Muscarinic-receptor antagonists, are therefore effective in preventing motion sickness and vomiting caused by gastric stimuli but not against vomiting caused by substances acting on the CTZ.

Emetic drugs

Stimulation of vomiting may be needed in certain circumstances, for example if a toxic substance has been ingested and gastric lavage is difficult. However, stimulation of emesis should not be tried if the substance is corrosive or if the patient is not fully conscious.

Ipecacuanha, or syrup of ipecac, is a gastric irritant and the most common drug used to induce vomiting. The active ingredients of this drug are emetine and cephaeline, which are alkaloids.

THE MOUTH, ORAL CAVITY AND OROPHARYNX

Anatomy

The oral cavity extends from the lips to the pillars of the fauces, which is the opening to the pharynx. It contains the tongue, alveolar arches (which anchor the teeth), gums, teeth and the openings of the salivary ducts (Fig. 2.6).

The blood supply of the oral cavity (as well as the oropharynx) comes from branches of the external carotid artery, such as the facial artery and lingual artery. Innervation comes from branches of the cranial nerves.

The oral cavity is lined with stratifed squamous epithelium with an underlying submucosa containing collagen, elastin and salivary glands.

Embryology and development

The head and neck derive primarily from the pharyngeal (branchial) arches, which are bars of mesenchymal tissue with an outer covering of ectoderm and inner

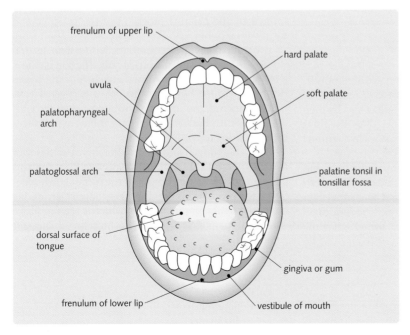

Fig. 2.6 The oral cavity. The lateral walls of the pillars of the fauces are composed of the palatoglossal arches (anterior) and the palatopharyngeal arches (posterior). The palatine tonsils lie between the two arches, covered with mucous membrane.

frenulum of upper lip

hard palate

uvula

soft palate

palatopharyngeal arch

palatoglossal arch

palatine tonsil in tonsillar fossa

dorsal surface of tongue

gingiva or gum

frenulum of lower lip

vestibule of mouth

covering of endoderm, separated by pharyngeal clefts and outpocketings called pharyngeal pouches.

Each pharyngeal arch contains neural crest cells, which contribute to skeletal components. Each also contains an arterial, cranial nerve and muscular component.

At about four and a half weeks of embryological development, the first and second arches form the mesenchymal prominences. The first pharyngeal arch consists of a dorsal and ventral portion called the maxillary and mandibular prominences, respectively. These fuse and develop with the frontonasal prominence to give rise to the mandible, upper lip, palate and nose. Failure to fuse results in abnormalities, such as cleft palate and cleft lip.

The lips

These mark the boundaries of the mouth. The outer surface of the lips is covered with skin containing hairs, sebaceous glands and sweat glands, while the inner surface is lined with non-keratinizing stratified squamous epithelium.

In between the inner and outer surfaces is the vermilion border. This is the transition zone. The epithelium resembles that of the inner surface, but has a rete ridge system with prominent blood vessels. It is these vessels which give the lips their red colour.

Deep to the epithelium, striated muscle is found arranged in a concentric fashion around the mouth. This is the orbicularis oris muscle which opens and closes the mouth.

The lips are supplied by the labial arteries, which come off the facial arteries. These form an arterial ring around the lips. Lightly pinching the lips with two fingers will allow their pulse to be felt.

The teeth

The primary teeth first erupt at around age 6–8 months and there are 20 in total. By age 18, however, eruption of the permanent teeth is normally complete and by then there are 32 teeth, 16 on each jaw (Fig. 2.7A). The third molars ('wisdom teeth') may or may not have erupted by that age.

Each tooth has three parts: the crown, the neck and the root (Fig. 2.7B). Histologically, most of the tooth is comprised of dentine. This is covered by enamel over the crown and cementum over the root. The root canal is the channel by which vessels and nerves enter the pulp cavity.

The palate

The hard and soft palates form the roof of the mouth and separate it from the nasal cavity. The former is

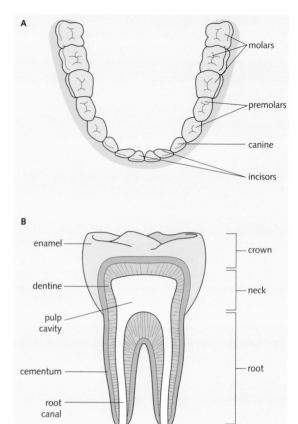

Fig. 2.7 (A) Adult human dentition. (B) The structure of a tooth.

formed by the palatine processes of the maxillae and the palatine bones.

The soft palate is posterior to the hard palate. Its oral surface contains many mucous glands. The soft palate is a mobile, muscular aponeurosis attached to the posterior border of the bony hard palate. It is covered with mucous membrane and is continuous laterally with the wall of the pharynx. Between the pillars of the fauces is the palatine tonsil.

The palatoglossal and palatopharyngeal arches join the tongue and the pharynx, respectively, to the soft palate. The curved free border of the soft palate lies between the oropharynx and the nasopharynx. From this hangs the uvula, in the midline, which is seen to move when a patient says 'aahh'. The muscles of the soft palate are:

- Levator veli palatini
- Tensor veli palatini
- Palatoglossus
- Palatopharyngeus
- Musculus uvulae.

All are supplied by the pharyngeal motor fibres of the vagus nerve via the pharyngeal plexus, except the tensor veli palatini, which is supplied by the mandibular nerve, a branch of the trigeminal nerve.

The tongue

Anatomy

The tongue is a muscular structure and its dorsum (upper surface) is divided into anterior (two thirds) and posterior (one third) by a V-shaped border-line – the sulcus terminalis. At the apex of the sulcus terminalis is the foramen caecum, which is the remnant of the embryonic thyroglossal duct opening.

The tongue consists of four pairs of intrinsic muscles (superior and inferior longitudinal, transverse and vertical), which have no attachments outside the tongue itself. These muscles are involved with changing the shape of the tongue.

The extrinsic muscles originate outside the tongue and attach to it. They act to control movement of the tongue. The extrinsic muscles are:

- Genioglossus – a fan-shaped muscle that attaches to the mandible in the midline
- Hyoglossus – attaches to the hyoid bone
- Styloglossus – attaches to the styloid process and its fibres interdigitate with the hyoglossus
- Palatoglossus – originates in the soft palate and enters the lateral part of the tongue.

Clinical Note

Paralysis or total relaxation of the genioglossus muscle, such as with general anaesthesia, allows the tongue to fall posteriorly and obstruct the airways, causing suffocation. Anaesthetized patients are always intubated to prevent this happening.

The palatoglossus muscle is innervated by the fibres from the cranial root of the accessory nerve (XIth cranial nerve), through the pharyngeal branch of the vagus nerve. The other lingual muscles are innervated by the hypoglossal nerve (XIIth cranial nerve). The nerve supply of the tongue is summarized in Fig. 2.8.

The arterial supply to the tongue is from the lingual artery (a branch of the external carotid). The lingual vein drains the tongue. Lymph drains to the deep cervical, submandibular and submental nodes.

HINTS AND TIPS

The function of the hypoglossal (XIIth cranial) nerve can be tested by asking the patient to protrude the tongue. A lesion in one of the hypoglossal nerves paralyses it, and the tongue will deviate towards the affected side when protruded because of the unopposed action of the contralateral genioglossus muscle.

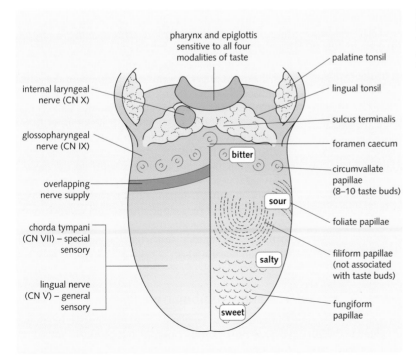

Fig. 2.8 The tongue, showing its innervation, the arrangement of the taste receptors and the areas most sensitive to the different types of taste.

Histology

The dorsal surface is covered with small papillae, especially the anterior two-thirds. Filiform papillae, which look like short bristles, are the most numerous and are found mainly in the middle of the tongue. Fungiform papillae, which are red and globular, are found among the filiform papillae and on the tip of the tongue.

Circumvallate papillae are found just anterior to the sulcus terminalis and most of the taste buds are located in the circular trenches surrounding these papillae (Fig. 2.8). The posterior third contains the lingual tonsil. Very rudimentary foliate papillae may also be found, although these are more numerous and developed in some animals.

The four basic tastes detected by taste buds are sweet, sour, salty and bitter. Taste receptors (also called taste buds) sensitive to a particular taste are found in different areas of the tongue (Fig. 2.8).

Embryology and development

Development of the tongue begins at the end of the 4th week of gestation. The tongue mucosa develops from the endoderm of the pharyngeal floor. The anterior two thirds of the tongue develop primarily from the lateral lingual swellings and the median tongue bud (or tuberculum impar), all of which are derived from the 1st pharyngeal arch.

The posterior third is formed by the growth of the hypopharyngeal eminence (a structure formed from the 3rd and 4th pharyngeal arches) over the copula, a midline structure formed by mesoderm of the 2nd, 3rd and part of the 4th arches.

The muscles of the tongue, except palatoglossus, are formed from mesoderm derived from the myotomes of the occipital somites, and are supplied by the hypoglossal nerve.

The muscles of mastication, and their actions are:

- Masseter – elevates and protrudes jaw, closing it
- Temporalis – elevates mandible; retrudes mandible after protrusion
- Lateral pterygoids – protrude mandible
- Medial – help elevate mandible, closing the jaw.

These develop from the mesoderm of the 1st pharyngeal (branchial) arch. Their motor nerve supply is from the mandibular branch of the trigeminal nerve. They all arise from the skull and insert into the mandible, causing movement of the mandible and the temporomandibular joint (Fig. 2.9).

Salivary glands

There are three pairs of large salivary glands (the parotid, submandibular and sublingual glands) and numerous smaller glands, scattered throughout the mouth (Fig. 2.10).

The parotid gland is formed from a tubular ectodermal outgrowth at the inner surface of the cheek. The submandibular and sublingual glands are formed in a similar fashion from invaginations of the endoderm of the floor of the mouth.

The salivary glands consist of parenchymal (functional) and stromal (support) components. Each parenchymal unit is called a salivon, which consists of an acinus (from the Latin word for grape) and a duct (Fig. 2.11). The duct of the salivon modifies the secretions of the acinus.

Acini consist of serous or mucous cells. The parotid gland has only serous acini, the sublingual gland contains mostly mucous acini and the submandibular gland contains predominantly serous acini. The minor salivary glands are mucous, except for von Ebner's glands and those in the tip of the tongue, which are serous.

The parotid gland

This is the largest salivary gland and it produces serous saliva. It lies between the ramus of the mandible and the mastoid and coronoid processes, and its anterior border overlies the masseter. An accessory lobe may be found above this muscle. The parotid gland is covered with a fibrous capsule that is continuous with the deep investing fascia of the neck. The facial nerve (VIIth cranial nerve) passes through the parotid gland.

The parotid duct is about 5 cm long. It pierces the buccinator muscle and opens into the mouth opposite the second upper molar tooth. This opening can be felt with the tongue.

The parotid gland is supplied by branches of the external carotid artery; venous blood drains to the retromandibular vein. It is innervated by both the sympathetic and parasympathetic systems. Parasympathetic innervation is secretomotor (causing production of saliva); sympathetic innervation is vasoconstrictor (causing a dry mouth).

Parasympathetic fibres are carried from the glossopharyngeal nerve through the otic ganglion and auriculotemporal nerve. Sympathetic fibres from the superior cervical ganglion pass along the external carotid artery.

Lymph from the superficial part of the gland drains to the parotid nodes and from the deep part to the retropharyngeal nodes.

The submandibular gland

The submandibular gland lies in the floor of the mouth covered by a fibrous capsule, and produces mixed serous and mucous secretions. Both its superficial and

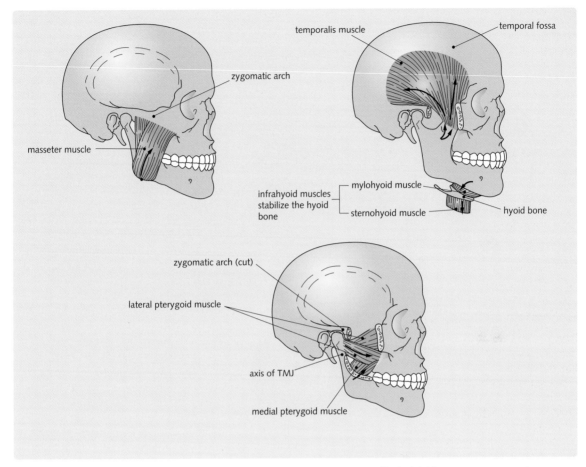

Fig. 2.9 The muscles of mastication and infrahyoid muscles. (TMJ = temporomandibular joint.)

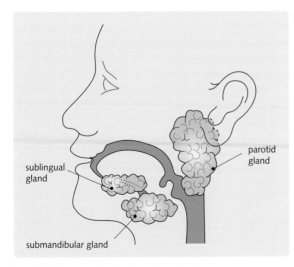

Fig. 2.10 The main paired salivary glands.

deep parts communicate around the posterior border of the mylohyoid muscle.

Its duct passes forwards between the mylohyoid and hyoglossus muscles to open onto sublingual papillae at the base of the frenulum. The lingual nerve crosses the duct.

The gland is supplied by the facial and lingual arteries (branches of the external carotid arteries); venous drainage is by the facial and lingual veins.

It is innervated by both the parasympathetic and sympathetic systems. Parasympathetic fibres are conveyed from the facial nerve through the chorda tympani and submandibular ganglion. Sympathetic innervation is from the superior cervical ganglion, with fibres passing along the arteries of the gland.

Lymphatic drainage is to the submandibular lymph nodes, which are partly embedded in the gland and partly lie between it and the mandible.

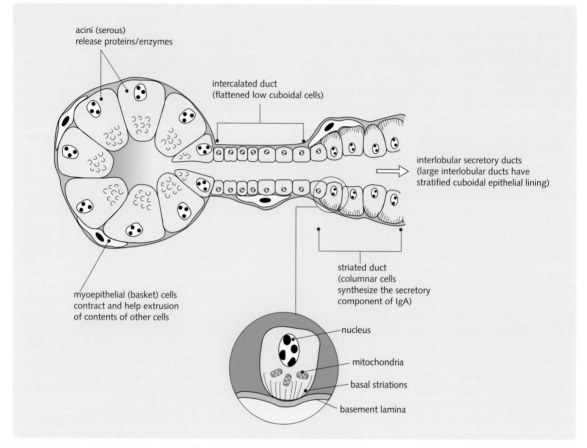

acini (serous)
release proteins/enzymes

intercalated duct
(flattened low cuboidal cells)

interlobular secretory ducts
(large interlobular ducts have
stratified cuboidal epithelial lining)

striated duct
(columnar cells
synthesize the secretory
component of IgA)

myoepithelial (basket) cells
contract and help extrusion
of contents of other cells

nucleus

mitochondria

basal striations

basement lamina

Fig. 2.11   The components of a salivon, the secreting unit of a salivary gland.

The sublingual gland

This is the smallest and also the most deeply situated of the paired salivary glands. It is almond-shaped and found below the mucous membrane of the floor of the mouth. It produces mainly mucous secretions, which either pass into numerous small ducts (10–20) that open into the floor of the mouth, or pass into the submandibular duct. The innervation, blood supply and venous and lymphatic drainage are similar to the submandibular gland.

Pharynx

The pharynx is a fibromuscular tube, approximately 15 cm long, that extends from the base of the skull to the inferior border of the cricoid cartilage anteriorly, and to the inferior border of C6 vertebra posteriorly. It communicates with the nose, middle ear (by the auditory tube), mouth and larynx.

It conducts food and fluids to the oesophagus and air to the larynx and lungs (however, some air is swallowed with food).

The pharynx can be split into three functional parts: the nasopharynx, the oropharynx and laryngopharynx. Its walls have mucous, submucous and muscular layers. The muscular layer of the pharynx consists of:

* Superior, middle and inferior constrictors
* Salpingopharyngeus
* Stylopharyngeus
* Palatopharyngeus.

The cricopharyngeus muscle forms the upper oesophageal sphincter (Fig. 2.12). Stylopharyngeus is supplied by the glossopharyngeal nerve, but all the other muscles of the pharynx are supplied by the vagus nerve through the pharyngeal plexus on the outer surface of the middle constrictor.

Superior to the superior constrictor muscle, the submucosa thickens to form the pharyngobasilar membrane, which blends with the buccopharyngeal fascia to form the pharyngeal recess.

The pharyngeal tonsils, or adenoids, lie submucosally in the nasopharynx. The epiglottis, a flap of cartilage

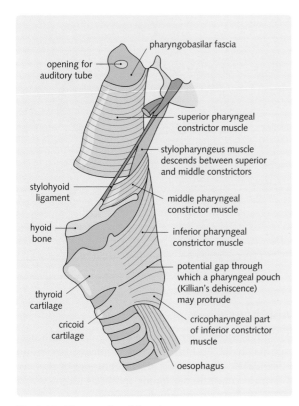

Fig. 2.12   The muscles of the pharynx.

covered with mucous membrane, lies posterior to the tongue in the laryngopharynx and closes the entrance to the larynx during swallowing. On either side of the epiglottis lie the piriform fossae – a common site for fish bones to lodge!

The pharynx is supplied by branches of the ascending pharyngeal, superior thyroid, maxillary, lingual and facial arteries. Venous drainage is to the internal jugular vein, via the pharyngeal venous plexus. Lymph from the nasopharynx drains to the retropharyngeal lymph nodes. The rest of the pharyngeal lymph drains to the deep cervical nodes.

Together with the lingual tonsils, the palatine tonsils and other smaller aggregations, the pharyngeal tonsils form a protective ring around the oro- and nasopharynx, called Waldeyer's ring. These lymphoid tissues are also described as mucosa-associated lymphoid tissue (MALT).

Histologically, the pharyngeal mucosa is continuous with that of the nose, oral cavity, auditory tube, larynx and oesophagus. The nasopharynx is lined with respiratory epithelium (ciliated mucous membrane with goblet cells).

The oropharynx and laryngopharynx are lined with stratified squamous epithelium to withstand abrasion from the passage of food.

DISORDERS OF THE MOUTH AND OROPHARYNX

Congenital abnormalities

Cleft lip and cleft palate are common defects, which present with abnormal facial appearance and defective speech. They occur in about every 1 out of every 700 live births and are more common in males. A lateral cleft lip (hare lip) may result from incomplete fusion of the maxillary and medial nasal prominences, and a cleft palate from failure of fusion of the palatine shelves. Cleft lip and palate may also occur together (Fig. 2.13).

The palatine shelves in the female fetus fuse about 1 week later than they do in the male; hence cleft palate on its own is more common in female babies. Of every nine affected babies, two have a cleft lip, three a cleft palate and four have both. About 20% of babies with cleft lip or palate also have other malformations.

Median cleft lip is much rarer and is caused by incomplete fusion of the two medial nasal prominences in the midline. Infants with midline clefts often have brain abnormalities, including loss of midline structures. These defects occur early in neurilation (days 19–21). The infants usually have severe learning difficulties.

Failure of the maxillary prominence to merge with the lateral nasal swelling causes an oblique facial cleft, exposing the nasolacrimal duct.

Repair is surgical and is normally carried out after 3 months in the case of cleft lip and about 1 year in cleft palate. Genetic and environmental factors have been identified. Trisomy 13 (Patau's syndrome) and a number of teratogens (most notably anticonvulsants such as phenytoin and phenobarbital and also folic acid antagonists) are associated with both cleft lip and cleft palate.

Infectious and inflammatory disease

The oral cavity and its mucosa are the target of many insults: infections, chemicals and physical agents. The oral mucosa is, therefore, affected by a number of inflammatory disorders, either restricted to the mouth, or as part of a systemic disease.

Herpes simplex virus

Herpes simplex virus 1 (HSV-1) infection usually affects the body above the waist and herpes simplex virus 2 (HSV-2) below it. Changes in sexual practices, however, have led to an increase in HSV-2 infections above the waist.

Fig. 2.13 Congenital abnormalities of the mouth and oropharynx. These result in variations of cleft palates and cleft lips. (A) Normal. (B) Unilateral cleft lip extending into the nose. (C) Unilateral cleft lip involving the lip and jaw and extending to the incisive foramen. (D) Bilateral cleft lip involving the lip and jaw. (E) Isolated cleft palate. (F) Cleft palate combined with unilateral anterior cleft.

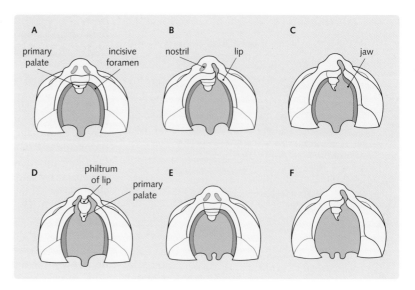

The primary infection may be asymptomatic or produce a severe inflammatory reaction. Presentation is usually with fever and painful ulcers in the mouth, which may be widespread and confluent.

The virus can remain latent in the trigeminal ganglia, but it may be reactivated by stress, trauma, fever and UV radiation. This recurrent form of the disease presents as cold sores.

About 70% of the population are infected with HSV-1 and recurrent infections are found in one third of those affected. Complications of HSV-1 include spread to the eye and acute encephalitis.

HSV infection in the immunocompromised, such as those undergoing cytotoxic chemotherapy for cancer, or those with human immunodeficiency virus (HIV) infection, is very dangerous. The infection can spread easily, leading to death in severe cases. Treatment for HSV involves topical or systemic administration of aciclovir, an antiviral drug.

Oral candidiasis (thrush)

Candidiasis is a fungal infection caused by the yeast *Candida albicans*; it looks similar to leucoplakia (see later), but unlike leucoplakia it can be scraped off with a spatula. Usually candidiasis is found in neonates, secondary to immunosuppression or a disturbance in the natural flora (e.g. after broad-spectrum antibiotic therapy). Therefore, these commensals can act as opportunists.

Candidiasis is common in acquired immune deficiency syndrome (AIDS) patients, in whom it may also cause lesions in the oesophagus.

Oral infections respond well to nystatin, or oral fluconazole. Systemic infections require parenteral therapy with amphotericin or ketoconazole for up to 3 weeks.

Aphthous ucers

Aphthous ulcers have a grey/white centre with a haemorrhagic rim, and usually heal spontaneously within a few days. Ulcers can occur for a number of reasons. The most common are minor aphthous ulcers, which recur, but have an unknown aetiology.

Sometimes nutritional deficiencies are found, such as iron, folic acid or vitamin B_{12} (with or without gastrointestinal disorders). Trauma to the oral mucosa, infections and some drugs, e.g. antimalarials and methyldopa can also cause ulcers. Ulceration is also associated with inflammatory bowel disease and coeliac disease.

Glossitis

Glossitis is inflammation of the tongue. It may occur in anaemia and certain other deficiency states, most notably vitamin B_{12} deficiency. It also occurs after trauma to the mouth from badly fitting dentures, jagged teeth, burns or the ingestion of corrosive substances.

The combination of glossitis, iron deficiency anaemia and an oesophageal web causing dysphagia occurs in Plummer–Vinson syndrome (Paterson–Brown–Kelly syndrome), most commonly seen in women with iron deficiency.

Sialadenitis

Sialadenitis is inflammation of the salivary glands. This uncommon condition may be caused by infection or obstruction of salivary ducts. Mumps (infectious parotitis) can also be the cause. Individuals with reduced amounts of saliva, e.g. in Sjögren's syndrome are at increased risk of sialadenitis due to saliva's antibacterial properties.

Oral manifestations of systemic disorders

Many infections, dermatological conditions, haematological diseases and other disorders can present with oral manifestations.

As previously mentioned, ulcers can be indicative of inflammatory bowel disease. Other systemic diseases presenting this way include systemic lupus erythematosus, Behçet's disease, cyclic neutropenia and immunodeficiency disorders.

Neoplastic disease

Premalignant and benign neoplasms of the mouth

These include:

- Leucoplakia (hyperkeratosis and hyperplasia of squamous epithelium) – a premalignant condition that takes its name from the Greek for 'white patches' and is associated with excess alcohol, poor dental hygiene and, in particular, smoking
- Erythroplakia (dysplastic leucoplakia) – lesions which have a higher malignant potential than leucoplakia
- Squamous papilloma (nipple-like growth) and condyloma acuminatum (raised wart-like growth) – these are both associated with human papilloma viruses 6 and 11 and they are largely benign.

Leucoplakia and erythroplakia are more common in men, particularly those aged between 40 and 70 years.

Malignant tumours of the mouth

In the UK, malignant tumours of the mouth account for 1% of all malignancies. Squamous cell carcinoma is by far the most common malignant tumour (95%); however, adenocarcinoma, melanomas and other malignant tumours may occur.

Alcohol and smoking predispose to squamous cell carcinoma; chewing tobacco even more so. Mouth cancer is twice as common in men as in women. The risk of a drinker who smokes developing squamous cell carcinoma is about 15 times that of the rest of the population. Cancers are commonly found on routine dental examination.

Squamous cell carcinoma may arise in areas of leucoplakia and also on the lip, where it is associated with exposure to sunlight.

Lesions are investigated with a biopsy, and treatment is by radiotherapy and/or surgery.

Neoplasms of the salivary glands

Neoplasms of the salivary gland account for 3% of all tumours, worldwide. The majority occur in the parotid gland and pleomorphic adenomas are the most common, accounting for two thirds of all salivary tumours. An adenoma is a benign epithelial growth derived from glandular tissue. Only 15% of pleomorphic adenomas (mixed tumours) become malignant.

Warthin's tumour (an adenolymphoma) is a tumour of the parotid salivary gland. It contains both epithelial and lymphoid tissues, with cystic spaces. It accounts for 5–10% of all salivary gland neoplasms.

THE OESOPHAGUS

The oesophagus is a fibromuscular tube, approximately 25 cm in length, extending from the pharynx to the stomach. It is composed of two layers; an outer longitudinal layer and an inner circular muscular layer. Its primary function is to convey food and fluids from the pharynx to the stomach during swallowing. It has cervical, thoracic and abdominal parts.

Anatomy

The oesophagus begins in the neck, at the inferior border of the cricoid cartilage, where it is continuous with the pharynx (Fig. 2.14). Initially it inclines to the left, but is moved medially by the aortic arch at the level of T4. Inferior to the arch, it inclines to the left and passes through the diaphragm just left of the median plane.

In the superior mediastinum, it lies anterior to the first four thoracic vertebrae and posterior to the trachea, left main bronchus and the left recurrent laryngeal nerve.

At the level of T5, the oesophagus moves forward and to the left, accompanied by the right and left vagi to descend behind the fibrous pericardium and in front

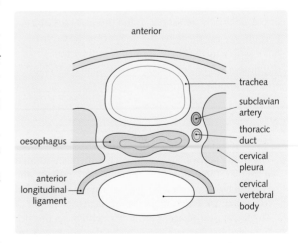

Fig. 2.14 Cross-section of the cervical region of the oesophagus, showing related structures at that level.

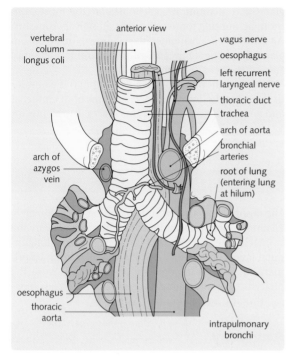

anterior view

vertebral column
longus coli

vagus nerve
oesophagus
left recurrent laryngeal nerve
thoracic duct
trachea
arch of aorta
bronchial arteries
root of lung (entering lung at hilum)

arch of azygos vein

oesophagus
thoracic aorta

intrapulmonary bronchi

Fig. 2.15 Anterior view of the oesophagus, in relation to the other thoracic viscera.

of the descending aorta. The oesophagus enters the abdomen through the oesophageal hiatus in the muscular part of the diaphragm, at the level of T10.

The abdominal part of the oesophagus is only about 2 cm long. It joins the stomach at the cardiac orifice, at the level of T11 (Fig. 2.15) and just posterior to the 7th costal cartilage. This part is also covered by peritoneum and encircled by the oesophageal plexus of nerves.

HINTS AND TIPS

Impressions or constrictions in the thoracic part of the oesophagus are made by the arch of the aorta, the point where the left main bronchus crosses the diaphragm as it passes through the oesophageal hiatus. This is a popular exam question!

The oesophagus has two sphincters:

- The upper oesophageal sphincter, which is a striated muscular (anatomical) sphincter and part of the cricopharyngeus muscle. It is normally constricted to prevent air entering the oesophagus
- The lower oesophageal sphincter, which is a physiological sphincter and made up of the lower 2–3 cm of oesophageal smooth muscle. This is the intra-abdominal segment of oesophagus. It acts as a flap

valve and with the muscosal rosette formed by folds of gastric mucosa, helps to occlude the lumen of the gastro-oesophageal junction.

Clinical Note

Apart from the physiological lower oesophageal sphincter, the other factors which help prevent reflux of gastric contents are the abdominal pressure acting on the intra-abdominal part of the oesophagus, the valve-like effect of the oblique angle between the oesophagus and the stomach, the pinch-cock effect of the diaphragm on the lower oesophagus and the plug-like action of the mucosal folds.

Blood supply

Blood supply is from the inferior thyroid artery, branches of the thoracic aorta and branches of the left gastric artery and left inferior phrenic artery (both ascend from the abdominal cavity).

Venous drainage

Venous drainage is to both the systemic circulation (by the inferior thyroid and azygos veins) and the hepatic portal system (by the left gastric vein). It is a site of portosystemic anastomosis (see later).

Innervation

The oesophagus is supplied by the vagus nerve and the splanchnic nerves (thoracic sympathetic trunks).

Striated muscle in the upper part is supplied by somatic motor neurons of the vagus nerve from the nucleus ambiguus, without synaptic interruption.

The smooth muscle of the lower part is innervated by visceral motor neurons of the vagus nerve that synapse with postganglionic neurons, whose cell bodies lie in the wall of the oesophagus and the splanchnic plexus. The oesophagus is also encircled by nerves of the oesophageal plexus.

Embryology and development

At about 4 weeks of gestation, the respiratory diverticulum (lung bud) begins to form at the ventral wall of the foregut. The diverticulum becomes separated from the dorsal part of the foregut by the oesophagotracheal septum (Fig. 2.16).

The dorsal portion of the foregut becomes the oesophagus, which, although short initially, lengthens with the descent of the heart and lungs. The ventral portion becomes the respiratory primordium and the surrounding mesenchyme forms the oesophageal muscle layers.

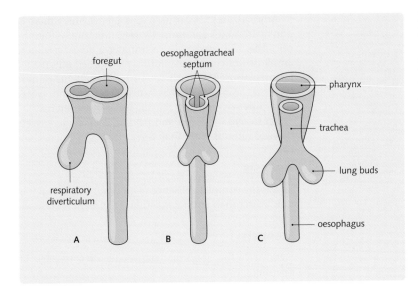

Fig. 2.16 The development of the pharynx and oesophagus. (A) Development byend of week 3 of gestation. (B and C) Development in the course of week 4. Abnormalities at this stage of development can lead to atresia and fistulae, which can result in death for the infant.

Histology

The layers of the oesophagus are essentially the same as in other parts of the gastrointestinal tract (Fig. 2.17).

The serosa covers the oesophagus inside the abdominal cavity. In the neck and thorax it is referred to as the adventitia, and blends with the surrounding connective tissue. The muscularis externa consists of an outer longitudinal and an inner circular layer, like the rest of the gastrointestinal tract.

The upper third of the oesophagus is striated muscle (a continuation of the muscular layer of the pharynx – the lowest part of cricopharyngeus forms the upper oesophageal sphincter). Striated muscle predominates here as the buccal phase of swallowing is voluntary, unlike the subsequent phases. The middle third is made up of both striated and smooth muscle, while the lower third is entirely smooth muscle.

The submucosa contains numerous branched tubular glands, more abundant in the upper region, which produce mucus to lubricate the oesophagus. These are seromucous glands which are similar to the salivary glands. The submucosa also contains blood vessels, lymphatics and nerves in abundance.

The mucosa is lined by thick, non-keratinized stratified squamous epithelium and has a lamina propria similar to that in other parts of the body, but the muscularis mucosae is thicker than in the rest of the digestive tract. When relaxed, the mucosa is heavily folded. This allows for a great degree of distension when food is swallowed.

In the abdominal part, the mucosa is lined by columnar epithelium similar to that of the gastric cardiac region. This is the squamo-columnar junction. In reflux disease (see later), where the squamous epithelium of the lower oesophagus is exposed to gastric acid, the squamo-columnar junction moves higher up the oesophagus.

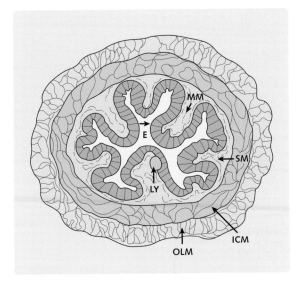

Fig. 2.17 Cross-sectional view of oesophageal tissue. (LY = lymphoid nodule; E = epithelium; MM = muscularis mucosae; SM = submucosa; ICM = inner circular muscle layer; OLM = outer longitudinal muscle layer.)

DISORDERS OF THE OESOPHAGUS

Congenital abnormalities

Atresia and tracheo-oesophageal fistulae

Atresia is the congenital absence or narrowing of a body opening. A fistula is an abnormal connection between two epithelial-lined surfaces (Fig. 2.18).

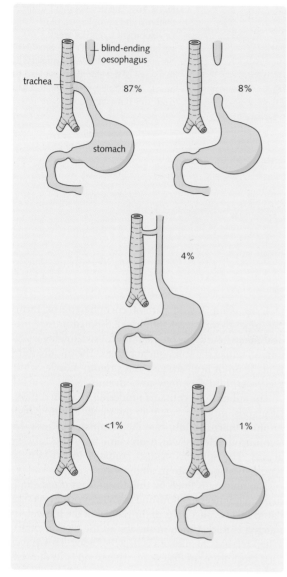

Fig. 2.18 Different forms of oesophageal atresia and fistulae and their frequencies.

Atresia is a common condition, affecting 1/3000 births, and is caused by a failure of the oesophageal endoderm to grow quickly enough when the embryo elongates in week 5.

In 90% of cases, oesophageal atresia and tracheo-oesophageal fistula occur together, but either may occur without the other.

In the most common form of atresia, the upper part of the oesophagus has a blind ending but the lower end forms a fistulous opening into the trachea. This means that the infant cannot swallow milk or saliva and the diagnosis becomes apparent shortly after birth. The infant is at risk of aspiration pneumonia and of fluid and electrolyte imbalances.

Atresia should be suspected in a fetus where there is polyhydramnios (abnormally large amounts of amniotic fluid, i.e. over 2 L). Normally a fetus swallows amniotic fluid and some fluid is reabsorbed into the fetal circulation. Where there is atresia, the fetus cannot swallow, amniotic fluid is not reabsorbed and excess fluid thus accumulates, causing a distended uterus.

Treatment of atresia and fistulae is by surgery, with survival rates of more than 85%.

Agensis

This is the complete absence of an oesophagus and it is much rarer than atresia or fistula. Treatment is surgical.

Stenosis

Stenosis is the abnormal narrowing of a passage or opening.

Congenital stenosis may occur, but acquired stenosis is more common (see later). Congenital stenosis is caused by incomplete recanalization during week 8, or from failure of development of blood vessels to the affected area. Usually the distal third is affected.

Inflammatory disease

Oesophagitis (inflammation of the oesophagus) usually presents as heartburn, and may be acute or chronic. Chronic oesophagitis is usually due to gastro-oesophageal reflux disease (GORD), which is common.

Acute oesophagitis

Acute oesophagitis is more common in immunocompromised individuals, for example in HIV infection.

Oral and oesophageal candidiasis are common in AIDS patients, and may cause dysphagia or retrosternal discomfort. They give rise to white plaques with haemorrhagic margins.

Other causes are HSV and cytomegalovirus (CMV), which may also cause focal or diffuse ulceration of the gut. HSV ulceration is more common at the upper and lower ends of the gastrointestinal tract while CMV lesions are more common in the bowel, but either may affect any part of the tract from the mouth to the anus.

Acute oesophagitis may also be caused by the deliberate or accidental swallowing of corrosive substances.

Gastro-oespophageal reflux disease (GORD)

Gastro-oesophageal reflux disease (GORD) is the reflux of acidic gastric content through the lower oesophageal sphincter. As mentioned earlier, it is the commonest cause of chronic oesophagitis and is highly prevalent, occurring in 30% of the general population.

Aetiology

Factors associated with GORD are:

- Pregnancy or obesity
- Fat, chocolate, coffee or alcohol ingestion
- Large meals
- Cigarette smoking
- Anticholinergic drugs, calcium channel antagonists and nitrate drugs
- Hiatus hernia (see later).

Pathophysiology

One or more of the following mechanisms implicate the pathogenesis:

- The resting LOS tone is low or absent
- The LOS tone fails to increase when lying flat, or when the intra-abdominal pressure has increased, e.g. during pregnancy or while wearing tight clothing
- Poor oesophageal peristalsis leads to reduced clearance of acid in the oesophagus
- A hiatus hernia can impair the function of the LOS and the diaphragm closure mechanism, as the pressure gradient between the abdominal and thoracic cavities is diminished
- Delayed gastric emptying increases the chance of reflux.

Clinical features

Most patients will complain of heartburn and 'acid regurgitation'. Some patients may be woken up at night if refluxed fluid irritates the larynx. Dysphagia and chest pain may be other presenting symptoms.

Investigations

In most cases, the diagnosis can be made clinically and no investigation is required. In atypical cases or if there is dysphagia, gastroscopy is the investigation of choice. Other options include a barium swallow and oesophageal pH monitoring may be required in exceptional circumstances.

Treatment

Treatment for GORD includes losing weight, raising the head of the bed at night so that the patient does not lie flat, and taking antacids. A reduction in the consumption of alcohol or other foods which precipitate an attack, as well as cessation of smoking is usually advised too.

The reduction of acid production can be achieved by using proton pump inhibitors and H2-receptor antagonists (see Chapter 3).

Metoclopramide, a motility stimulant (see Chapter 5), may enhance peristalsis and help acid clearance in the oesophagus.

Antireflux surgery (fundoplication) may be carried out in patients who fail to respond to medical treatment.

Complications

The squamous mucosa of the lower oesophagus is not designed to cope with acid. Therefore, reflux causes injury to, and desquamation of, oesophageal cells. Normally the cells shed from the surface of the epithelium are replaced by basal cells, which mature and move up through the layers of squamous epithelium. Increased loss due to reflux is compensated for by a proliferation of basal cells (basal cell hyperplasia) (Fig. 2.19).

Ulcers form if basal cell formation cannot keep pace with cell loss. These may haemorrhage, perforate, or heal by fibrosis (sometimes forming a stricture) and epithelial regeneration. The premalignant disorder, Barrett's oesophagus (described in neoplastic disease), may also result.

Diseases associated with motor dysfunction

Motor dysfunction may be caused by:

- A failure of innervation
- A defect in the muscle wall of the oesophagus
- A combination of the two above.

Achalasia

Achalasia is an uncommon condition (prevalence 1/100 000 in Western populations) which can present at any age, but it is rare in childhood. It involves the loss of coordinated peristalsis of the lower oesophagus and spasm of the lower oesophageal sphincter, thereby preventing the passage of food and liquids into the stomach.

The aetiology is unknown. It may be caused by damage to the innervation of the oesophagus, for example in Chagas' disease, where trypanosomes invade the wall of the oesophagus, damaging the intrinsic plexuses.

Degenerative lesions are found in the vagus nerve with a loss of ganglionic cells of the myenteric nerve plexus in the oesophageal wall. Two thirds of patients with achalasia have autoantibodies to a dopamine-carrying protein on the surface of the cells in the myenteric plexus.

Diagnosis is by radiography. A barium swallow shows dilatation of the oesophagus, with a beak deformity at the lower end, caused by a failure of relaxation of the lower oesophageal sphincter. Manometry shows an absence of peristalsis and a high resting lower oesophageal sphincter pressure.

The patient usually has a long history of sporadic dysphagia for both solids and liquids. Regurgitation of food is common, especially at night. Retrosternal chest pain is felt, due to the vigorous non-peristaltic contractions of the oesophagus.

Treatment consists of endoscopic balloon dilatation of the lower oesophageal sphincter or surgery (Heller's

Fig. 2.19 Cell desquamation and proliferation in the normal oesophagus and in gastro-oesophageal reflux (GORD). Oesophagitis can be graded from I to IV; I being mild and IV being serious with danger of perforation. Often ulceration is seen with oesophagitis, and the premalignant disorder called Barrett's oesophagus may result.

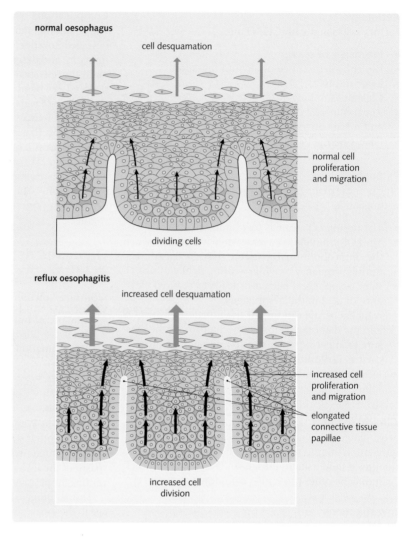

cardiomyotomy/operation) to weaken the sphincter. Reflux is common after surgery unless a fundoplication is also performed.

Achalasia is a risk factor for squamous carcinoma of the oesophagus.

Hiatus hernia

Hiatus hernia describes the herniation of part of the stomach through the diaphragm. It is a common condition, occurring in 30% of those over the age of 50, most frequently in parous women.

Hernias can be sliding, where the gastro-oesophageal junction slides through the hiatus and lies above the diaphragm, or rolling (para-oesophageal), where a part of the fundus of the stomach rolls up through the hernia next to the oesophagus (Fig. 2.20). Sliding hernias are more common.

Symptoms are usually associated with reflux, but many are asymptomatic.

Rolling hernias usually require surgical correction to prevent strangulation.

Diverticula

Diverticula (out-pouchings) may form in the proximal or distal oesophagus, particularly where there is a disorder of motor function in the oesophagus. They may be due to pulsion, where pressure is raised due to muscle spasm, or to traction, where the diverticula result from 'pulling' due to fixation to other structures.

Pharyngeal pouches are more common in elderly men. Food may collect in the pouch and later be regurgitated. Dysphagia (see Chapter 8) is common. A swelling may be felt in the neck. Pharyngeal pouches are the only common diverticula of the oesophagus. Diagnosis is by barium swallow and treatment is surgical.

A traction diverticulum, which is very rare, may form in the lower oesophagus, particularly where fibrosis of the lower oesophagus has occurred.

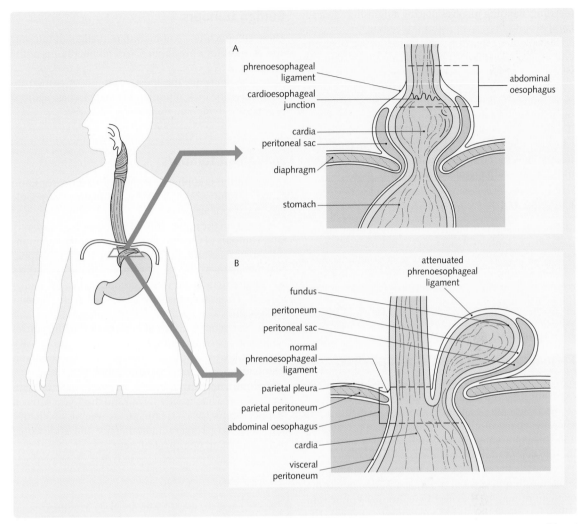

Fig. 2.20 Sliding (A) and rolling (B) hiatus hernias. The sliding hernia is more common, especially in people over 50 years old, and can exacerbate reflux.

Vascular disorders

Oesophageal varices

Oesophageal varices are dilated veins at the junction of the oesophagus and the stomach. This is a site of a connection between the systemic and portal venous systems (portosystemic anastomosis; see Chapter 6).

Normally, the connections are closed, but in patients with cirrhosis of the liver and portal hypertension the raised pressure in the portal system causes them to open up and enlarge.

The enlarged veins protrude into the lumen of the lower oesophagus (visible on endoscopy). They may burst, resulting in haematemesis, which may rapidly be fatal. Oesophageal varices account for 10% of upper gastrointestinal bleeding but a higher proportion of associated mortality.

Cirrhosis is the cause of 90% of varices in the UK, but schistosomiasis (bilharzia) causing non-cirrotic pre-hepatic portal hypertension is the major worldwide cause. Portal vein occlusion associated with pancreatitis or umbilical vein sepsis results in left-sided portal hypertension.

The management of acute variceal bleeding requires resuscitation involving restoring blood volume and taking measures to stop the bleeding. Urgent endoscopy is required and vasoconstrictor drugs (e.g. terlipressin and octreotide, a somatostatin analogue) can be given.

Sclerotherapy and elastic band ligation are widely used techniques to stem the loss of blood. Both are performed by endoscopy and can help prevent rebleeding. Sclerotherapy involves injecting the varices with a sclerosing agent to produce vessel thrombosis and arrest bleeding. Banding involves placing a tight-fitting elastic band around the varix to stop it bleeding.

Patients are often put on a beta-blocker (e.g. propranolol or carvedilol), a prophylactic measure to prevent further variceal bleeds by lowering portal blood pressure and reducing portal blood flow.

Prognosis following bleeding varices is dependent on aetiology and liver function: excellent in portal vein thrombosis and poor for Child's C cirrhosis particularly when jaundice, ascites, encephalopathy or hypoalbuminaemia may be present. Overall, mortality from a first bleed from oesophageal varices is 40%.

Mallory–Weiss syndrome

Mallory–Weiss syndrome is haematemesis from a tear at the gastro-oesophageal junction (a Mallory–Weiss tear). It is caused by prolonged retching or coughing and a sudden increase in intra-abdominal pressure. It is most common following violent retching associated with binge drinking.

Neoplastic disease

Premalignant – Barrett's oesophagus

Barrett's oesophagus is a premalignant condition resulting from prolonged reflux of the acid contents of the stomach into the oesophagus through an incompetent lower oesophageal sphincter. It occurs in approximately 15% of symptomatic cases of reflux and is most commonly seen in middle-aged men.

Normally the epithelium of the lower oesophagus is squamous but in cases of prolonged injury the normal epithelium may be replaced by columnar epithelium, which is covered by mucin (a metaplastic change). This is believed to occur as an adaptation to prolonged injury to the lower oesophagus. This metaplastic change may be followed by dysplastic change, which predisposes to malignant transformation. It is a histological diagnosis made on biopsies taken at endoscopy.

Endoscopy is the investigation of choice to visualize the columnar epithelium, with biopsies taken to confirm the diagnosis histalogically.

Treatment is with proton pump inhibitors long term to prevent acid reflux. Patients are offered regular endoscopies for surveillance, and if high-grade dysplasia persists then an oesophagectomy is often recommended. For patients who are unfit for surgery they may be offered epithelial laser ablation or photodynamic therapy.

Adenocarcinoma is 30–40 times more likely to occur in patients with Barrett's oesophagus.

Benign tumours

These are much less common than malignant tumours and account for only about 5% of all neoplasms of the oesophagus.

Leiomyomas are the most common of benign tumours but fibromas, lipomas, haemangiomas, neurofibromas and lymphangiomas may also arise.

Malignant tumours

Cancer of the oesophagus is the eighth most common cancer in the world. It is found mainly in people 60–70 years of age.

Cancers in the upper third of the oesophagus are very rare. Tumours of the middle third are mainly squamous cell carcinomas and these account for 40% of oesophageal malignancy (Fig. 2.21). Tumours in the lower third are adenocarcinomas, which comprise 45% of malignancies. These have usually developed from Barrett's oesophagus.

Clinical manifestations of oesophageal malignancies begin with persistent dysphagia, which is progressive from liquids to solids, and weight loss. Anorexia and lymphadenopathy are also common.

Unfortunately, by the time symptoms are present, the carcinoma has usually spread and the 5-year survival is only about 5%. Treatment is mainly palliative and consists of surgery, radiotherapy and endoscopic placement of an oesophageal stent.

Fig. 2.21 Causes of squamous carcinoma of the oesophagus.

Oesophageal disorders
Chronic oesophagitis
Achalasia
Plummer–Vinson syndrome

Predisposing factors
Coeliac disease
Ectodermal dysplasia, epidermolysis bullosa
Tylosis
Genetic predisposition

Dietary
Vitamin deficiency (A, C, riboflavin, thiamine, pyridoxine)
Mineral deficiency (zinc, molybdenum)
Fungal contamination of foodstuffs
Nitrites/nitrosamines in foodstuffs

Lifestyle
Alcohol
Smoking

After reading this chapter, you should be able to:

- Describe the anatomy of the stomach, with regard to its macroscopic structure, relations, arterial supply, venous and lymphatic drainage and nerve supply
- Outline the embryological development of the stomach
- Describe the functions of the stomach
- List the substances secreted by the stomach and their functions
- Describe the mechanisms controlling gastric secretion, gastric motility and emptying
- Describe how the gastric mucosa is protected from autodigestion
- Describe how the stomach protects itself from infection and how the bacterium *Helicobacter pylori* overcomes these protective factors
- Outline the following types of gastric disorders: congenital abnormalities, infections and inflammatory disease, vascular disease and neoplastic disease

OVERVIEW

The stomach is a mobile, muscular organ that mixes food with digestive juices to form chyme. It receives food and fluid from the oesophagus, and releases its contents into the duodenum. Gastric contents are broken down both by the churning action of the stomach and by being squirted through the narrow pylorus.

The stomach acts as a reservoir for food as it is very distensible, with a capacity of up to 2–3 L. The wall of the stomach is impermeable to most substances, but alcohol, water, salts and some drugs may be absorbed through it. Most other substances are absorbed from more distal parts of the gastrointestinal tract.

ANATOMY

The stomach lies between the oesophagus proximally and the duodenum distally. It is J-shaped normally and varies widely in size and shape depending on body habitus, the food content and the posture of the body.

Anatomically, the stomach is divided into four parts (Fig. 3.1):

- Cardia – the region around the oesophagus. The cardiac orifice normally lies posterior to the 7th left costal cartilage at the level of T10 or T11 vertebra
- Fundus – the superior part of the stomach, it lies above the imaginary horizontal plane passing through the cardiac orifice. Usually it is found posterior to the left 5th rib in themid-clavicular line

- Body – this lies between the fundus and the antrum, and is the largest part of the stomach
- Pyloric part – this comprises the pyloric antrum and the narrower pyloric canal. It lies in the imaginary transpyloric plane at the level of L1 vertebra to the right of the angular notch (incisura angularis), which is the junction between the body and the pyloric part.

There are two sphincters at each of the gastric orifices. The physiological lower oesophageal sphincter (LOS) protects the oesophagus from reflux of the acidic gastric contents. The anatomical pyloric sphincter controls the flow of gastric contents into the duodenum.

The cardiac (gastro-oesophageal) orifice of the stomach lies behind the 7th left costal cartilage about 2–4 cm to the left of the median plane. The pylorus, which is the distal sphincteric region, has a variable location from L2–L4 vertebrae, but usually lies 1 cm to the right of the midline, in or below the transpyloric planes. It is joined to the cardiac orifice by the lesser curvature. The position of the greater curvature varies greatly. Fig. 3.2 shows the surface markings of the stomach.

Relations

The anterior surface is in contact with:

- The diaphragm (in the fundal region)
- The anterior abdominal wall
- The left lobe of the liver.

The spleen lies posterolateral to the fundus.

Fig. 3.1   Structure of the stomach.

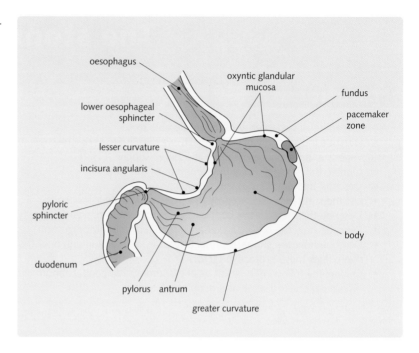

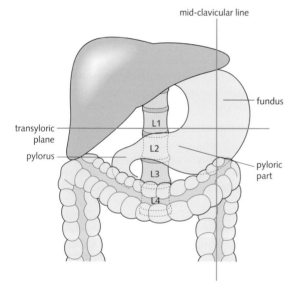

Fig. 3.2   Surface markings of the stomach.

The diaphragm, left adrenal gland, upper part of the left kidney, splenic artery, pancreas, transverse mesocolon and, in some people, the transverse colon lie posteriorly forming the stomach bed. They are separated from the stomach by the omental bursa (lesser sac of the peritoneum).

The omenta

The anterior and posterior surfaces of the stomach meet at the greater and lesser curvatures. The surfaces are covered by peritoneum except where blood vessels run on the curvatures and in a small area posterior to the cardiac orifice. The peritoneum is reflected at the greater curvature as the greater omentum. This is a fat-laden, apron-like double layer of peritoneum hanging off the stomach and the inferior border of the first part of the duodenum. It has a remarkable ability to stick to damaged or perforated parts of the gastrointestinal tract, sealing off leaks and giving some protection against peritonitis.

Excess fat may be stored in the greater omentum, especially in men, who have different distributions of fat from women. This is how the infamous beer belly came to be!

The lesser omentum is made up of peritoneum reflected at the lesser curvature to extend to the liver. The mucosa of the stomach is folded into large longitudinal rugae, which can be seen on radiographs after a barium meal. These permit the stomach to distend.

Blood supply

There is a rich blood supply to the stomach (Fig. 3.3), derived from three branches of the coeliac trunk:

- The left gastric artery supplies both anterior and posterior surfaces of the stomach, running along the lesser curvature
- The splenic artery follows a tortuous route across the posterior abdominal wall along the upper border of the pancreas. It gives rise to the left gastroepiploic (gastro-omental) artery, which runs along the

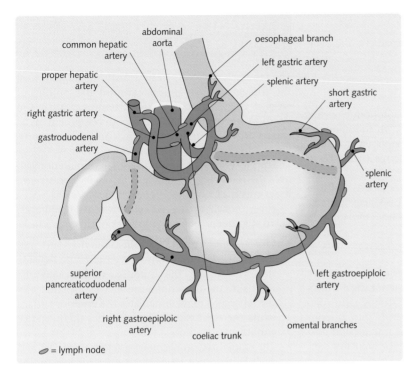

Fig. 3.3 The blood supply and lymphatic drainage of the stomach. The lymphatics follow the arteries. The lymphatics following the right gastric artery drain to the pyloric, hepatic and left gastric nodes. Those following the right gastroepiploic artery drain to the right gastroepiploic and pyloric nodes. Those following the left gastroepiploic and splenic arteries drain to the pancreaticosplenic nodes, and those following the left gastric artery drain to the left gastric nodes.

greater curvature and anastomoses with the right gastroepiploic artery. Additionally, short gastric arteries to the fundus arise from the distal end of the splenic artery

- The common hepatic artery gives rise to the right gastric artery and the gastroduodenal artery. The gastroduodenal artery passes behind the first part of the duodenum and gives rise to the right gastroepiploic and the superior pancreaticoduodenal arteries.

Venous drainage

The stomach drains, like most of the alimentary system, to the hepatic portal system. The gastric veins accompany the arteries, and drainage of specific veins is as follows:

- The right and left gastric veins drain into the portal vein itself
- The short gastric and left gastroepiploic veins drain into the splenic vein and its tributaries

- The right gastroepiploic vein usually drains into the superior mesenteric vein
- Oesophageal tributaries of the left gastric vein form an important porto-caval anastomosis with tributaries of the azygos vein in the thorax.

Lymphatic drainage

The lymphatics also follow the distribution of the arteries. There are four major groups of lymph nodes:

- The left gastric nodes
- The pancreaticosplenic nodes
- The right gastroepiploic nodes
- The pyloric nodes.

Lymph drains from the anterior and posterior surfaces of the stomach towards its curvatureswhere many of the gastroepiploic nodes are situated.

These nodes all drain to the coeliac nodes and then to the cisterna chyli. From the cisterna chyli, lymph drains to the thoracic duct, which is the largest lymphatic vessel in the body.

Nerve supply

The stomach is supplied by both sympathetic and parasympathetic systems.

Sympathetic supply

The sympathetic supply is from the autonomic coeliac plexus through the periarterial plexus, which runs along the arteries of the stomach. Presynaptic sympathetic fibres come from the splanchnic nerves (from T6 to T9 of the spinal cord).

It causes vasoconstriction of the gastric blood vessels, relaxation of the gastric muscles and decreased activity of gastric glands. These also carry pain fibres from the stomach.

Parasympathetic supply

The parasympathetic supply is from the vagus nerve (Xth cranial nerve). Anterior and posterior vagal trunks from the oesophageal plexus pass through the diaphragm with the oesophagus and divide into anterior and posterior gastric branches on the anterior and posterior surfaces of the stomach. Posterior branches contribute to the coeliac plexus.

Gastric branches form Auerbach's and Meissner's intrinsic plexuses (described in the section on gastric histology). Up-regulation of parasympathetic innervation causes an increase in gastric motility and secretion.

EMBRYOLOGY AND DEVELOPMENT

The stomach develops from a fusiform dilatation of the foregut, which appears around the middle of week 4 of gestation (Fig. 3.4). Its appearance and position change greatly during development as it rotates around both a longitudinal and an anteroposterior axis.

The posterior wall grows faster than the anterior wall over the following 2 weeks and forms the greater and lesser curvatures.

The stomach rotates 90° clockwise as it enlarges. There are three major consequences of this rotation:

- The greater curvature shifts to the left and the lesser curvature shifts to the right. The left side therefore forms the anterior surface and the right side the posterior surface. This explains why the left vagus nerve innervates the anterior surface while the right vagus nerve supplies the posterior surface
- The cranial region becomes situated at the left and slightly inferiorly, while the converse is true for the caudal region. Before rotation, both the cranial and caudal ends are in the median plane
- The long axis of the stomach becomes almost parallel with the long axis of the body.

Fig. 3.4 Development of the stomach. The stomach rotates 90° around its longitudinal axis, causing the left vagus to innervate the left, anterior, surface and the right vagus to innervate the right, posterior, surface. The longitudinal rotation also causes the formation of the space behind and to the left of the stomach, called the omental bursa (lesser sac), which is continuous with the coelomic cavity behind the stomach.

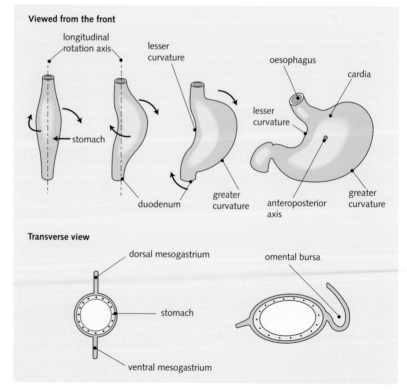

HISTOLOGY

All parts of the stomach have the same basic structural layers (Fig. 3.5):

* Mucosa
* Submucosa
* Muscularis externa
* Serosa.

Mucosa

The mucosa and submucosa are folded into longitudinal rugae when the stomach is empty. The mucosal surface is lined with simple columnar epithelium (which has a lifespan of about 1 week) and forms numerous gastric pits which are openings for the gastric glands. The mucous cells lining the gastric lumen secrete mucus as well as bicarbonate ions (HCO_3^-).

The depth of the gastric mucosa is divided into three histological zones

* A superficial zone (including the isthmus of the gland)
* A neck zone
* A deep zone.

The upper superficial zone is composed of surface mucous cells with openings to the gastric pits, while the gland isthmus comprises mainly parietal cells.

The neck zone, between the superficial and deep zones, is composed of mostly immature stem cells, but has some neck mucous cells and parietal cells. The immature stem cells eventually proliferate and move upwards to replace mucous cells in the superficial zone.

> **HINTS AND TIPS**
>
> Stem cells are very important in the cell regeneration and healing of a gastric ulcer.

In the deep zone, glands are found. While the basic structure of any gastric gland is broadly similar, they also vary in structure according to where they are situated. Each of the three main areas of the stomach – the cardiac, fundus and body and the pyloric regions – have their own arrangement of gland. The predominant cell types also vary according to region:

* Cardiac glands are predominantly composed of mucus-secreting cells
* Glands in the fundus and body consist mostly of acid-secreting parietal cells and pepsin-secreting chief cells, along with some mucus-secreting cells
* Pyloric glands are mostly composed of mucus-secreting cells and neuroendocrine cells which secrete the hormone gastrin.

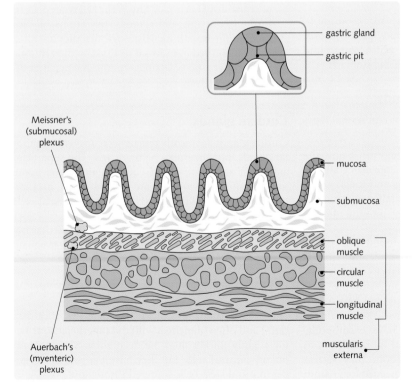

Fig. 3.5 Cross-section of the stomach wall.

Submucosa

This is made up of collagen, fibroblasts and acellular matrix with blood vessels, nerves and lymphatics. It also contains autonomic ganglion cells and lymphoid aggregates, which make up the gut-associated lymphoid tissue (GALT). This structure is consistent throughout the digestive tract.

Muscularis externa

Unlike the rest of the GI tract where the muscularis externa consists of two muscular coats, the gastric muscularis externa is comprised of three layers of smooth muscle:

- An outer longitudinal muscle layer (absent from much of the anterior and posterior surfaces of the stomach)
- A middle circular muscle layer (poorly developed in the paraoesophageal region)
- An inner oblique muscle layer.

Serosa

This consists of an inner layer of connective tissue and an outer layer of simple squamous epithelium. It is also known as the visceral peritoneum and allows for frictionless movement of organs within their cavities.

Gastric glands

As mentioned above, gastric glands vary according to their location, there are three main types (gastric glands, cardiac glands and pyloric glands) which correspond roughly to the anatomical regions of the stomach.

Gastric (body or fundic) glands

These are the most numerous and contain several types of cell:

- *Mucous neck cells* – These are found just below the gastric pits and contain numerous mucigen granules, a well-developed Golgi apparatus and rough endoplasmic reticula (RER). They are tall and columnar in shape, and secrete HCO_3^- ions into the mucous lining of the stomach wall
- *Parietal (oxyntic) cells* – These are found deeper than mucous neck cells and are most plentiful in the gland isthmus. They are pyramidal cells which look triangular or rounded in section, with the apex pointing towards the gland lumen, and have a central spherical nucleus, which gives them a 'fried-egg' appearance. Parietal cells have eosinophilic cytoplasm and contain numerous mitochondria to provide energy for HCl production. They secrete HCl and intrinsic factor, which is needed for vitamin

B_{12} absorption. Parietal cells are absent in achlorhydria ('absence of acid'); thus, no intrinsic factor is produced in this condition, which if prolonged will cause vitamin B_{12} deficiency and a macrocytic anaemia. Their internal appearance changes when food has been eaten (Fig. 3.6)

- *Chief (zymogen) cells* – These are found in the deepest part of gastric glands and are typical protein-secreting cells. They secrete pepsinogen, the inactive precursor of pepsin (a proteolytic enzyme), which is converted to pepsin by acid. They are rich in mitochondria, Golgi bodies and RER, which are required for the production of pepsinogen. Histologically, they have condensed nuclei which are basally located, and highly basophilic cytoplasm due to their numerous ribosomes
- *Neuroendocrine (enteroendocrine) cells* – These are also called APUD cells (amine precursor uptake and decarboxylation cells) and are part of the diffuse neuroendocrine system. They are found on the epithelial basement membrane and secrete peptide hormonal substances, such as vasoactive intestinal polypeptide (VIP) and somatostatin. In the gastric region, the most common type of endocrine cell is the enterochromaffin-like (ECL) cell. These are 20 times smaller than parietal cells and secrete histamine into the lamina propria of the mucosa
- *Undifferentiated stem cells* – Stem cells are precursors of all the mucosal epithelial cells. When undifferentiated, they show no cytoplasmic specialization and are capable of becoming any of the cell types present in the gastric mucosal glands. They are usually located in the neck zone. Histologically, they are most easily identified in mucosal sections by their mitotic figures after mucosal damage, as this is when they divide most actively.

Cardiac glands

Cardiac glands are mostly mucus-secreting, coiled tubular glands, but they may be branched. The superficial and deep zones are about equal in thickness. Some undifferentiated stem cells are present in the neck region. Neuroendocrine (APUD) cells and parietal cells are scattered throughout, increasing in number nearer the junction with the body. The muscularis mucosae below the cardiac glands are thick and often interdigitate with the glands.

Pyloric glands

The pyloric glands are coiled (but less so than cardiac ones) and often branched, with the superficial zone being slightly thicker than the deep zone. They contain mainly mucous cells, but they have parietal, enteroendocrine and stem cells scattered throughout.

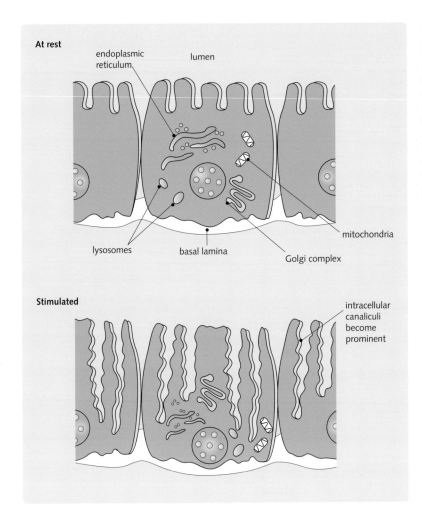

Fig. 3.6 Morphological changes in parietal cells. At rest, the parietal cells have numerous tubulovesicles derived from smooth endoplasmic reticulum (SER). These contain H+ pumps and do not connect with the apical surface membrane. After stimulation of acid secretion, the tubulovesicles merge and become deep trough-like invaginations of the apical surface, called secretory canaliculi. These communicate with the lumen of the gland. The surface area is also increased by numerous microvilli.

In particular, the enteroendocrine cells secrete gastrin in this area. These cells are called G cells, because they secrete gastrin. D cells, another type of enteroendocrine cell, secrete somatostatin in paracrine fashion. Nearer the pyloric sphincter, parietal cells become more numerous. The cell types found in each region of the stomach are summarized in Fig. 3.7.

Nerve fibres

There are two major networks of intrinsic nerve fibres:

- Auerbach's (myenteric) plexus, between the inner oblique and the middle circular muscle layer
- Meissner's (submucous) plexus, between the inner oblique muscle layer and the mucosa.

Both plexuses are interconnected and contain nerve cells with processes that originate in the wall of the gut or mucosa. The mucosa has mechanoreceptors and chemoreceptors, which are sensitive to stretch of the gut wall and composition of the stomach contents, respectively.

Nerve cells innervate hormone-secreting cells (see next section) and all the muscle layers in the mucosa.

FUNCTIONS AND PHYSIOLOGY

Storage of food

The stomach acts as a reservoir for food, releasing the gastric contents into the duodenum at a steady rate. Relaxation of the LOS and arrival of food in the stomach is followed by a receptive relaxation of the fundus and body of the stomach.

This is mediated by a vagal reflex, which inhibits the smooth muscle tone in this area (via the vagal inhibitory fibres with release of VIP and nitric oxide). The vagal inhibitory fibres cause relaxation by inducing hyperpolarization.

Fig. 3.7 Types of gastric cell. (APUD cells = amine precursor uptake and decarboxylation cells; VIP = vasoactive intestinal polypeptide).

Cell type	Area of stomach		Function
Mucous cells	Cardiac	Many	Secrete mucus to protect the epithelium from acid secretions
	Gastric	Fewer	
	Pyloric	Many	
Parietal cells (oxyntic cells)	Cardiac	Few	Secretion of HCl and intrinsic factor (for vitamin B_{12} absorption)
	Gastric	Many	
	Pyloric	More near the pyloric sphincter	
Chief cells (zymogen cells)	Cardiac	Many	Secretion of pepsinogen, the precursor of pepsin, a proteolytic enzyme
	Gastric	Few	
	Pyloric		
Enteroendocrine (APUD cells)	Cardiac	Few	Secretion of protein hormones such as VIP and somatostatin. (gastrin is secreted in the pyloric region)
	Gastric	Many	
	Pyloric	Few	
Stem cells	Cardiac	Present	These give rise to new cells to replace the old mucosal and glandular epithelial cells
	Gastric	Present	
	Pyloric	Present	

The muscle wall is thinner in the fundus and body, resulting in generally weaker muscle contractions than in the antral area. These factors allow the fundus and body of the stomach to store food and accommodate up to 1.5 L without a marked increase in intragastric pressure.

The muscles in the antral region contract vigorously, mixing the food with gastric secretions to continue digestion.

Food may remain in the stomach, unmixed, for up to 1 hour. Fats form an oily layer on top of other gastric contents. A fatty meal delays gastric emptying but liquids generally empty more quickly.

Gastric secretions

The average adult produces 2–3 L of gastric juice every 24 hours. Gastric juice contains mucus, digestive enzymes (pepsinogen and lipase), HCl and intrinsic factor.

Resting juice

Resting juice is an isotonic juice secreted by the *surface cells*. It is similar to plasma, but it has an alkaline pH of 7.7 and a higher concentration of HCO_3^-.

Mucus

Mucus is secreted by *goblet cells* of the surface epithelium and *mucus neck cells*, especially in the pyloric antrum.

The alkaline mucus of the stomach is a thick, sticky mucopolysaccharide. It is secreted with HCO_3^- ions, which are exchanged for Cl^- ions by the epithelial cells. It plays an important role in the protection of the stomach against its acid contents.

Mucus forms a water-insoluble gel that adheres to the surface of the stomach lumen. It reduces the flow of H^+ ions and acts as a barrier to pepsin. Although pepsin can degrade mucus, the HCO_3^- secretions increase the pH and make the enzyme less active.

Pepsin

Pepsin is secreted from the *chief cells* in the gastric pits in the form of its precursor, pepsinogen. HCl activates pepsinogen by cleaving off nine amino acid residues to form pepsin. Pepsin is a proteolytic enzyme that acts on proteins and polypeptides, by hydrolysing internal peptide bonds.

Lipase

Gastric lipase is an enzyme that acts on triglycerides to produce fatty acids and glycerol. It is useful in facilitating subsequent hydrolysis by pancreatic lipases, but it is of little physiological importance except in pancreatic insufficiency.

Intrinsic factor

Intrinsic factor (IF) is made in the *parietal cells* of the stomach; it is a glycoprotein vital for the absorption of vitamin B_{12} via receptors for IF-B_{12} in the terminal ileum. Without intrinsic factor, vitamin B_{12} is digested in the intestine and not absorbed.

R-proteins in the saliva and stomach protect vitamin B_{12} until it is absorbed. Upon absorption, it is bound to transcobalamin II, which serves to transport it in plasma.

Most diets contain excess vitamin B_{12} and stores are built up in the liver. These stores last for 2–3 years; thus, it takes considerable time for a dietary deficiency to produce symptoms.

Hydrochloric acid

HCl is produced by the parietal (oxyntic) cells. The concentration of HCl depends on:

- The rate of HCl secretion
- The amount of buffering provided by the resting juice, ingested food and drink and the alkaline secretion of the pyloric glands, duodenum, pancreas and bile
- Gastric motility
- The rate of gastric emptying
- The amount of diffusion back into the mucosa.

The pH of the contents of the stomach after feeding is normally about 2–3.

Gastric HCl provides a defence mechanism that is non-specific in killing ingested microorganisms. It also aids protein digestion (by enabling the activation of pepsin from pepsinogen) and stimulates the flow of bile and pancreatic juice.

The secretion of HCl by parietal cells is stimulated by histamine, acetylcholine and gastrin (Fig. 3.8). It is also stimulated by caffeine, through the activation of cyclic AMP. Both H^+ and Cl^- are actively transported by different ion pumps in the parietal cell membrane.

Clinical Note

Because alcohol and caffeine are substances which promote the secretion of HCl, patients with peptic ulcers or underlying gastric hypersecretion should avoid beverages which contain these two chemicals.

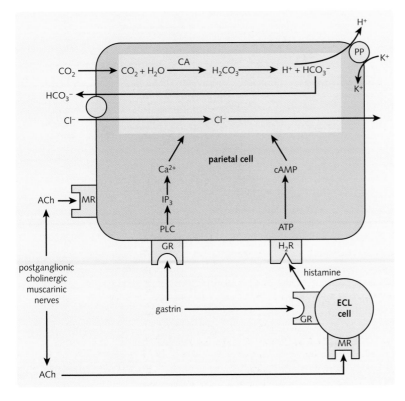

Fig. 3.8 Stimulation of secretion of HCl by parietal cells. (ACh = acetylcholine; AC = adenylate cyclase; ECL = enterochromaffin-like; IP_3 = inositol triphosphate; PLC = phospholipase C; cAMP = cyclic AMP; ATP = adenosine triphosphate; GR = gastrin receptor; MR = muscarinic receptor; H_2R = histamine-2 receptor.)

Secretion is inhibited by vagotomy (which removes acetylcholine stimulation) and pharmacologically, the latter of which is covered in the next section.

Pharmacology of gastric acid secretion

The key points to note are:

- The three main factors which stimulate acid production are gastrin, histamine and acetylcholine
- Acid secretion can be modified by extrinsic neural factors (vagus nerve) and intrinsic neural reflexes
- The terminal step in the pathway is H^+/K^+-ATPase.

As such, these factors, or their receptors, are possible sites of action for drugs which inhibit gastric acid secretion. There are also drugs which act to neutralize secreted acid.

However, no drugs which act on muscarinic or gastrin receptors are currently licensed for clinical use to inhibit gastric acid secretion, although a muscarinic blocker such as atropine will have this effect. Fig. 3.9 summarizes the relevant gastric pharmacology.

Proton-pump inhibitors (PPIs)

PPIs are irreversible inhibitors of H^+/K^+-ATPase, also known as the proton pump. As stated above, the proton pump is the final step in the acid-secretory pathway. PPIs are so far the most effective and powerful drugs in reducing gastric acid secretion. Examples of PPIs are omeprazole, lansoprazole and pantoprazole.

PPIs are weak bases inactive at neutral pH, and they therefore accumulate and are activated in the acidic environment of the parietal cell canaliculi. This preferential accumulation causes PPIs to have a specific

Fig. 3.9 Sites and mechanisms of action of drugs which inhibit gastric acid secretion and drugs which protect the gastric mucosa. (GR = gastrin receptor; H_2R = histamine-2 receptor; MR = muscarinic receptor; PP = proton pump; cAMP = cyclic AMP; ATP = adenosine triphosphate.)

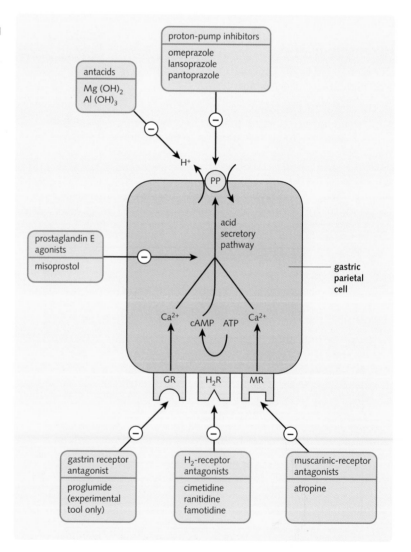

effect on the parietal cells. They are the drug of choice in drug-resistant peptic ulceration and in hypersecretion.

H2-receptor antagonists

These block H2-receptors on the gastric parietal cell, preventing intracellular cAMP synthesis and thus reducing acid secretion. Additionally, they also inhibit gastrin-stimulated acid secretion and decrease acetylcholine-stimulated secretion, as a result of which pepsin secretion also decreases due to the reduction in volume. Common examples of H2-receptor antagonists are cimetidine, ranitidine, nizatidine and famotidine.

Antacids

Antacids neutralize gastric acid and therefore cause a rise in gastric pH. They thus cause inhibition of peptic activity, as secretion ceases at pH 5. Common antacids are salts of aluminium and magnesium, for example aluminium hydroxide and magnesium hydroxide.

Alginates may be combined with antacids, an example of which is Gaviscon. These are used in oesophageal reflux. The alginic acid, when combined with saliva, forms a raft which floats on the gastric contents, thus protecting the oesophageal mucosa during reflux.

Control of gastric secretion

The control of gastric secretion is brought about by a combination of nervous, hormonal and paracrine messages. There are three phases of stimulation (Fig. 3.10):

- The cephalic phase
- The gastric phase
- The intestinal phase.

The cephalic phase

The cephalic phase is the shortest phase and is initiated by the sight, smell and taste of food. It usually begins before the meal and lasts up to 30 minutes into the meal. This allows the stomach to prepare itself for the imminent arrival of food.

It is mediated entirely by the vagus nerve, hence vagotomy of the stomach leads to cessation of the cephalic phase and was performed in the past to reduce acid secretion before pharmacological means were available.

Acid secretion is up-regulated by acetylcholine (ACh) released from neurons of the intramural plexus acting:

- Directly, by stimulation of the parietal cells
- Indirectly, by causing release of gastrin from antral G cells, which stimulates the parietal cells too. The mediator at the G cell is gastrin-releasing peptide (GRP)
- Indirectly, by causing the release of histamine from ECL cells, which also up-regulates acid production.

The gastric phase

This is the longest phase, lasting for up to 2½ hours after the start of the meal. It is triggered by the presence of food causing distension of the stomach, and the presence of amino acids and peptides (products of pepsin degradation). Alcohol and caffeine are also pro-secretory factors. Most acid secretion in response to a meal takes place during the gastric phase.

Distension of the body or antrum of the stomach stimulates mechanoreceptors that cause local (enteric) and central vago-vagal cholinergic reflexes.

Amino acids and peptides activate vagal chemoreceptors and also antral G cells, which are sensitive to peptides. These secrete gastrin in response. Gastrin and acetylcholine then activate ECL cells to produce histamine, which further increases acid secretion from the parietal cells.

> **HINTS AND TIPS**
>
> Vago-vagal reflexes, as found in the gastric phase of the control of gastric secretions, are so named because both afferent and efferent impulses are carried by neurons in the vagus nerve.

The intestinal phase

The intestinal phase is brought about by the presence of chyme in the duodenum. It has both excitatory and inhibitory components. In the excitatory component, amino acids and peptides in chyme stimulate intestinal gastrin release. This is carried via the blood to the stomach and thus contributes to serum gastrin levels during a meal.

The inhibitory phase, however, predominates, as the same factors, i.e. acid (with a pH < 2), fat, hypertonicity and distension have the following effects in the duodenum:

- Somatostatin is released from D cells. This acts directly on the parietal cells to inhibit acid secretion
- Acid mediates the release of secretin into the bloodstream. This inhibits the release of gastrin by G cells and reduces the response of parietal cells to gastrin
- Fatty acids (from triglyceride digestion) in the duodenum and proximal jejunum cause the release of gastric inhibitory polypeptide (GIP) and cholecystokinin (CCK), which both act to inhibit secretion of acid by parietal cells. GIP also suppresses gastrin release.

Secretin, GIP and CCK are collectively called enterogastrones, because they have an inhibitory effect on gastric secretion. Hypertonic solutions in the duodenum also suppress gastric secretion. This is mediated by an unidentified enterogastrone. The inhibition of gastric

A

phase	stimuli	mechanism
cephalic	sight, smell and taste of food	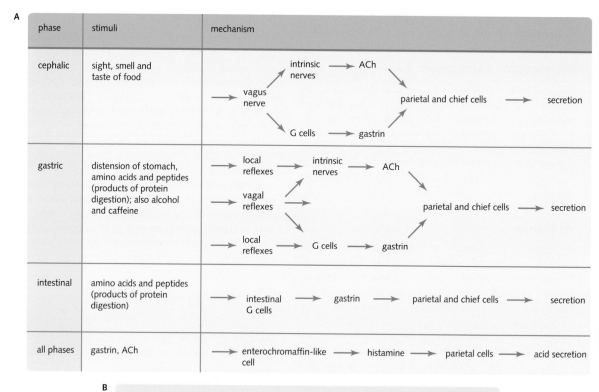
gastric	distension of stomach, amino acids and peptides (products of protein digestion); also alcohol and caffeine	
intestinal	amino acids and peptides (products of protein digestion)	
all phases	gastrin, ACh	

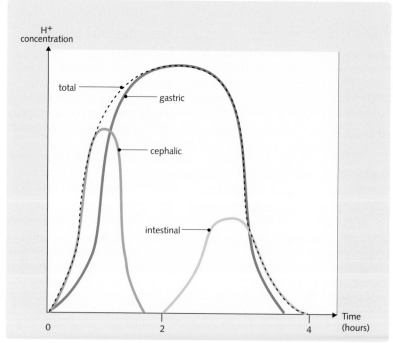

Fig. 3.10 The three phases of gastric secretion. (A) Control mechanisms for each phase of gastric secretion. (ACh = acetylcholine.) (B) Graphical representation of the three stages.

Fig. 3.11 Mechanisms for inhibiting gastric acid secretion.

Stimulus	Mediator	Action
Acid (pH <2)	Somatostatin	Directly inhibits parietal cells
	Secretin	Inhibits gastrin release. Decreases response of parietal cells to gastrin
	Enteric reflex	Directly inhibits parietal cells
Fatty acids	Gastric inhibitory peptide (GIP)	Directly inhibits parietal cells. Inhibits gastrin secretion from G cells
	Cholecystokinin (CCK)	Adds to the inhibition of parietal cells
Hypertonic solutions	Unidentified enterogesterone	Inhibits acid secretion
	Enteric reflex	Inhibits acid secretion
Distention of duodenum	Mechanoreceptor initiated enteric reflex	Decreases acid secretion
Emptying of stomach	Enteric reflex	Decreases acid secretion

secretions is also controlled by an enteric reflex, which is integrated with higher controls from the medulla oblongata.

The loss of volume in the stomach and the distension of the duodenum (as chyme passes from one to the other), both activate the local enteric reflex, via mechanoreceptors. Chemoreceptors in the duodenum can also activate the reflex ion response to irritants, reduced pH and hypertonic solutions. The mechanisms for inhibiting acid secretion are summarized in Fig. 3.11.

Gastric motility and emptying

Gastric motility and emptying are carefully regulated to ensure that chyme is delivered to the duodenum at a rate at which it can be absorbed.

Gastric motility

Motility in the stomach is initially brought about by reflex receptive relaxation, which allows food to enter from the oesophagus. This process is mediated by vagal inhibitory fibres.

Mixing of the food with gastric secretions follows and takes place in the distal body and antrum of the stomach (the caudal region). The muscularis externa is thicker in this area of the stomach. The contractions involved in mixing and emptying the stomach contents are brought about by the three smooth muscle layers, which are coordinated by intrinsic and extrinsic nerves.

The most prominent plexus is Auerbach's plexus, situated in a three-dimensional matrix between the layers of smooth muscle in the stomach wall. It receives innervation from both sympathetic and parasympathetic systems. Axons from the plexus innervate both muscle fibres and glandular cells.

Interneurons connect intrinsic afferent sensory fibres with efferent neurons of smooth muscle and secretory cells, to ensure that gastric activity is fully coordinated, even in the absence of external innervation. Cholinergic (parasympathetic) stimulation from the vagus increases gastric motility and secretion, but adrenergic (sympathetic) stimulation in the coeliac plexus has the opposite effect.

The mechanics of gastric motility

When the stomach is full of food, it undergoes a 'lag' phase. During this time, the stomach is not contracting, but intense secretions are digesting the food down to basic components to form chyme. Once the lag phase is over, there is a reversal of vagal discharge. There is an up-regulation in vagal excitatory fibre activation and a decrease in vagal inhibitory fibre activation.

The contractions break off small boluses of food, carrying them towards the pylorus. Large pieces of food are refluxed back towards the gastric body for further degradation. This process is termed retropulsion and allows for the thorough mixing and mechanical breakdown of solid food material (Fig. 3.12).

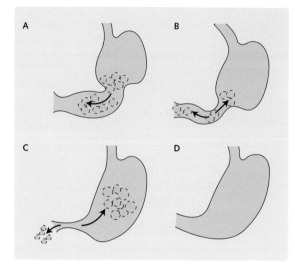

Fig. 3.12 Effects of gastric peristaltic contractions on intraluminal contents. (Redrawn with permission from Johnson LR. Physiology of the Gastrointestinal Tract, 4th edn. New York: Raven Press, 2000.)

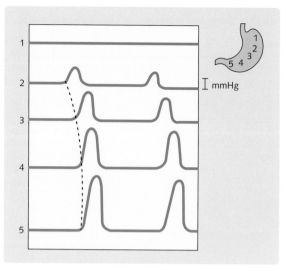

Fig. 3.13 Intraluminal pressures recorded from five areas in the stomach. (Redrawn with permission from Johnson LR. Physiology of the Gastrointestinal Tract, 4th edn. New York: Raven Press, 2000.)

The force and frequency of contractions depends on:

- The neural activity of intrinsic and extrinsic nerves
- The myogenic properties of smooth muscle
- The properties of paracrine and endocrine agents (gastrin and motilin up-regulate the force of gastric contraction, but secretin inhibits it).

HINTS AND TIPS

The cephalad region of the stomach (fundus and corpus) is the area for storage and the caudad region (distal corpus and antrum) is the area for mixing food.

The basic electrical rhythm of the stomach

The pacemaker zone of the stomach is located in the fundus on the greater curvature. The cells in the pacemaker zone spontaneously depolarize, setting the basic electrical rhythm (BER) of the stomach. This depolarization occurs continuously. Depending on the excitability of the gastric smooth muscle at the time, the BER may trigger large peristaltic contractions. These sweep down towards the antrum where the amplitude of contraction is greatest, due to its thicker muscle layers. The contractions occur at a rate of three per minute, and last between 2 and 20 seconds (Fig. 3.13).

Gastric emptying

Emptying of gastric contents into the duodenum is part of the continuum of gastric motility. As retropulsion occurs,

the pyloric sphincter opens by a coordination of antral and duodenal contractions. Small digested particles are squirted through the sphincter into the duodenum.

The rate at which the stomach empties depends on:

- *The type of food eaten.* Carbohydrates are emptied most quickly, proteins more slowly and fatty foods even more so to ensure that food is released into the duodenum at a rate at which it can be absorbed. Fatty acids or monoglycerides in the duodenum decrease the rate of gastric emptying by increasing the contractility of the pyloric sphincter. The presence of acidic contents with a pH of less than about 3.5 in the duodenum also slows gastric emptying
- *The osmotic pressure of the contents of the duodenum.* Duodenal osmoreceptors initiate a decrease in gastric emptying in response to hyperosmolar chyme
- *Vagal innervation.* Antral and duodenal overdistension activates mechanoreceptors that stimulate a vagovagal reflex. This acts to inhibit gastric contractile activity by vagal inhibitory fibres. Vagotomy results in a marked decrease in the rate of gastric emptying
- *The release of somatostatin, secretin, CCK and GIP by the duodenum,* in response to the presence of chyme. These all inhibit gastric emptying.

Protection of the gastric mucosa

The gastric mucosa is frequently subjected to the corrosive secretions of HCl and pepsin. Several mechanisms exist to prevent tissue damage by the gastric juices:

- *Mucus,* secreted by neck and surface mucous cells in the body and fundus and similar cells elsewhere in the stomach, forms a water-insoluble gel that coats the mucosa. Prostaglandins stimulate mucus production

- *The surface cells secrete HCO_3^- which, together with the mucus, forms an adherent layer. This raises the pH around the mucus layer, thus making pepsin less active and preventing the enzymes degrading the mucus*
- *The surface membranes of the mucosal cells, the tight junctions between them and the ability to form a fibrin coat* protect the cells
- *Prostaglandins*, especially those of the E and I series, inhibit acid secretion by enhancing blood flow to the mucosa which in turn encourages mucus production.

Several factors cause a breakdown of the mucosal protection or an increase in acid production and predispose to gastric irritation and peptic ulceration:

- Acid secretion (from the parietal cells) is stimulated by histamine, acetylcholineand gastrin (Fig. 3.8)
- *Non-steroidal anti-inflammatory drugs (NSAIDs) and aspirin* reduce mucus secretion and decrease bicarbonate secretion by inhibiting prostaglandin production
- In the Zollinger–Ellison syndrome, gastrin-secreting adenomas result in marked hyperacidity. The adenomas are usually found in the pancreas and present as gastric or duodenal ulcers. The syndrome is rare.
- *Helicobacter pylori* (see below)
- *Hyperparathyroidism* predisposes to ulcer formation because increased levels of calcium stimulate acid production
- Chronic exposure to nicotine from smoking causes an increase in acid secretion.

Pharmacology of gastric mucosal protection

As mentioned above, prostaglandins are protective against gastric mucosal ulceration. Prostaglandin analogues have the same effect. Misoprostol, which is a stable analogue of PGE1, protects the mucosa by inhibiting gastric acid secretion, enhancing or maintaining the blood flow to the mucosa and increasing the secretion of bicarbonate and mucus. It is used to prevent gastric

ulceration due to long-term use of non-steroidal anti-inflammatory drugs (NSAIDs), which also act through the arachidonic acid/prostaglandin pathway.

Sucralfate is a complex of sulphated sucrose and aluminium hydroxide. In acidic conditions under pH 4, it forms a polymerized gel with mucus. The gel is believed to decrease mucus degradation as well as limit hydrogen ion diffusion. In addition, it stimulates mucus and bicarbonate production as well as prostaglandin secretion.

Bismuth chelate protects the mucosa by coating the bases of peptic ulcers, adsorbing pepsin and increasing bicarbonate and prostaglandin secretion. More importantly, it has toxic effects on *H. pylori* and may be used as part of triple therapy to eradicate the bacterium.

Gastric defences against infection

The stomach has a number of defence strategies. Gastric acid and pepsin secretions act to kill aerobic microorganisms and other ingested bacteria, preventing infection of the gastric mucosa. Other factors preventing infection include:

- Mucus production
- Peristalsis and fluid movement
- Seamless epithelium with tight junctions
- A fast cell turnover
- IgA secretions at mucosal surfaces.

DISORDERS OF THE STOMACH

Congenital abnormalities

Diaphragmatic hernia

The diaphragm develops from:

- The septum transversum
- The pleuroperitoneal membranes
- The dorsal mesentery of the oesophagus
- Muscular components of the body wall.

The pleuroperitoneal folds appear at the beginning of week 5. They fuse with the septum transversum and the oesophageal mesentery in week 7, separating the abdominal and thoracic cavities. This primitive diaphragm then fuses with a ring of muscle that develops from the body wall.

If there is incomplete fusion, the contents of the abdomen may push up into the pleural cavity, forming a diaphragmatic hernia (usually on the left side), pushing the heart forwards and compressing the lungs. The incidence is about 1 in 2000 births and treatment is surgical.

Hypertrophic pyloric stenosis

Pyloric stenosis (narrowing) occurs in about 1 in 150 male infants and 1 in 750 female infants. A genetic factor is involved.

Stenosis is caused by hypertrophy of the circular muscles of the pylorus, obstructing the pyloric canal and the flow of contents from the stomach into the duodenum. Typically, it presents 4–6 weeks after birth with projectile vomiting within half an hour of a feed. Note that there is no bile in the vomit because the obstruction is proximal to the ampulla of Vater.

Peristaltic waves are visible in the child, a sausage-shaped mass (the enlarged pylorus) can be felt in the right upper quadrant and the hypertrophied pyloric muscle can be observed using ultrasonography. Treatment is surgical.

Stenosis may also be acquired in adult life, usually caused by scarring from peptic ulceration or because of malignancy obstructing the outflow. It is diagnosed by barium meal and gastroscopy.

> **Clinical Note**
>
> When treating a patient who is vomiting, always test the vomit for the presence of bile. Bile joins the intestinal contents at the ampulla of Vater. Vomit will only contain bile if the lesion is below the ampulla.

Gastritis

Gastritis (inflammation of the stomach) may be acute or chronic.

Acute gastritis

This involves an acute inflammatory reaction at the superficial mucosa, with the infiltration of neutrophils.

Acute gastritis is almost always caused by drugs (especially NSAIDs such as aspirin) or by alcohol (the most common cause) causing chemical exfoliation of the surface epithelial cells and decreasing the secretion of protective mucus.

The causative drugs or chemicals often inhibit prostaglandins, which protect the gastric mucosa by stimulating mucus and HCO_3 production and inhibiting acid secretion (despite their role in inflammation). The degree of damage ranges from erosions (acute erosive gastritis, see below) to ulcers (involving the full thickness of the mucosa). *H. pylori* has been implicated in both acute and chronic gastritis.

Acute erosive gastritis is typified by a partial loss of gastric mucosa. It is caused by shock, severe burns and toxic substances and alcohol as mentioned above. Discomfort (dyspepsia), epigastric pain and vomiting are typical symptoms.

> **Clinical Note**
>
> NSAIDs, such as aspirin, inhibit the enzyme cyclooxygenase (COX), which is necessary for prostaglandin production. Concurrent therapy with a proton-pump inhibitor can prevent gastritis and ulcer formation.

Chronic gastritis

Chronic inflammatory changes in the mucosa cause atrophy and epithelial metaplasia. It can be classified according to aetiology.

- Autoimmune
- Bacterial infection
- Reflux.

Autoimmune

Inflammation is mediated by antibodies against gastric parietal cells (90%) and intrinsic factor (60%). Intrinsic factor is needed to absorb vitamin B_{12}. In its absence, macrocytic anaemia develops once liver stores of vitamin B_{12} have been used up.

Pernicious anaemia occurs where autoimmune gastritis and macrocytic anaemia exist together. It is associated with other autoimmune diseases such as thyroid disease, vitiligo, Addison's disease and myxoedema. Pernicious anaemia is a risk factor for carcinoma of the stomach.

The body of the stomach is always affected and often this type of gastritis involves the entire stomach.

> **Clinical Note**
>
> Vitamin B_{12} is needed for the synthesis of DNA. Normally, the nucleus is extruded from red blood cells before they are released into the peripheral blood from the bone marrow. In vitamin B_{12} deficiency, however, maturation of the nucleus is delayed relative to the cytoplasm and macrocytic or megaloblastic blood cells with nuclei are seen in the peripheral blood.

Bacterial infection

Helicobacter pylori infection is present in about 90% of cases of active chronic infective gastritis. It provokes an acute inflammatory response and the release of proteases, which destroy gastric glands, leading to atrophy. There is a mixed acute and chronic inflammatory reaction in the epithelium and lamina propria.

Infective gastritis usually begins in the antrum, but it may cause atrophy, fibrosis and intestinal metaplasia of the entire stomach, where the normal gastric mucosa is replaced with epithelium similar to that found in the small intestine.

Reflux

Reflux is also known as reactive gastritis. This is caused by regurgitation of duodenal contents into the stomach through the pylorus and is more common where pyloric or duodenal motility has been compromised, for example after surgery to the pyloric part. This type of gastritis is caused by irritants such as NSAIDs, alcohol and biliary reflux, and may present with dyspepsia and bilious vomiting.

Helicobacter pylori

Helicobacter pylori is a Gram-negative spiral-shaped bacillus with the ability to penetrate the gastric mucus lining. It is a common pathogen, with more than half of adults over the age of 50 in the UK being infected, but the incidence in younger groups is falling. In developing countries the infection rate is far higher, with rates of up to 90% in some countries. However, most infected patients are asymptomatic.

The bacterium is highly pathogenic and has many virulence factors which allow it to survive in the hostile environment of the stomach:

- Its *motility* allows it to penetrate close to the epithelium, where the pH is near-neutral
- It produces the enzyme *urease*, which converts urea to ammonia, which buffers the gastric acid with the concurrent production of carbon dioxide. This is a highly effective virulence factor, as urea channels in the inner cell membrane of the bacterium open at pH levels less than 6.5, delivering urea to the bacterial urease. The activity of *H. pylori* urease is the basis for the urea breath test to detect the bacterium
- The *vacuolating toxin* (VacA) alters intracellular vesicular trafficking in gastric cells, leading to the formation of large vacuoles
- The *cytotoxin-associated antigen* (CagA) is an immunodominant antigen which elicits a strong serological response. It has been shown to be involved in pathogenesis via the insertion of pathogenicity islands
- Other virulence factors include *adhesin, phospholipases and porins*.

Fortunately, *H. pylori* can be eradicated pharmacologically with triple therapy treatment. This consists of a PPI with two antibiotics, currently a combination of clarithromycin with either amoxicillin or metronidazole. This generally has a 90% success rate, and in those patients in whom triple therapy is unsuccessful, quadruple therapy, with the addition of bismuth chelate should be offered.

> **HINTS AND TIPS**
>
> When prescribing metronidazole, advise patients to avoid alcohol. Metronidazole has a disulfiram-like effect and patients will feel severely ill if they drink alcohol at the same time. Disulfiram inhibits acetaldehyde dehydrogenase, an enzyme in the pathway for alcohol metabolism. In this situation acetaldehyde builds up which can cause unpleasant flushing and nausea. Unless they are warned, they will understandably think the symptoms are caused by the drug and stop taking it.

Peptic ulcer disease

Ulcers arise when damaging factors, particularly gastric secretions, overwhelm the natural protection of the mucosal lining of the gastrointestinal tract. They can result from a decrease in protective factors, an increase in damaging factors, or both.

Peptic ulcers can be divided into acute and chronic forms. The former are usually caused by the same factors as acute erosive gastritis, and in the same locations. Severe stress and trauma, such as after burns (Curling's ulcer), head trauma (Cushing's ulcer) and ischaemia of the gastric mucosa are other causes.

Chronic peptic ulcers occur in the upper gastrointestinal tract where gastric acid and pepsin are present. They are caused by hyperacidity, *H. pylori* infection (the commonest cause), reflux of duodenal contents, NSAIDs and smoking. Genetic factors play a role, as peptic ulceration is more common in patients with blood group O and first-degree relatives of people with duodenal ulcers are three times more likely to develop them themselves. Males are three times more likely to develop chronic ulcers than females. They are an example of a chronic inflammatory process (Fig. 3.14).

The two main types of peptic ulcers are duodenal ulcers and gastric ulcers (especially at the junction of the antrum and the body). Other sites include the distal oesophagus, particularly in Barrett's oesophagus, a Meckel's diverticulum and where a gastroenterostomy has been performed.

There is an increase in incidence of peptic ulcer above the age of 45 years. Both duodenal and gastric ulcers are common in the elderly.

Fig. 3.14 Structure of a peptic ulcer. The interplay between the opposing forces of continuing tissue damage and healing with scar formation is the cause of chronic inflammation. (Redrawn with permission from Stevens A, Lowe J. Human Histology, 2nd edn. Edinburgh: Mosby, 1997.)

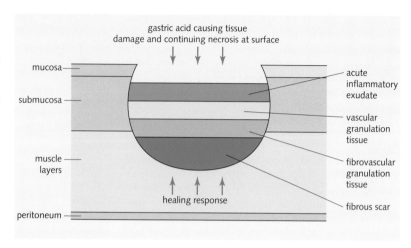

Epigastric pain is the main presenting symptom, with endoscopy and tests for the presence of *H. pylori* being the usual investigations when peptic ulcer disease is suspected.

Treatment for peptic ulcers include proton pump inhibitors for at least 2 months, and triple therapy for the eradication of *H. pylori* if necessary. If possible, patients are advised to stop taking NSAIDs or use the lowest dose possible for symptom control.

Duodenal ulcers

Duodenal ulcers (DU) are two to three times more common than gastric ulcers (GU), occurring in about 15% of the population. Approximately 90% of DU are associated with *H. pylori*.

Classically the epigastric pain is said to be relieved by food or antacids, and exacerbated by hunger.

Gastric ulcers

Seventy per cent of GU are associated with *H. pylori*, with the rest mainly associated with NSAID treatment. Gastric ulcers may also occur in response to acute gastritis or extreme hyperacidity, as in Zollinger–Ellison syndrome.

The epigastric pain is characteristically associated with food.

Zollinger–Ellison syndrome is a rare condition due to gastrin-secreting pancreatic adenomas causing excess acid production. It can lead to acute ulcers in the antrum, duodenum and, in severe cases, the jejunum.

Complications of chronic peptic ulcer include:

- Haemorrhage
- Perforation, leading to peritonitis
- Penetration, where the ulcer penetrates through the stomach or duodenal wall into underlying tissue. Usually it is the pancreas or liver which is affected

- Stricture, causing acquired pyloric stenosis in the stomach, or oesophageal stricture which is more common
- Malignant change, which is rare.

Vascular disorders

Angiodysplasia

Angiodysplasia is a rare cause of upper gastrointestinal bleeding, which may range in severity from occult to massive. It is a condition found in elderly patients where there is one or more malformed blood vessels (typically veins) in the mucosa or submucosa.

These can be found anywhere in the gastrointestinal tract. The vessels are dilated, thin-walled and look like 'cherry spots'. They are normally asymptomatic.

Gastric varices

Gastric varices are uncommon, but they may occur in submucosal veins below the gastro-oesophageal junction as a result of portal hypertension.

Like oesophageal varices, they should never be biopsied or they will haemorrhage with potentially fatal consequences.

Treatment includes injecting with a sclerosing agent, or thrombin to arrest bleeding by thrombosis.

Delayed gastric emptying

Gastric emptying can be delayed by mechanical or non-mechanical obstructions.

Mechanical obstructions include tumours, duodenal, gastric or pyloric stenosis, and bezoars (a mass of swallowed foreign material, which has collected and is obstructing emptying).

Non-mechanical delayed gastric emptying is known as gastroparesis. This is an uncommon complication of diabetes, but it can also occur due to gastric arrhythmias, myotonic dystrophy, collagen-vascular diseases, neuropathies and after vagotomy.

Mechanical delayed gastric emptying must be excluded before non-mechanical aetiologies can be explored. Quite often, the cause is unknown and the problem is called idiopathic gastroparesis, but is probably due to gastric arrhythmias.

Diabetic gastroparesis is associated with peripheral neuropathy.

Patients can be asymptomatic, or they may have a combination of symptoms, including bloating, abdominal pain, persistent belching, nausea (with or without vomiting), anorexia, early satiety and weight loss. Treatment includes:

- Nutritional supplementation
- Prokinetic drugs, e.g. metoclopramide – see Chapter 5
- Surgery.

Neoplastic disease

Benign neoplasms

These include:

- Gastrointestinal stromal tumour (GIST, formerly called leiomyoma), arising from smooth muscle, which may bleed from ulceration. These are the most common benign gastric tumours
- Adenomas (benign tumours of glandular origin) make up 5–10% of polypoid lesions in the stomach and may contain proliferative dysplastic epithelium with the potential for malignant transformation. They are much more common in the colon but, if present in the stomach, are usually in the antrum. They may be pedunculated (with a stalk) or sessile (without a stalk) and are more common in males. The incidence of adenomas increases with age
- Hyperplastic polyps (regenerative polyps) are elongated gastric pits separated by fibrous tissue, usually found in association with H. pylori infection in the antrum
- Simple fundic polyps (glandular cystic dilatation in the body of the stomach)
- Hamartomas (overgrowth of mature tissue, displaying disordered arrangement and proportion) are most commonly seen in Peutz–Jeghers syndrome, a hereditary disorder
- Ectopic (heterotopic) pancreatic tissue
- Fibromas and neurofibromas, which are connective tissue tumours
- Haemangiomas, which are highly vascular in nature.

Malignant neoplasms

Aetiology

In the UK, approximately 15 in 100 000 people are affected each year with gastric carcinoma and the incidence increases with age, affecting men more than women. It is the fifth biggest cause of death due to malignancy. The incidence is falling in both Europe and the USA, although it remains high in the Far East, for which dietary factors have been implicated.

Adenocarcinoma is the most common gastric neoplasm and accounts for 90% of all malignant neoplasms in the stomach. Malignant lymphomas account for 5% of gastric malignant neoplasms, and other malignancies such as carcinoid and malignant spindle cell tumours occur rarely.

A number of conditions are premalignant, such as atrophic gastritis, some chronic gastric ulcers, pernicious anaemia, and post-gastrectomy (carcinomas often develop 15–20 years after surgery).

Genetic factors may be involved, as the incidence is slightly higher in blood group A as well as in patients with hereditary non-polyposis colorectal cancer, but a decrease in gastric acid secretion and corresponding increase in bacteria (which are normally killed by gastric acid), particularly H. pylori, are common predisposing factors.

Helicobacter pylori infections cause chronic gastritis, which occasionally becomes atrophic gastritis, leading to metaplasia, dysplasia and ultimately carcinoma.

Dietary factors may act to initiate or promote carcinogenesis. A diet high in salt increases the risk. Also, dietary nitrates are converted to carcinogenic nitrosamines by bacteria. Therefore, diets high in nitrates predispose to carcinoma. The incidence is high in Japan but much lower amongst Japanese living in the USA. Diets high in fruit and vegetables can help protect against cancer because of the antioxidants they contain.

Pathology

Four different macroscopic appearances may be recognized:

- *Malignant ulcers* with raised, everted edges
- *Polypoid tumours* – these tend to present early with discomfort, as they protrude into the lumen and so are subject to trauma. It has the best prognosis of all the pathological types as it is most suitable for surgical excision
- *Colloid tumours* – these are large tumours which appear gelatinous
- *Diffuse infiltrative tumours* (linitis plastica, or 'leather bottle' stomach, so named because the stomach becomes small, thick and contracted) – these present very late and so have a poor prognosis. Unfortunately, they comprise a third of all gastric carcinomas.

Histology shows sheets of anaplastic cells, many with a single vacuole displacing the nucleus to one side, giving them the name 'signet-ring cells'.

Carcinomas may spread through the lymphatic system, the bloodstream and direct spread locally.

Metastases can occur in the liver, bone, brain and lung. Through peritoneal seeding, metastases can also be found in the ovary (Krukenberg tumour).

Clinical features

Presentation is often late, with a correspondingly poor prognosis due to metastatic spread. Signs and symptoms include:

- Epigastric pain
- Nausea and vomiting (especially if the tumour is at the pylorus, causing obstruction)
- Anorexia
- Anaemia, most likely iron-deficient from occult bleeding
- Haematemesis
- Weight loss, often profound
- Palpable epigastric mass (in 50% of patients)
- Signs of metastatic spread such as ascites, hepatomegaly and jaundice.

Clinical Note

Never ignore it if one of the supraclavicular lymph nodes on the left side of the body is enlarged. Lymph from the cardiac region of the stomach drains to these nodes and they may become enlarged due to metastatic spread from gastric carcinoma (Virchow's node, also called Troisier's sign).

Diagnosis

Endoscopy is the investigation of choice. All gastric ulcers should be biopsied to exclude malignancy. Patients should have a follow-up endoscopy in 6 weeks to confirm ulcer healing. Computed tomography (CT) scan is usually performed to look for any metastatic spread.

Prognosis and treatment

Generally, the 5-year survival rate is less than 10%, but it is much better for diagnosis of early carcinoma, i.e. neoplasms confined to the mucosa and submucosa.

Treatment includes radiotherapy and surgery to excise the tumour and any affected lymph nodes. Partial or total gastrectomy may be necessary in some cases.

The small intestine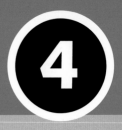

● **Objectives**

After reading this chapter, you should be able to:
- Describe the anatomy of the small intestine with regard to its macroscopic structure, relations, arterial supply, venous and lymphatic drainage, and nerve supply
- Outline the embryological development of the small intestine
- Describe the histological structure of the small intestine
- Outline the functions of the small intestine, and the mechanisms controlling small intestinal motility
- Describe the process of digestion and absorption in the small intestine
- Outline the following types of small intestinal disorders: congenital abnormalities, malabsorption and neoplastic disease

OVERVIEW

The small intestine extends from the stomach to the ileocaecal valve, where it joins the colon. It is approximately 6–7 metres long and is the main site for the digestive and absorptive processes.

ANATOMY

The small intestine consists of three parts: the duodenum, jejunum and ileum (Fig. 4.1).

Duodenum

The duodenum is about 25 cm in length and extends from the pylorus to the duodenojejunal flexure. It is C-shaped and snakes around the head of the pancreas beginning 2–3 cm on the right side of the median plane and ending an equal distance from the median plane, but to the left. It lies in the umbilical region and except for the first 2.5 cm, it is retroperitoneal and hence is the most fixed part of the small intestine.

The first 2 cm of the duodenum is called the duodenal cap. Only the proximal half has mesentery, which allows mobility. The greater omentum and hepatoduodenal ligament are attached proximally. The remainder of the duodenum has no mesentery and is therefore immobile.

The first part of the duodenum is about 5 cm long, and is related to the following structures:

- Anteriorly: the peritoneum, gall bladder and quadrate lobe of the liver

- Posteriorly: the gastroduodenal artery, inferior vena cava, portal vein and bile duct
- Inferiorly: the neck of the pancreas.

The second, retroperitoneal section is about 10 cm in length and descends to the right side of L3. The common bile duct and pancreatic duct open into the posteromedial wall, coming together to form the ampulla of Vater (hepatopancreatic ampulla) about two thirds along its length (Fig. 4.2). This opens at the major duodenal papilla.

The relations of the second part are:

- Anteriorly: the transverse colon, mesocolon and coils of the small intestine
- Posteriorly: the hilum of the right kidney, its renal vessels, the right ureter and the psoas major muscle
- Medially: the head of the pancreas and the bile and pancreatic ducts.

The third, horizontal section of the duodenum is also retroperitoneal, and is approximately 10 cm in length. This passes to the left, anterior to L3, before turning upwards. It is adherent to the posterior abdominal wall, and is related to:

- Posteriorly: the right psoas major muscle, right ureter, the abdominal aorta and inferior vena cava
- Anteriorly: the coils of the small intestine and the superior mesenteric artery
- Superiorly: the superior mesenteric vessels and the head of the pancreas.

The fourth ascending part is 3 cm in length and ascends to the duodenojejunal flexure to the left of L2. The duodenum becomes the jejunum at the ligament of Treitz, a fibromuscular band, which is also called

Fig. 4.1 The position of the small and large intestines.

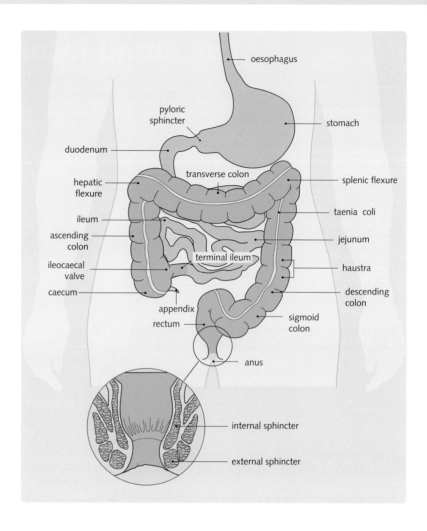

the suspensory muscle of the duodenum. The relations of the final part are:

- Anteriorly: the coils of jejunum and the beginning of the root of the mesentery
- Posteriorly: the left psoas major muscle and the left margin of the aorta
- The head and body of the pancreas lie medially and superiorly to D4, respectively.

Jejunum

The jejunum begins at the duodenojejunal flexure and makes up about two fifths of the small intestine. It is about 2.5 m long and lies mostly in the umbilical region. The jejunum has large and well-developed mucosal plicae circulares (circular folds).

Ileum

The ileum, which is about 3.5 m long, constitutes the rest of the small intestine. There is no clear demarcation between it and the jejunum, but the ileum is paler, thinner-walled and less vascular than the jejunum. These differences, especially the fact that it is less vascular, are important surgically.

It is situated in the suprapubic and inguinal regions. Its terminal part lies in the pelvis major, ascending over the right psoas muscle and the right iliac vessels to join with the caecum at the ileocolic junction. The plicae circulares are small in the superior part of the ileum and absent in the terminal end.

Mesentery

The small intestine has a fan-shaped mesentery, which suspends it from the posterior abdominal wall and allows the jejunum and ileum to be mobile. The root of the mesentery is about 15 cm long and this moves from left to right in an oblique and inferior direction. It begins on the left side of L2 and ends at the right sacroiliac joint, passing the following structures:

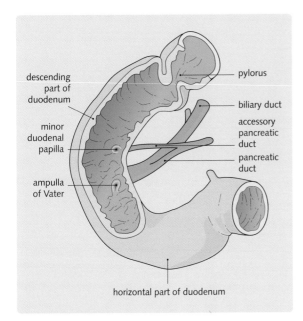

descending part of duodenum

minor duodenal papilla

ampulla of Vater

pylorus

biliary duct

accessory pancreatic duct

pancreatic duct

horizontal part of duodenum

Fig. 4.2 The second (descending) part of the duodenum, showing the periampullar structures.

- The horizontal part (D3) of the duodenum
- The aorta
- The inferior vena cava
- The right psoas major muscle
- The right ureter
- The right testicular (or ovarian) vessels.

Blood supply

The proximal half of the duodenum is a foregut structure and so is supplied by the coeliac trunk through the gastroduodenal artery and its branch, the superior pancreaticoduodenal artery. The distal half of the duodenum is a midgut structure. It is supplied by the inferior pancreaticoduodenal artery, which is a branch of the superior mesenteric artery.

The superior and inferior pancreaticoduodenal arteries form anastomoses called the anterior and posterior arcades. These lie in between the duodenum and the pancreas.

As they are midgut structures, the jejunum and ileum are supplied by the superior mesenteric artery, which arises from the abdominal aorta at the level of L1. Some 15–18 jejunal and ileal branches arise from the left side of the superior mesenteric artery and pass between the two layers of the mesentery, forming arches or loops called arcades. The arterial supplies of the jejunum and ileum are compared in Fig. 4.3.

Straight arteries called vasa recta branch off from the arcades and do not anastomose in the mesentery. Many blood vessel anastomoses are found within the walls of the intestines.

The last ileal branch from the superior mesenteric artery anastomoses with a branch of the ileocolic artery.

Venous drainage

The venous drainage follows the arterial supply of the small intestine. From the duodenum, blood drains into the portal venous system, via the superior mesenteric vein. Drainage occurs in three ways:

- Direct drainage to the portal vein
- Indirect drainage, via small veins, to the pancreaticoduodenal veins
- Indirect drainage, via the prepyloric veins, to the right gastric vein.

In the jejunum and ileum, all the tributaries of the superior mesenteric vein run alongside the branches of the superior mesenteric artery.

Lymphatic drainage

In the duodenum, the anterior and posterior surface lymphatics anastomose. The anterior vessels drain to the pyloric and pancreaticoduodenal lymph nodes, which then drain to the coeliac lymph nodes. The posterior vessels drain to the superior mesenteric nodes.

In the jejunum and ileum, the lymphatics are present in the villi as lacteals. The lymph vessels drain into the mesenteric lymph nodes close to the intestinal wall, along the arterial arcades and along the proximal section of the superior mesenteric artery.

The terminal ileal lymph vessels drain to the ileocolic lymph nodes, which run with the ileal branch of the ileocolic artery.

Innervation

Duodenal innervation comes from the vagus and sympathetic nerves via nerve plexuses on the pancreaticoduodenal arteries.

The jejunum and ileum are also supplied by the vagus and splanchnic nerves. These travel through the coeliac ganglion and form plexuses around the superior mesenteric artery.

> **HINTS AND TIPS**
>
> The superior mesenteric nerve plexus, supplying the small intestine, receives sympathetic and parasympathetic supplies from the superior mesenteric ganglion and coeliac division of the vagal trunk, respectively.

Fig. 4.3 Arteries of the gastrointestinal tract.

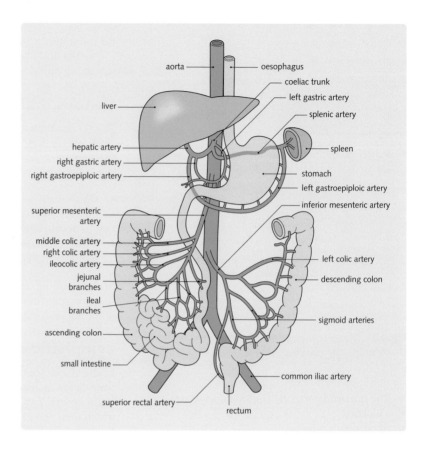

EMBRYOLOGY AND DEVELOPMENT

The proximal portion of the small intestine (from the pylorus to the duodenal papilla) develops from the foregut. The remainder of the intestine develops from the midgut and hindgut. Rapid elongation of the midgut, to form the primary intestinal loop, occurs from 5 weeks of embryonic life.

The midgut gives rise to the remainder of the duodenum (that part distal to the duodenal papilla) and to the proximal two thirds of the transverse colon. The duodenum is, therefore, supplied by branches of the artery of the foregut (the coeliac artery) and the superior mesenteric artery (which supplies the midgut).

The midgut is suspended from the dorsal abdominal wall by a mesentery. It communicates with the yolk sac through the vitelline duct. A small portion of the vitelline duct persists in 2% of individuals and forms an outpouching of the ileum known as Meckel's diverticulum.

During development, the liver and primitive gut grow so rapidly that there is not enough room in the fetal abdominal cavity, and the midgut herniates outside the abdominal cavity at about the 6th week. It develops in the umbilical cord until the end of the 3rd month, when it begins to return to the abdominal cavity.

While outside the abdomen, the primary intestinal loop rotates approximately 270° around the superior mesenteric artery. Viewed from the front, the rotation is anticlockwise (Fig. 4.4).

The jejunum and ileum form a number of coiled loops but the large intestine remains uncoiled. The jejunum is the first portion of gut to return to the abdominal cavity.

HISTOLOGY

The tissue layers of the small intestine are essentially the same as those found elsewhere in the gastrointestinal tract (see Fig. 1.2), consisting of a mucosa, submucosa, muscularis externa and serosa.

The mucosa

The mucosa consists of an epithelial layer, the lamina propria and the muscularis mucosae. It is the main site

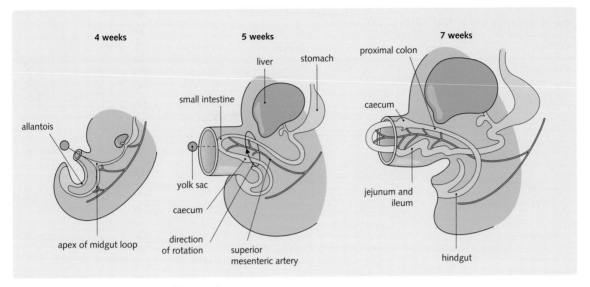

Fig. 4.4 Rotation and herniation of the developing gut.

of absorption for the digestion of products, such as amino acids, fats and sugars and so it, as well as the submucosa, is specialized to allow maximum absorption.

The mucosa has a much greater surface area than other parts of the gastrointestinal tract due to:

- The length of the small intestine
- Plicae circulares
- Numerous villi
- A striated border of microvilli.

These factors together produce a 600-fold increase in the absorptive area of the small intestine. Plicae circulares are folds in the mucosa and submucosa, arranged on a circular fashion around the lumen of the small intestine. They are most prominent in the jejunum, but absent in the distal part of the small intestine.

Intestinal glands (crypts of Lieberkühn) are found throughout the length of the small intestine. They are simple tubular glands extending through the thickness of the mucous membrane and opening into the intestinal lumen at the base of the villi (Fig. 4.5).

Villi

The villi change in shape along the length of the small intestine. In the duodenum they are broad, but they become leaf-like further down the tract. In the terminal ileum, villi are finger-like projections.

They consist of an epithelial cover and a lamina propria with a centrally placed lymphatic capillary (lacteal) that drains into the large lymphatic vessels in the

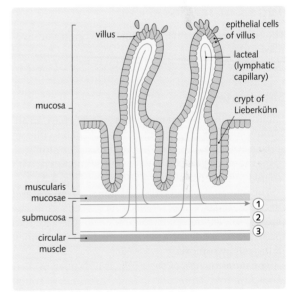

Fig. 4.5 Cross-section of small intestinal villi. Drainage is to the hepatic portal vein (1), branches of superior mesenteric artery (2) and the lymphatic system (3).

submucosa (Fig. 4.5). Lacteals dilate after a meal, but they are collapsed in the fasting state.

HINTS AND TIPS

Villi are projections consisting of a series of epithelial cells; microvilli are smaller protrusions from individual epithelial cells.

Fig. 4.6 Cells of the small intestinal mucosa and their functions.

Cell type	Function
Enterocytes	Intestinal absorptive cells. These tall columnar cells have microvilli and absorb water andnutrients from the lumen of the gut
Goblet cells	These produce mucus and are found on the villi. They are least numerous in the duodenum and most numerous in the erminal ileum
Paneth cells	These are phagocytic cells and contain lysozyme granules. They are found deep in the intestinal glands
Membranous microfold 'M' cells	Epithelial cells, which overlie Peyer's patches and allow for entry of antigen
Undifferentiated (stem) cells	These give rise to enterocytes, goblet cells and enteroendocrine cells. They are located in the lower thirds of the crypts
Enteroendocrine (APUD) cells	These cells secrete hormones and neuropeptides, such as somatostatin, 5-HT, secretin and gastrin. They are found in the crypts of the small intestine and have microvilli at their luminal apices

Types of mucosal cell

The cell types of the small intestinal mucosa are summarized in Fig. 4.6.

Enterocytes

Enterocytes are the most numerous cells and have an absorptive function. They are found chiefly on the villi and surface of the small intestine and, in smaller numbers, in the intestinal glands. They are tall columnar cells with striated microvilli and irregular outlines (Fig. 4.7).

The cells absorb water from the lumen of the gut, and the paracellular spaces contain ATPases (membrane pumps) which transport sodium from the cell into the spaces, drawing the water absorbed from the lumen of the cell by osmosis.

The ultrastructure of these cells is indicative of their absorptive role. They contain large quantities of rough endoplasmic reticulum (RER), mitochondria and Golgi bodies. Many ribosomes are present.

The microvilli are covered by a protein coat, the glycocalyx. This contains many enzymes (e.g. lactase, alkaline phosphatase, lipases), which are involved in digestion and transport.

Goblet cells

Goblet cells (Fig. 4.8) in the intestine produce mucus, as they do in other epithelia. They are packed with mucin and their cytoplasm has abundant RER, reflecting their secretory role.

They are interspersed between the enterocytes and are most numerous on the villi and in the superior two thirds of the crypts.

Goblet cells are least numerous in the duodenum, but they increase in frequency along the length of the small intestine, being most populous in the terminal ileum.

Paneth cells

Paneth cells are found in the deepest part of the intestinal glands. They synthesize and secrete large amounts of protein, and thus have cytoplasm rich in RER. The secreted proteins are defensins which protect against infection by regulating the gut flora.

They are also phagocytic and contain granules of lysozyme, an enzyme that digests the walls of certain bacteria.

Stem cells

Stem (undifferentiated) cells are located in the lower third of the crypts of Lieberkühn. They replenish all the other cells of the small intestine.

Approximately 1.7 billion enterocytes are shed from the adult intestine each day, being replaced by undifferentiated cells migrating up from the bases of the crypts. The turnover of enterocytes takes about 5 days.

Enteroendocrine cells

The enteroendocrine (amine precursor uptake and decarboxylation, APUD) cells situated in the crypts of the small intestine are very similar to those found in

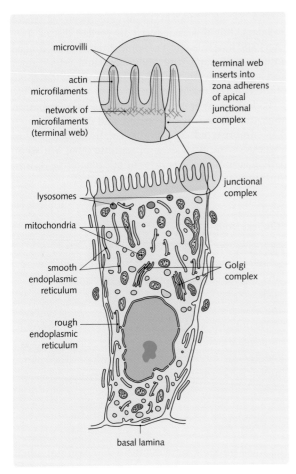

Fig. 4.7   An enterocyte.

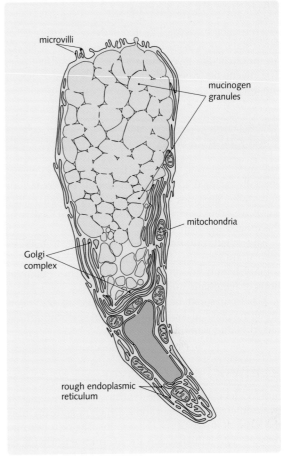

Fig. 4.8   A goblet cell.

the stomach. They are triangular-shaped with the luminal apex displaying microvilli, and contain neuroendocrine granules.

They secrete hormones and neuropeptides, including somatostatin, 5-hydroxytryptamine (serotonin), secretin, gastrin, motilin and vasoactive intestinal polypeptide.

Peyer's patches

Peyer's patches are present in the mucosa of the ileum, extending into the submucosa, and are characteristically found opposite the attachment of the mesentery. They consist of aggregations of lymphoid nodules and form part of the mucosa-associated lymphoid tissue (MALT) system. The Peyer's patches contain three types of cell:

- Membranous microfold 'M' cells, which allow antigen to enter
- Dome cells, which are rich in MHC class II and present antigen to lymphocytes
- Lymphocytes (B and T) found in the follicular zone.

Lamina propria

The lamina propria of the small intestine is made up of a glycosaminoglycan (GAG) matrix, fibroblasts, collagen, reticulin and smooth muscle fibres.

It also contains capillaries, lymphatics, nerves and diffuse lymphoid tissue.

Submucosa

The submucosa contains the submucosal (Meissner's) plexus as well as a large quantity of mucosa-associated lymphoid tissue (MALT) and lymphatics. It is vascular and extends into the plicae circulares.

In the duodenum, compound tubular Brunner's glands are also present. They secrete mucus, bicarbonate and growth factors such as epidermal growth factor. The last of these promotes the growth and regeneration of tissues. Brunner's glands also secrete urogastrone, an inhibitor of acid secretion.

Muscularis externa

The muscularis externa, like that of the rest of the gastro-intestinal tract, is made up of two smooth muscle layers: an inner circular layer and an outer longitudinal one. The myenteric (Auerbach's) plexus is located between the muscle layers.

PHYSIOLOGY

The small intestine has a very large surface area and is specially adapted to digest and absorb nutrients, salt and water. Enzymes and hormones produced in the small intestine complete the digestion that began in the mouth and stomach.

The small intestine has immunological defences against antigens that have been ingested consisting of solitary lymph nodules and Peyer's patches (aggregations of lymphatic nodules).

Gastrointestinal hormones produced in the small intestine play an important role in gastrointestinal secretion and motility.

Epithelial cell turnover

Enterocytes have a high rate of turnover and are replaced by undifferentiated (stem) cells, which migrate up from the bases of the crypts of Lieberkühn. The cells become partially differentiated and they continue to divide as they migrate upwards from the bottom of the crypts (Fig. 4.9).

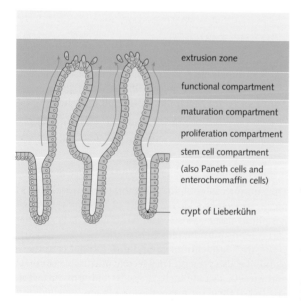

extrusion zone

functional compartment

maturation compartment

proliferation compartment

stem cell compartment
(also Paneth cells and enterochromaffin cells)

crypt of Lieberkühn

Fig. 4.9 Cell turnover and migration of stem cells in the small intestine.

The average lifespan of an enterocyte is about 2–3 days, but this is reduced in coeliac disease (see later) and as a side effect of some drugs, e.g. prolonged anticancer therapy. The undifferentiated cells cannot keep up with the increased loss, resulting in a flattening of the villi and malabsorption.

Radiotherapy may have a similar effect (radiation enteritis) depending on the dose and the site at which it is administered. Symptoms usually resolve within 6 weeks of the final dose of radiotherapy, but some patients experience chronic radiation enteritis (symptoms persisting for more than 3 months).

Clinical Note

In coeliac disease, which is caused by an allergy to gluten in wheat, the surface of the jejunum is flattened and there is extensive loss of villi. This causes malabsorption, as the loss of villi results in a decrease in the available absorptive area.

This loss of villi also results in an increased enterocyte turnover and thus an increase in stem cell numbers, as the stem cells try to replenish the lost cells. There is further information later in the chapter.

Secretions

The small intestine secretes mucus and gastrointestinal hormones.

- Mucus is produced by the goblet cells (Fig. 4.8), which are most numerous on the villi. The mucus lubricates the mucosal surface and protects it from trauma as particles of food pass through it
- The gastrointestinal hormones which affect the small intestine are summarized in Fig. 4.10.

The epithelial cells secrete an aqueous solution during the course of digestion but, under normal conditions, they absorb slightly more than they secrete.

Defence

The defences of the small intestine are in the most part due to T and B lymphocytes.

T lymphocytes account for 75% of all lymphocytes, and are made in the thymus gland, following which they migrate into encapsulated peripheral tissues such as those of the spleen and lymph nodes. T lymphocytes also migrate to non-encapsulated lymphoid tissue known as mucosa-associated lymphoid tissue (MALT). This gives protection against antigens entering the body through mucosal epithelial surfaces.

Fig. 4.10 The main hormones acting on the small intestine and their functions.

Hormone	Gastrointestinal source	Signal for release	Action
CCK	Enteroendocrine (APUD) cells in upper intestine	Peptides and amino acids and fats, elevated serum Ca^{2+} in duodenum	Contracts gall bladder and relaxes sphincter of Oddi; causes secretion of alkaline enzymatic pancreatic juice, inhibits gastric emptying, exerts trophic effect on pancreas, acts as a satiety hormone, stimulates glucagon secretion and contracts the pyloric sphincter
Secretin	S cells in upper small intestine	Acid and products of fat digestion in duodenum	Increases secretion of HCO_3^- by the pancreas and biliary tract, decreases acid secretion, contracts the pyloric sphincter and augments CCK's stimulation of pancreatic secretions
Gastrin	G cells in antrum	Peptides and amino acids, distension, vagal stimulation, blood-borne calcium and epinephrine	Acid and pepsinogen secretion, trophic to mucosa of stomach and small and large intestines, increases gastric motility, may close LOS, stimulates insulin and glucagon secretion after protein meal. Inhibits gastric emptying
Somatostatin	D cells of pancreatic islets, intestinal cells	Glucose, amino acids, free fatty acids, glucagon and β-adrenergic and cholinergic neurotransmitters	Inhibits secretion of insulin, glucagon, acid, pepsin, gastrin, secretin and intestinal juices, decreases gastric, duodenal and gall bladder motility

The majority of MALT is present as gut-associated lymphoid tissue (GALT); smaller amounts are present in the bronchi, skin and genitourinary tract.

T cells are divided into:

- Helper (CD4) cells, which enhance the reaction of the immune system following the presentation of antigen to T helper cells by antigen-presenting cells, via MHC class II receptors
- Cytotoxic (CD8) cells, which are capable of killing other cells, e.g. cancer cells and cells that have been infected with viruses, and can also down-regulate the immune response. They are activated via an endogenous antigen–MHC class I complex.

B lymphocytes are made in the bone marrow and, in the fetus, in the liver. They also migrate to peripheral tissues, including MALT. B cells produce antibody and, once they have encountered a particular antigen, form memory cells, which can undergo clonal expansion (multiplication to form large numbers of identical B cells). They then differentiate to form plasma cells, which have a relatively short half-life but which produce large numbers of specific antibody to particular antigens. Scattered lymphoid cells are also found in the mucosa of the small intestine.

The main type of antibody produced by intestinal B cells is IgA, the major immunoglobulin of external secretions. There are approximately 10^{10} plasma cells per metre of small intestine, the majority of which (70–90%) produce IgA. IgA dimers are transported across the glandular epithelium into the gut lumen by binding to a receptor on the epithelial surface. The IgA–receptor complex is endocytosed and transported across the cell into the lumen. Part of the receptor (the secretory component) remains attached to the IgA and protects IgA from proteolytic enzymes in the lumen.

IgA prevents microorganisms from entering as it binds and neutralizes them directly without the need for other effector systems. A much smaller amount of IgM is also secreted by the intestinal B cells.

Specialized M cells (so named because of the numerous microfolds on their luminal surface) overlie the Peyer's patches and they absorb, transport, process and present antigens to the lymphoid cells lying between them.

Motility

Motility in the small intestine facilitates three main functions:

- Mixing of intestinal contents
- Bringing the contents into contact with the absorptive surfaces of the small intestine
- Forward propulsion of the contents.

Chyme takes between 2 and 3 hours to pass through the small intestine, which is the site at which most digestion and absorption of nutrients takes place. There are two main types of contraction seen in the fed state: segmentation and peristalsis.

Segmentation mixes the digested food and exposes it to the absorptive surfaces. It is a discontinuous, oscillating contraction resulting in alternating contracted and relaxed areas, the latter containing chyme. Although the movement is mainly in a forwards-and-backwards

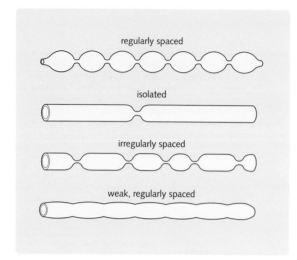

Fig. 4.11 Segmentation in the small intestine.

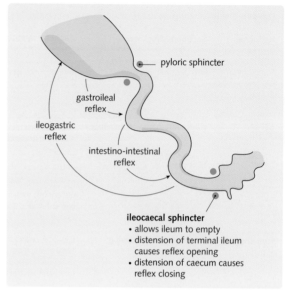

ileocaecal sphincter
- allows ileum to empty
- distension of terminal ileum causes reflex opening
- distension of caecum causes reflex closing

Fig. 4.12 Control of small intestine motility.

direction, there is a slow net movement towards the anus as the frequency of the contractions decreases down the length of the small intestine (Fig. 4.11).

Peristaltic contraction brings about rapid propulsion of the intestinal contents towards the anus, at a rate of 2–25 cm/s. It involves contraction of the longitudinal muscles and is a reflex initiated by local distension caused by the bolus of food. Peristalsis moves chyme more quickly towards the colon and does not mix it as efficiently as segmentation.

Motility in the fasting state is due to migrating motor complexes (MMC) which occur every 90–120 min. The MMC involves high-frequency bursts of powerful contractions, beginning in the stomach and moving towards the terminal ileum. The pyloric sphincter is open wide during the MMC.

The MMC has a number of functions:

- It moves indigestible food, e.g. tomato skins, nuts, sweetcorn into the lower bowel
- It allows for the removal of dead epithelial cells
- It prevents bacterial overgrowth
- It prevents colonic bacteria entering the small intestine.

Control of intestinal motility

The motility of the small intestine is controlled by nervous, hormonal and local factors which coordinate the various intestinal reflexes (Fig. 4.12). Of importance is the gastroileal reflex, which causes ileal segmentation in response to gastrin secreted due to the presence of chyme in the stomach.

Vagal stimulation is required to maintain the fed motor pattern. Segmentation is coordinated by the myenteric plexus, and circular muscle contraction is brought about by acetylcholine and substance P.

The peristaltic reflex occurs by the simultaneous oral (proximal) contraction and anal (distal) relaxation, either side of the bolus. The contraction is mediated by vagal excitatory contractions, via substance P and acetylcholine.

The relaxation is mediated by vagal inhibitory contractions, via nitric oxide (NO) and VIP. Movement of the bolus into the next section of the intestine triggers the next reflex.

In the fasting state, the MMC is coordinated by the enteric nervous system. It is initiated by vagal stimulation and motilin. During an MMC, plasma motilin concentrations increase, but they decrease on the arrival of food in the stomach.

Control of the ileocaecal valve

The incompetent ileocaecal valve (see Chapter 5) separates the terminal ileum from the colon and is normally closed. However, it opens in response to:

- Distension of the terminal ileum (by a reflex mechanism)
- Short-range peristalsis in the terminal ileum
- Gastroileal reflex (which enhances emptying of the ileum after a meal).

The intestinal circulation

The intestinal circulation is part of the splanchnic circulation, which supplies the lower oesophagus, stomach, liver, gall bladder, pancreas, spleen and intestines.

At rest, approximately 10–30% of the cardiac output flows to the digestive organs and three quarters of this is required by the mucosa and submucosa for facilitation of absorption and transport. The remaining quarter is utilized by the smooth muscle layer of the bowels.

This circulation is named the intestinal counter-current system, and is very similar to that seen in the loop of Henle in the kidney. In the mucosal villi, the blood vessels are arranged in a network of hairpin loops.

The arteriole enters at the base of the villus and divides into a capillary network at the tip of the villus, just deep to the epithelial lining of the villus. The arteriole and venule are only 20 mm apart and lipid-permeable molecules, such as oxygen, can pass from one vessel to the other.

The blood flows are opposite in direction (hence 'counter-current'). This facilitates some of the dissolved oxygen in the plasma to move along its diffusion gradient from the arteriole to the venule, without entering the capillary network.

When intestinal blood flow is low, this shunting of oxygen can cause death to the epithelial cells at the villus tip. Necrosis of enterocytes at the villus tip is a sign of severe intestinal ischaemia.

The most important function of the counter-current blood flow is to produce a region of hyperosmolarity in the villus tip by means of a multiplier system (Fig. 4.13). Hyperosmolarity is achieved by the following mechanisms:

- Na^+ ions are pumped into the subepithelial extracellular fluid by the enterocytes and taken up in the capillary network. As blood flows down into the venule, Na^+ ions diffuse across to the capillary, which returns the Na^+ ions to the villus tip. This results in a hyperosmolar region at the tip, which draws in water molecules from the intestinal lumen
- Water molecules may also be drawn into the descending capillaries from the arterial vessel, if there is an increased Na^+ concentration. This also results in the delivery of hyperosmolar blood to the villus tip.

Control of the intestinal circulation

Nerves, hormones and local factors control the intestinal circulation.

A change in the cardiac output, arterial pressure or blood volume will have the same effect on this circulation as on the general systemic circulation. For example, massive haemorrhage will result in a decreased venous return to the heart, decreased cardiac output and a drop in arterial blood pressure. This activates baroreceptors to bring about the sympathetic reflex of vasoconstriction in precapillary vessels.

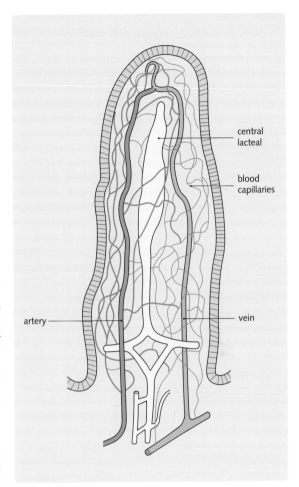

Fig. 4.13 The counter-current mechanism in the villi of the small intestine. This enables absorption of electrolytes and water.

Autonomic nervous control regulates the blood flow by:

- Parasympathetic nerves, which are vasodilators, via acetylcholine and VIP
- Sympathetic nerves, which are vasoconstrictors, via adrenaline (epinephrine) and noradrenaline (norepinephrine) (acting on β2-adrenoreceptors)
- Enteric nerves, which are vasodilators, via acetylcholine and VIP
- Primary sensory nerves (C fibres), which are vasodilators, via NO, substance P and calcitonin gene-related peptide (CGRP)
- Endocrine and paracrine controls can also regulate the intestinal circulation.

Metabolites in the gut after a meal can act as vasodilators. Glucose and fatty acids cause postprandial hyperaemia, which is mediated by VIP release from the enteric nervous system.

DIGESTION AND ABSORPTION

Digestion begins in the mouth and continues in the stomach, but most digestion and absorption takes place in the small intestine. For food to be absorbed, it must be broken down into small particles that can be transported across the epithelial cells of the gastro-intestinal tract and into the bloodstream. Substances are then carried to the liver via the hepatic portal system.

As elsewhere in the body, molecules may be transported across the epithelial cells by simple diffusion, facilitated diffusion and primary or secondary active transport. The properties of these different types of transport are shown in Figs 4.14 and 4.15.

Factors which control absorption by the small intestine

A number of factors control absorption by the small intestine:

- Adequate blood supply
- Carrier molecule density and availability at the brush border
- Cell maturation rate
- Number of transporting cells

Fig. 4.14 Cellular transport mechanisms. (Courtesy of Dr MA Rattray, UMDS, London.)

Type of transport	Proteins required	Transport against or with concentration gradient	Energy required
Passive diffusion	No	With	No
Facilitated diffusion	Yes	With	No
Primary active transport	Yes	Against	Yes: hydrolysis of ATP
Secondary active transport	Yes	Against	Yes: electrochemical gradient

Fig. 4.15 Absorption in the small intestine. For simplicity, all digested foods are shown in the lumen of the small intestine, even though some are digested by brush-border enzymes. (Redrawn with permission from Berne RM, Levy MN. Principles of Physiology, 3rd edn. St Louis: Mosby, 2000.)

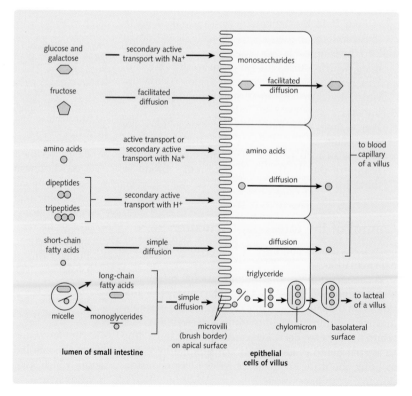

- Passive permeability and the intracellular concentrations of molecules
- The electrochemical gradient for Na+
- Sympathetic innervation and epinephrine in the plasma both increase the absorption of Na^+ and Cl^- (and therefore water)
- Parasympathetic stimulation decreases the absorption of these substances.

Digestion and absorption of different components of the diet

Carbohydrates

Carbohydrates provide most of the calories in the average diet, the majority being in the form of starch (a polymer of glucose).

Starch contains α-1,4 and α-1,6 linkages: the former are hydrolysed by amylase in saliva(ptyalin) and in pancreatic secretions (pancreatic amylase).

This produces maltose and maltotriose (together known as malto-oligosaccharides), comprising 70% of the breakdown products, and α-limit dextrans (the remaining 30%).

Starch is therefore partially digested in the mouth and its digestion continues in the duodenum, as salivary amylase is inactivated in the stomach by gastric acid.

Other enzymes exist in the brush border of the duodenum, and these complete the digestion of starch. These enzymes further breakdown starch into the monosaccharides glucose and galactose, which are actively taken up with sodium. Carbohydrates are only absorbed as monosaccharides through the gut mucosa.

Glucose and galactose then cross the basal membrane into the capillaries by facilitated transport and simple diffusion (Fig. 4.16).

Another monosaccharide, fructose, is also produced and taken up by a sodium-independent mechanism.

A deficiency of enzymes in the digestive system can result in carbohydrate malabsorption. The most common

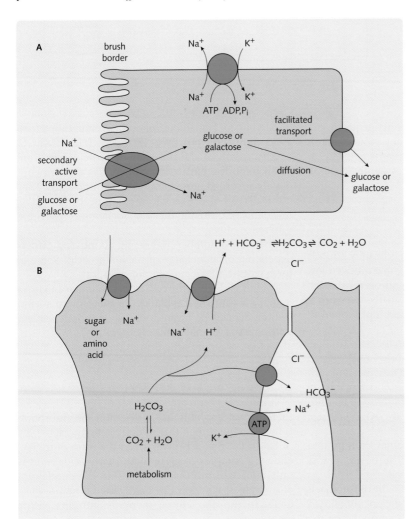

Fig. 4.16 (A) Sugar and (B) ion transport in the small intestine. ([A] Redrawn with permission from Nature 330: 379; London: Macmillan Magazines Ltd, 1986.)

Fig. 4.17 Digestion of carbohydrates.

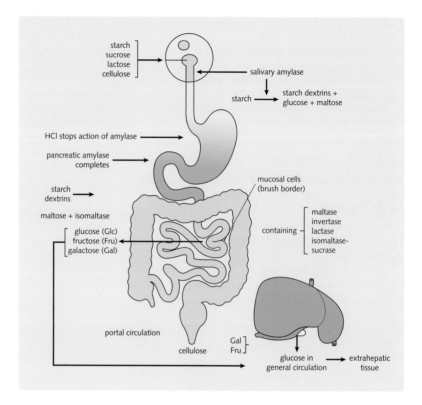

deficiency is lactase deficiency. This is often acquired, and results in lactose intolerance in about 50% of adults worldwide. Congenital lactase deficiency is rare.

The digestion of carbohydrates is summarized in Fig. 4.17.

Protein

The protein requirement of a normal healthy adult is about 40 g/day (to replace the 5–7 g/day nitrogen lost as urea in the urine and so maintain nitrogen balance). In the Western world, meat eaters usually exceed this, but in the developing world the amount of protein in the diet is less.

We do not have a store of protein in the body (unlike, for example, carbohydrate which is stored as glycogen). Every protein in the body performs a function and proteins are in a constant state of flux (1–2% of total body protein is turned over daily), being synthesized by ribosomes and then degraded in the body. We synthesize about 300 g/day.

Protein in the intestinal lumen comes from protein eaten in the diet and also from cell turnover, almost all of which are digested and absorbed.

Digestion of dietary protein begins in the stomach (pepsin hydrolyses about 15% of dietary protein to amino acids and small peptides). It continues in the duodenum and small intestine where pancreatic proteases continue the process of hydrolysis (Fig. 4.18).

Absorption of the products of protein digestion: small peptides, particularly dipeptides and tripeptides are absorbed more rapidly than amino acids. They are transported across the membrane by an active mechanism utilizing the electrochemical potential difference of Na^+.

There are a number of different amino acid carriers depending on the charge of the amino acid. Some of these require a Na^+ gradient for transport.

Amino acids enter the cells from the lumen and leave it to pass into the capillaries by three mechanisms: sodium-dependent transport, sodium-independent transport and simple diffusion.

Defects of amino acid absorption are rare.

Fat

Fat is not water-soluble and its digestion and absorption is more complex than that of other substances.

Fat in the diet is principally in the form of triglycerides (a complex of glycerol and fatty acids) and is only released from the stomach into the duodenum at the rate at which it can be digested. The presence of fat in the duodenum, therefore, inhibits gastric emptying.

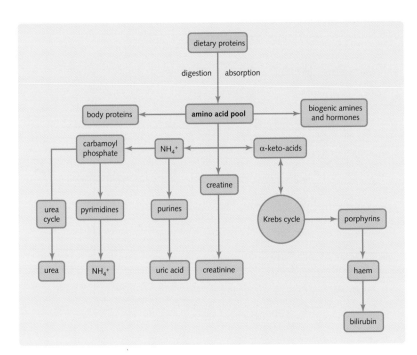

Fig. 4.18 Digestion of protein.

Gastric lipase begins the hydrolysis of triglycerides, although it is not significant unless pancreatic lipase is deficient.

In the duodenum, bile acids, aided by lecithin, emulsify fat to form micelles by their detergent action. A minimum concentration of bile acids is needed to form micelles (the critical micelle concentration). Micelles consist of 20–30 molecules, arranged so that lipid (non-polar) molecules lie in the centre, surrounded by conjugated bile acids and water-soluble molecules. They increase the surface area for enzymatic digestion by pancreatic lipase.

Pancreatic lipase is inactivated by acid and so is ineffective if excess acid is produced by the stomach. This occurs in the Zollinger–Ellison syndrome, where fat malabsorption occurs.

Absorption of the products of fat digestion: the products of fat digestion, being lipids, diffuse across the lipid membrane of the brush border of the small intestine. Different components are absorbed at different rates. Free fatty acids diffuse across rapidly, cholesterol more slowly. The micelles, therefore, become more concentrated in cholesterol as they move along the small intestine.

Under normal conditions, most dietary fat is absorbed before the contents reach the end of the jejunum and any fat in the stools (in the absence of steatorrhoea) is from desquamated epithelial cells and from bacterial flora in the gut.

Once inside the epithelial cells, lipid is taken into the smooth endoplasmic reticulum where much of it is re-esterified.

Some lipid is also synthesized in the epithelial cells. Dietary and synthesized lipids are then incorporated into chylomicrons and, provided α-lipoprotein is present, the chylomicrons are exocytosed into lateral intercellular spaces to enter the lacteals. Having reached the lymphatic system, they travel up the thoracic duct and enter the venous circulation.

Apolipoproteins are an important constituent of chylomicrons. They are made by hepatocytes and the epithelial cells of the intestine. Their absence leads to the accumulation of lipid in intestinal epithelial cells.

Chylomicrons consist mainly of triglyceride with a phospholipid coat studded with apolipoproteins. They contain small amounts of cholesterol and cholesterol esters in the centre, and their overall size depends on the amount of fat in the diet. Following a high fat intake, chylomicrons may have a diameter of up to 750 nm, in low-fat diets they may be as small as 60 nm.

Abetalipoproteinaemia is a rare inborn error of metabolism inherited as a recessive trait, characterized by failure of chylomicron formation and an accumulation of dietary fat within enterocytes.

A diagrammatic representation of the digestion and absorption of fat is shown in Fig. 4.19.

HINTS AND TIPS

Remember that bile is not enzymatic; its acids emulsify fats via a detergent action and do not hydrolyse it.

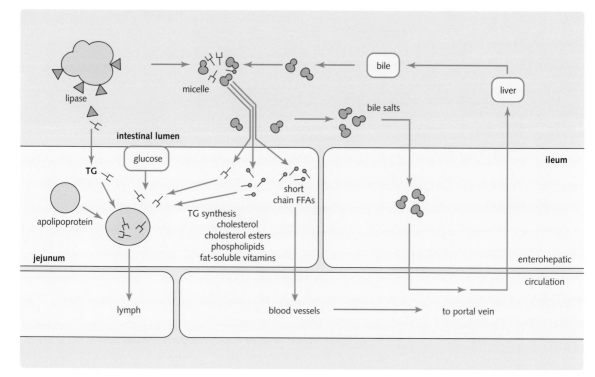

Fig. 4.19 Cellular uptake of free fatty acids and chylomicrons. (TG = triglyceride; FFA = free fatty acid.)

Vitamins

Fat-soluble vitamins

Absorption of the fat-soluble vitamins A, D, E and K depends on the absorption of fat and any condition in which fat digestion and absorption is decreased will eventually lead to a deficiency of these vitamins.

Water-soluble vitamins

At the concentrations present in a normal diet, most of these are taken up by specific transport mechanisms, many of which are sodium-dependent.

An important example of a water-soluble vitamin is vitamin B_{12}. On ingestion, it is bound to R protein found in saliva and in gastric secretions, which protects it from digestion in the stomach. Once vitamin B_{12} has been separated from R protein in the duodenum by the action of pancreatic proteases, vitamin B_{12} binds to intrinsic factor (IF) secreted by gastric parietal cells.

Receptors for the IF–B_{12} dimer are present in the membranes of the epithelial cells of the terminal ileum, which bind the complex and allow uptake of vitamin B_{12}.

Vitamin B_{12} is then transported across the basal membrane of the epithelial cells into the portal blood (Fig. 4.20). It is then bound to transcobalamin II and

Fig. 4.20 Vitamin B_{12} absorption in the terminal ileum. (IF = intrinsic factor.)

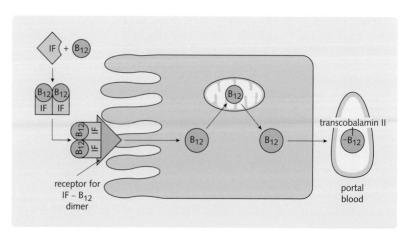

taken up by the liver, kidney, spleen, heart, placenta, reticulocytes and fibroblasts.

The presence of autoantibodies against IF causes malabsorption of vitamin B_{12} and macrocytic anaemia. The resulting disease is called pernicious anaemia.

Clinical Note

Treatment of vitamin B_{12} deficiency is by intramuscular injections of hydroxocobalamin (one of the forms of vitamin B_{12}) every 2–3 days until six injections have been given. If the cause of the deficiency remains uncorrected, injections should continue to be given at 3-monthly intervals.

Water

The normal daily intake of water is about 1.5 L/day. However, up to 9 L water per day are absorbed from the gastrointestinal tract (through the reabsorption of secretions) under normal circumstances, most of it from the small intestine, especially the jejunum (Fig. 4.21).

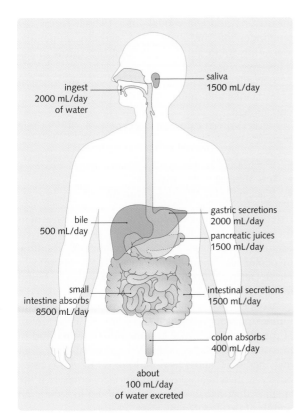

saliva
1500 mL/day

ingest
2000 mL/day
of water

bile
500 mL/day

gastric secretions
2000 mL/day

pancreatic juices
1500 mL/day

small
intestine absorbs
8500 mL/day

intestinal secretions
1500 mL/day

colon absorbs
400 mL/day

about
100 mL/day
of water excreted

Fig. 4.21 Fluid secretion and absorption in the gastrointestinal tract.

Electrolytes

Sodium
Almost all of the Na^+ in the gastrointestinal tract is reabsorbed (about 99%), mostly from the jejunum in association with glucose, galactose and certain amino acids. Na^+ is transported across the epithelial cell membrane down its electrochemical gradient and pumped into the intercellular spaces in exchange for K^+.

Na^+ is absorbed against its electrochemical gradient in the ileum and the colon. Water follows the active pumping of Na^+ by $Na+/K^+$ ATPases through a transcellular or paracellular (tight junctions) route.

Potassium
K^+ is absorbed in the jejunum and ileum. It is secreted into the colon when K^+ concentrations in the lumen are less than 25 mmol/L.

Calcium
This is absorbed throughout the small intestine (especially in the duodenum and jejunum) although absorption is disrupted in vitamin-D-deficient states.

Ca^{2+} passes across the luminal membrane and into the cytoplasm, where it is bound to a protein and then transported across the basolateral membrane, some of it in exchange for Na^+.

Ca^{2+} deficiency is seen in vitamin D deficiency, for example in rickets. Vitamin D helps to regulate Ca^{2+} absorption and metabolism in the body.

Iron
Iron deficiency is relatively common, particularly in menstruating women. The total amount of iron in the body is only about 3–4 g, of which about two-thirds is in haemoglobin.

An average Western diet contains about 20 mg of iron a day, of which only about 10% can be absorbed.

Both males and females lose almost 1 mg of iron a day in the urine and desquamated cells, and females lose about 50 mg of iron a month in the menstrual flow.

Absorption is increased in iron deficiency and by increased erythropoietic activity. Growing children, pregnant women and people who have bled are thus able to absorb increased amounts of iron to compensate for their greater need.

Most dietary iron is in the form Fe^{3+}, which is reduced to Fe^{2+} by ascorbic acid in gastric secretions or ferrireductase in the mucosa and then absorbed. Anything that prevents this reduction decreases the absorption of iron, e.g. the production of an insoluble complex with other dietary compounds such as tannin (present in tea), phytate and certain fibres.

Fe^{2+} is taken across the enterocyte membrane of the small intestinal villi by a divalent metal transporter. In the enterocyte, Fe^{2+} is oxidized to Fe^{3+} and then either released into the plasma where it binds to a transferrin molecule or stored in the epithelial cells, bound to ferritin.

The proportion of iron released depends on the body's requirement. A larger amount remains in the cell bound to ferritin when dietary intake exceeds the body's requirement. This iron is then shed when the epithelial cell is desquamated and prevents iron overload.

Excessive amounts of iron are absorbed in haemochromatosis (see Chapter 6), an autosomal recessive condition.

Clinical Note

Haemochromatosis leads to the deposition of iron in the liver, heart, pancreas and pituitary. This results in damage to those organs. The disease is more common in men because premenopausal women are protected by menstruation and childbirth.

Stem cells in the crypts of Lieberkühn can be programmed to absorb more iron, e.g. following haemorrhage. An increase in absorption may be seen 3–4 days after trauma and in response to other events causing blood loss (the time taken for stem cells to mature and reach the tips of the villi where most iron absorption takes place).

THE FLORA OF THE SMALL INTESTINE

Bacteria may be commensal or pathogenic. Broadly, they may be classified as aerobic or anaerobic.

In health, most of these bacteria are commensal and many of them have important functions, particularly in protecting against colonization by pathogenic bacteria. However, flora which are harmless or even beneficial in one site may become pathogens in another part of the body.

Most of the gastrointestinal tract is heavily colonized with flora. Relatively sterile sites include the stomach (where the acid conditions are too hostile to support much flora), gall bladder and salivary glands. The small intestine is also fairly sterile.

The degree of colonization varies along its length. The duodenum has few microorganisms, mostly Gram-positive cocci and bacilli due to the acidic gastric juices and the alkaline biliary and pancreatic secretions. The jejunum has more bacteria than the duodenum. *Enterococcus faecalis*, lactobacilli and diphtheroids are found here.

The ileum has a large flora of 10^4–10^8 organisms per mL of fluid. The bacteria are obligate anaerobes and include *Bacteroides*, *Clostridium*, *Bifidobacterium* and Enterobactericeae.

DISORDERS OF THE SMALL INTESTINE

Only those disorders affecting only or primarily the small intestine will be covered here. Disorders and diseases which involve both the small and large intestines are discussed in Chapter 5.

Congenital abnormalities

Meckel's diverticulum

Meckel's diverticulum is the remnant of the vitelline duct present in embryonic life. It connects the developing embryo with the yolk sac.

In the embryo, the vitelline duct is found at the apex of the primary intestinal loop that forms when the midgut rapidly elongates (see Fig. 4.4). The long sides of the loop are known as the cephalic limb (which forms the duodenum, jejunum and part of the ileum) and the caudal limb (which forms the remainder of the ileum, the caecum, appendix, ascending colon and the proximal two thirds of the transverse colon).

Meckel's diverticulum, therefore, marks the junction of the cranial and caudal limbs of what was the embryonic midgut.

Meckel's diverticulum can be described with the 'rule of twos':

- It is present in 2% of the population
- It is about 2 inches long
- It is approximately 2 feet from the caecum.

Heterotopic gastric epithelium (normal tissue present in the wrong place) may sometimes be found in the diverticulum, including HCl-secreting oxyntic cells, resulting in peptic ulceration. Rarely, ulcers may perforate or bleed. Heterotopic pancreatic tissue may also be found there.

Acute inflammation of the diverticulum may occur, mimicking acute appendicitis. The mucosa at the mouth of the diverticulum may become inflamed and lead to intussusceptions and ossruction, or the diverticulum may perforate and cause peritonitis. In most cases, however, diverticula are asymptomatic, however if the vitelline duct remains patent throughout its length, an umbilical-ileo fistula may form.

Laporoscopic resection of the diverticulum is the treatment of choice.

Atresia and stenosis

Atresia is a failure of canalization and results in complete obstruction. Stenosis is a narrowing of the lumen and results in partial obstruction.

Atresia and stenosis may occur anywhere along the length of the gastrointestinal tract, but they are found most often in the duodenum and least often in the colon.

The incidence is 1 in 5000 births. They are diagnosed quickly after birth. The causes of atresia and stenosis range from lack of recanalization (in the proximal duodenum) to malrotation and gastroschisis (in the distal duodenum), leading to the cessation of the blood supply.

The loss of a blood supply results in complete tissue necrosis to that part of the bowel. The anus may be imperforate, with the anal canal ending blindly at the anal membrane, or a fistula may form between the rectum and perineum. Alternatively, the rectum may empty into the vagina forming a rectovaginal fistula or into the urethra, forming a urorectal fistula.

Malasorption syndromes

Malabsorption is the decreased absorption of nutrients which may be caused by a number of conditions, including biochemical disorders (such as absent or defective digestive enzymes) and disease of the small intestine. A simple classification is given in Fig. 4.22.

Causes and effects of malabsorption

The causes of decreased nutrient absorption include:

- Reduced small intestinal surface area
- Infection leading to damage of the mucosa and bacterial removal of nutrients
- Defective intraluminal hydrolysis or solubilization (due to lack of enzymes)
- Abnormalities of mucosal epithelial cells (involving loss of digestive enzymes or carriers)
- Drug-induced mechanisms
- Lymphatic obstruction
- Rapid transit though the small intestine
- Failure of nutrients to reach the small intestine, e.g. because of a fistula
- After surgical resection of gut and/or radiation therapy.

Whatever the cause, the results of malabsorption are essentially the same.

Patients complain of frothy, greasy stools, which are difficult to flush away (steatorrhoea), diarrhoea, weight loss and abdominal distension.

Anaemia may be due to deficiency of iron, folate or vitamin B_{12}. Vitamin K deficiency can lead to bleeding disorders, purpura (extravasation of red cells into the skin, characterized by red skin lesions, which do not blanch on pressure) and petechiae (flat, red or purple spots about the size of a pinhead in the skin or mucous membranes).

Fig. 4.22 Classification of malabsorption syndromes.

Cause of malabsorption	Mechanism
Defective intraluminal hydrolysis	Lack of enzyme production Dysfunctional enzymes
Primary mucosal cell abnormalities	Loss of enzymes in mucosa Loss of carrier molecules Damage to mucosa via drugs or inflammation
Decreased surface area of intestines	Inflammation Drug induced damage
Infection	Due to enterotoxic microorganisms in the food Due to external injury to the bowel Due to antibiotics
Iatrogenic	Antibiotics, leading to decreased commensals and increased opportunistic infection
Drug induced	Toxicity Increased motility Increased fluid secretion Carrier inhibition Decreased enzyme production No uptake of fats from lacteals
Unexplained	Unknown

Endocrine disorders may result from generalized malnutrition and deficiencies of vitamin A and B1 may lead to peripheral neuropathy.

Deficient absorption of amino acids can result in hypoalbuminaemia and oedema. Dermatitis and hyperkeratosis may also be evident in the skin. The musculoskeletal system may also be affected with osteopenia and tetany. Fig. 4.23 summarizes the systemic effects of malabsorption.

Coeliac disease

Coeliac disease is a chronic inflammatory disease of the small intestinal mucosa caused by an abnormal reaction to gluten, which is found in wheat.

It is most common in northern Europe, although it occurs worldwide. It has an average prevalence in the UK of 1 in 100 people. Many autoimmune diseases are associated with it, for instance dermatitis herpetiformis, type 1 diabetes mellitus and thyroid disease.

The disease causes damage to the enterocytes. The precise mechanism for this is unclear, although it is suggested that environmental factors allow gliadin, a protein found in gluten, to come into contact with tissue transglutaminase in the lamina propria. The gliadin is modified by TTG and is recognized as antigenic by $CD4^+$ T cells.

Stem cells are unable to keep up with the rate of loss of enterocytes. This results in villous atrophy and the presence of immature cells, which are unable to absorb nutrients normally on the flattened surface. This, in turn, causes malabsorption and an intolerance of lactose and other sugars because of a secondary disaccharide deficiency resulting from the loss of surface epithelial cells.

Patients commonly present with diarrhoea, abdominal pain and bloating which is often associated with particular foods, and any of the other features of malabsorption can be present. The diagnosis should also be considered in patients with weight loss, or iron-deficient anaemia.

Investigations include blood tests for antigliadin and anti-TTG assays. However, the gold standard for diagnosis is jejunal biopsy showing evidence of villous atrophy.

Treatment is a permanent gluten-free diet, the vast majority of patients showing a marked improvement

Fig. 4.23 Systemic effects of malabsorption.

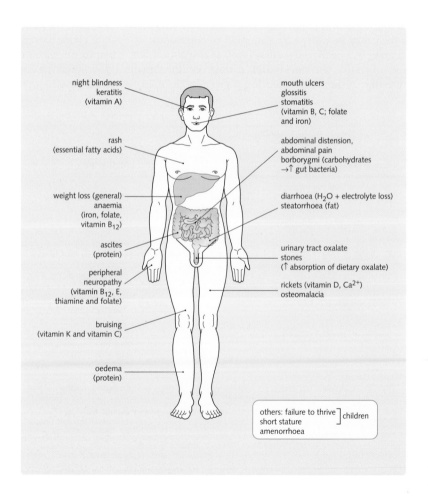

night blindness
keratitis
(vitamin A)

mouth ulcers
glossitis
stomatitis
(vitamin B, C; folate
and iron)

rash
(essential fatty acids)

abdominal distension,
abdominal pain
borborygmi (carbohydrates
→↑ gut bacteria)

weight loss (general)
anaemia
(iron, folate,
vitamin B_{12})

diarrhoea (H_2O + electrolyte loss)
steatorrhoea (fat)

ascites
(protein)

urinary tract oxalate
stones
(↑ absorption of dietary oxalate)

peripheral
neuropathy
(vitamin B_{12}, E,
thiamine and folate)

rickets (vitamin D, Ca^{2+})
osteomalacia

bruising
(vitamin K and vitamin C)

oedema
(protein)

others: failure to thrive ⎤ children
short stature
amenorrhoea

on dietary change. Gluten is present in wheat, barley, oats and rye and these must all be excluded. It is not, however, present in rice or maize.

The condition predisposes to T cell lymphomas in the small intestine (an unusual small bowel lymphoma among the non-coeliac population, in whom most small bowel lymphomas are B cells). There is also a higher incidence of other gastrointestinal cancers such as cancer of the stomach and oesophagus. Another common complication is osteoporosis.

Tropical sprue

Tropical sprue is a chronic, progressive malabsorption in patients from, or in, the tropics (mainly the West Indies and Asia) associated with abnormalities of small intestinal structure and function. It is thought to have an infective cause.

Symptoms include diarrhoea, abdominal distension, fatigue and weight loss. Megaloblastic anaemia caused by folate deficiency is common. Overgrowth of bacteria in the small intestine is frequently found.

Like coeliac disease, there is villous atrophy, although obviously a gluten-free diet is of no help.

Treatment is with broad-spectrum antibiotics, e.g. tetracycline.

Whipple's disease

This is a rare bacterial infection usually occurring in middle-aged men. It is ten times more common in men and is caused by the bacterium *Tropheryma whipplei* (a Gram-positive actinomycete).

Symptoms include weight loss and other abdominal symptoms, polyarthralgia, chronic cough and hyperpigmentation.

Diagnosis is by jejunal biopsy, which shows intact villi where the normal cells of the lamina propria have been replaced by 'foamy' macrophages containing PAS-positive glycoprotein granules. Similar cells may be found in lymph nodes, spleen and liver.

Treatment is with tetracycline.

Bacterial overgrowth

The small intestine normally supports a large number of flora but these are kept in check by peristalsis, the acidity of chyme leaving the stomach and the secretion of immunoglobulins into the intestinal lumen by the mucosal cells.

Where one or more of these factors is reduced, e.g. if there is a structural abnormality, bacterial overgrowth may occur. It may also occur in the elderly for unknown causes.

Jejunal biopsy may show a normal mucosa. Diagnosis is with the hydrogen breath test – an early rise in breath hydrogen levels is diagnostic. These organisms may inactivate bile acids in the lumen by dehydroxylation, leading to fat malabsorption. The gut flora may catabolize ingested protein, metabolize sugars and bind vitamin B_{12}, preventing its absorption. Vitamin K levels may, however, be raised as the bacteria may produce it.

Treatment is with antibiotics, such as tetracycline, metronidazole or ciprofloxacin.

Giardiasis

Giardiasis, prevalent in the tropics, is an important cause of traveller's diarrhoea. It is caused by the flagellate protozoan *Giardia lamblia*, which lives in the duodenum and jejunum and is transmitted by the faecal–oral route. Cases may also occur in Britain among people who have never been abroad.

Asymptomatic carriage may occur. Alternatively, symptoms of diarrhoea, malabsorption and abdominal pain or bloating may develop within 1 or 2 weeks of ingesting cysts.

Giardia lamblia exists as a trophozoite and a cyst, the cyst being the transmissible form. Intestinal damage varies from slight changes in villous architecture to partial villous atrophy with severe malabsorption.

Diagnosis is by stool microscopy. Both cysts and kite-shaped trophozoites may be found, but their absence does not exclude the diagnosis: in some cases they are only excreted at intervals. The parasite may also be seen in duodenal aspirates and in a jejunal biopsy.

Treatment is with metronidazole or tinidazole.

Neoplastic disease

Small intestinal tumours are much rarer that tumours of the large intestine and rectum. Patients generally present with iron-deficient anaemia, obstruction, bleeding or volvulus.

Benign tumours

These include:

- Lipomas
- Leiomyomas
- Adenomas (often benign)
- Hamartomas.

Malignant lesions

These include:

- Adenocarcinomas
- Carcinoid
- Lymphomas
- Metastases, from lung or melanoma.

Adenocarcinoma accounts for 50% of all tumours found in the small intestine. It is associated with both celiac and Crohn's disease, although the pathogenesis is unknown. Diagnosis is normally by abdominal CT scan or barium enema. Surgical resection is the treatment of choice.

Carcinoid tumours make up 10% of small intestinal malignant lesions. These are described in further detail in Chapter 5.

Intestinal lymphoma is rare, but more common in the small intestine than the large. They may be of B-cell or T-cell lineage. The majority are of the non-Hodgkin's B-cell type, which arise from mucosa-associated lymphoid tissue. T-cell lymphomas are associated with celiac disease and have a poorer prognosis. Treatment is with surgery followed by either radiotherapy or chemotherapy.

The large intestine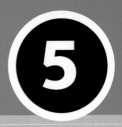

Objectives

After reading this chapter, you should be able to:
- Describe the anatomy of the large intestine, with regard to its macroscopic structure, relations, arterial supply, venous and lymphatic drainage, and nerve supply
- Outline the embryological development of the large intestine
- Outline the histological structure of the large intestine
- Describe the functions of the large intestine
- Describe the mechanisms controlling large intestinal motility and outline the process of defecation
- Outline the following types of large intestinal disorders: congenital abnormalities, infections, inflammatory bowel disease, diverticular disease, obstruction, vascular disorders, neoplastic disease, appendicitis and anorectal disorders

OVERVIEW

The large intestine extends from the ileocaecal junction to the anus, and is about 1.5 m in length. Its main role is to concentrate faeces by absorbing water, hence it also plays a role in water and electrolyte balance. It also has to transport faeces through the entire colon to the anus.

ANATOMY

The large intestine can be divided into seven sections (Fig. 5.1):

- The caecum and appendix
- The ascending colon
- The transverse colon
- The descending colon
- The sigmoid colon
- The rectum
- The anal canal.

The outer, longitudinal muscle forms three distinct bands visible at dissection called taenia coli. These bands are shorter than the circular muscle layer and gather the caecum and colon into a series of pouch-like folds called haustrations or sacculations.

HINTS AND TIPS

The haustra are visible on radiographs when an opaque medium is introduced through the rectum.

The outer surface of the large intestine has appendices epiploicae projecting from it. These are sacs of omentum distended with fat.

Clinical Note

The large intestine is easily distinguished from the small intestine as its haustra do not extend across the entire width, unlike the small intestine which has plicae circulares (also called valves of Kerckring or valvulae conniventes) visible across the whole width on radiographs.

Caecum

The caecum is a sac lying in the right iliac fossa. It is continuous with the ascending colon distally and the ileum proximally, with which it communicates through the ileocaecal valve (Fig. 5.2).

HINTS AND TIPS

The ileocaecal valve is incompetent. This is good, because it prevents the build-up of wind or stools in the colon and allows the easing of pressure across the valve.

It is covered entirely in peritoneum, but has no mesentery. The caecum is often attached by peritoneal caecal

Fig. 5.1 The large intestine.

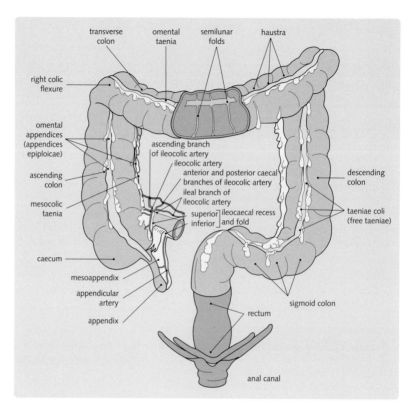

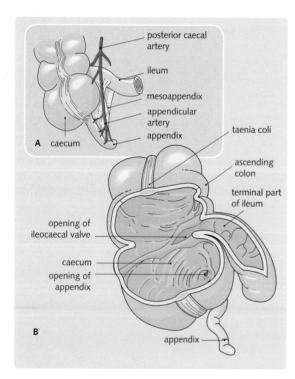

Fig. 5.2 The ileocaecal valve (exterior view (A) and cutaway view (B)) and the appendix.

folds to the iliac fossa to form the retrocaecal recess, a small peritoneal cavity in which the appendix lies.

The caecum is supplied by the ileocolic artery, a branch of the superior mesenteric artery. Venous blood from the caecum drains via the ileocolic vein into the superior mesenteric vein.

It is innervated via the superior mesenteric plexus.

Appendix

The (vermiform) appendix is about 8 cm in length and protrudes from the posterolateral wall of the caecum (Fig. 5.1). It has aggregations of lymphatic tissue and the three taenia coli of the caecum come together at the base of the appendix, forming an outer longitudinal muscle coat.

It is a blind-ending sac and so may become inflamed (appendicitis) if obstructed, e.g. by faecoliths, which are small, hard masses of faeces. This requires surgical removal of the appendix to prevent rupture and peritonitis.

The appendix is mobile as it has a mesentery, the mesoappendix. Because of this and the way it develops (see later), its position is variable. It usually lies behind the caecum or in the pelvis.

Blood supply and lymphatic drainage

The appendix is covered in peritoneum and supplied by the appendicular artery (a branch of the ileocolic artery), which lies in the mesentery that connects the appendix to the terminal ileum.

The ileocolic vein drains the appendix.

The lymphatic drainage and innervation for the caecum and appendix is the same. The lymph drains into the ileocolic lymph nodes (which lie along the ileocolic artery) and the lymph nodes in the mesoappendix.

Innervation

The innervation to the caecum and appendix comes from the coeliac and superior mesenteric plexuses.

Ascending colon

The ascending colon arises from the ileocaecal valve to the inferior surface of the liver, where it turns to the left forming the hepatic (right colic) flexure (Fig. 5.1).

It has no mesentery and lies retroperitoneally. However, it has peritoneum covering the lateral and anterior surfaces, which attaches it to the posterior abdominal wall. The peritoneum on the medial and lateral sides of the ascending colon forms the right paracolic gutter.

Anterior to the ascending colon lie the coils of the small intestine and the greater omentum. These separate it from the anterior abdominal wall.

Posteriorly are the iliacus, transversus abdominis and quadratus lumborum muscles, and the right kidney.

Blood supply and lymphatic drainage

The ascending colon, being a midgut structure, is supplied by the right colic artery and ileocolic artery, which are branches of the superior mesenteric artery.

Its venous drainage is via the right colic and ileocolic veins, which drain into the superior mesenteric vein.

Lymph from this region drains to the paracolic and epicolic lymph nodes. These drain into the superior mesenteric lymph nodes.

Innervation

Innervation to the ascending colon comes from the coeliac and superior mesenteric plexuses, like that of the caecum and appendix.

Transverse colon

The transverse colon extends from the hepatic (right colic) flexure to the splenic (left colic) flexure. It is the largest part of the large intestine and is about 45–50 cm in length.

The transverse colon is mobile due to its length and the presence of a mesentery (the mesocolon). This double layer of peritoneum is attached to the inferior border of the pancreas and greater omentum and allows the transverse colon to hang from the posterior abdominal wall, usually to the level of the umbilicus.

The splenic flexure is slightly more superior than the hepatic flexure, due to the spleen being smaller than the liver. The splenic flexure is attached to the diaphragm by the phrenicocolic ligament, a fold of peritoneum.

Blood supply and lymphatic drainage

The arterial blood supply is from the middle, right and left colic arteries (Fig. 4.3). The middle colic artery is the major arterial supply. It is a branch of the superior mesenteric artery, along with the right colic artery. These supply the proximal two-thirds of the transverse colon which is derived from the midgut.

The left colic artery is a branch of the inferior mesenteric artery supplying its distal, hindgut-derived third.

The superior mesenteric vein drains the transverse colon, and its lymph drains to the lymph nodes along the middle colic artery. These then drain into the superior mesenteric lymph nodes.

Innervation

Innervation to the transverse colon comes from the superior mesenteric plexus, which follows the path of the middle and right colic arteries.

The nerves from the inferior mesenteric plexus follow the path of the left colic artery. Both sympathetic and parasympathetic (vagal) nerves supply the transverse colon.

Descending colon

The descending colon is about 30 cm in length and is the narrowest part of the colon. It extends from the splenic flexure to the left iliac fossa at the pelvic brim, where it becomes the sigmoid colon.

The descending colon has no mesentery and lies retroperitoneally, attached to the posterior abdominal wall. Like the ascending colon, it has paracolic gutters medially and laterally.

The lateral border of the left kidney, the transversus abdominis and quadratus lumborum muscles lie posterior to the descending colon.

Blood supply and lymphatic drainage

The left colic and superior sigmoid arteries supply the descending colon. Both are branches of the inferior mesenteric artery.

Venous drainage is via the inferior mesenteric vein. The lymph drains to the intermediatecolic lymph nodes, which lie along the left colic artery.

Innervation

Parasympathetic innervation comes from the pelvic splanchnic nerves and sympathetic innervation is derived from the lumbar part of the sympathetic trunk and the superior hypogastric plexus.

Sigmoid colon

The sigmoid colon is S-shaped and lies in the left iliac fossa. It extends from the pelvic brim to join the rectum at the level of S3.

The sigmoid colon has a long mesentery; the sigmoid mesocolon. This has a V-shaped root attachment and somis very mobile.

It lies anterior to the left external iliac vessels, the left sacral plexus and the left piriformis muscle. Parts of it can also be found in the rectouterine pouch (of Douglas) in females or the rectovesical pouch in males.

Long appendices epiploicae hang from the external wall of the sigmoid colon. The position, size and shape of the sigmoid colon depend on how full of faeces it is. This is the main storage site of faeces, prior to defecation.

Clinical Note

The sigmoid colon is the part of the colon most prone to volvulus due to its length and high mobility. It is also the part most susceptible to perforation as it has the highest pressure in the colon and its walls are the weakest.

Blood supply and lymphatic drainage

The sigmoid colon is supplied by two or three sigmoid arteries. These descend to the left and divide into ascending and descending branches. The descending branch of the left colic artery anastomoses with the most superior sigmoid artery.

The inferior mesenteric vein drains blood from the sigmoid colon, while the lymph drains to the intermediate colic lymph nodes, as in the descending colon.

Innervation

The innervation is the same as that to the descending colon.

Rectum

The rectum is continuous with the sigmoid colon proximally and the anus distally.

It starts at the level of S3, in the posterior part of the pelvis and curves along the sacrum and coccyx, in an S-shaped course before widening to form the rectal ampulla. It has no mesentery and so is immobile.

Peritoneum covers the anterior and lateral surfaces in the superior third, and the anterior surface only in the middle third. The inferior third is not covered. In males, it is reflected from the bladder to form the rectovesical pouch while in women it is reflected from the vagina to form the rectouterine pouch (of Douglas).

The rectum has three flexures, the most important being the anorectal flexure. This is produced by the puborectalis muscle encircling the rectum at the junction with the anal canal to form a 'sling' and a 90° anorectal angle.

At each flexure is a transverse fold formed by infoldings of the rectal wall. They are maintained by the taeniae coli and partly close the lumen.

The relations of the rectum are different in the male and female. In the male, the bladder, prostate, seminal vesicles and vasa deferentia lie in front of it; in the female it is related anteriorly to the uterus and vagina.

Posterior to the rectum lie:

- The three inferior sacral vertebrae
- The coccyx
- The anococcygeal ligament
- The median sacral vessels
- Branches of the superior rectal artery
- The inferior ends of the sympathetic trunks and sacral plexuses.

The rectal ampulla stores faeces before defecation and is very distendable. It is supported by the levator ani muscles.

Blood supply and lymphatic drainage

The arterial supply to the rectum comes from a number of sources:

- The median sacral arteries
- The superior, middle and inferior rectal arteries which supply the corresponding parts of the rectum.

The rectal arteries anastomose with each other. The superior rectal artery is a continuation of the inferior mesenteric artery while the middle and inferior rectal arteries are branches of the internal iliac arteries and the internal pudendal arteries, respectively.

The superior, middle and inferior rectal veins drain the rectum. They anastomose to form internal and external venous plexuses.

The external plexus is outside the muscular wall and the internal plexus is just deep to the mucosa. The internal venous plexus communicates with the uterovaginal venous plexus in the female and the vesical venous plexus in the male.

The different areas of the rectal venous plexus drain into different vessels:

- The superior part drains into the superior rectal vein, then into the inferior mesenteric vein
- The middle part drains into the middle rectal vein, then into the internal iliac vein
- The inferior part drains into the internal pudendal vein.

The superior rectal veins drain into the portal system and the inferior rectal veins drain into the systemic circulation. The rectum is thus a site of a porto-systemic anastomosis (see Chapter 6).

The superior part of the rectum drains lymph into the pararectal lymph nodes, which then drain to the sigmoid mesocolon lymph nodes and inferior mesenteric lymph nodes. The inferior part of the rectum drains lymph into the internal iliac lymph nodes.

Innervation

The rectum receives sympathetic and parasympathetic innervation. Nerves from the inferior hypogastric plexus make up the middle rectal plexus.

Parasympathetic innervation is derived from S1, S3 and S4 nerves, which run with the pelvic splanchnic nerves, finally joining up with the inferior hypogastric plexus. Sensory fibres follow the sympathetic fibres and are stimulated by rectal distension.

Anus

The anal canal is continuous with the rectum and is about 3 cm long. It begins at the anorectal flexure and it is surrounded by the levator ani muscles, ending at the anus.

The anal canal descends between the perineal body and the anococcygeal ligament. The ischioanal fossae are two wedge-shaped spaces on either side of the anal canal.

The anus has an internal and an external sphincter (Fig. 5.3). The external sphincter surrounds the lower two thirds of the anal canal and is composed of striated

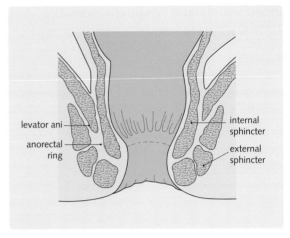

Fig. 5.3 The rectum and anal canal, showing the anal sphincters.

muscle. It is thus under voluntary control, allowing delay of defecation.

The internal sphincter surrounds the upper two thirds of the anal canal and is made up of involuntary circular smooth muscle continuous with that of the rectum. Both sphincters must relax for defecation to occur.

In the male, the anal canal lies behind the prostate and the bulb of the penis. The perineal body separates it from these structures, but a digital rectal examination can give important information about the prostate. In the female, the perineal body separates the anal canal from the vagina.

In the mucosa of the superior half are six to twelve longitudinal ridges called anal columns. They contain the terminal branches of the superior rectal artery and vein.

The superior ends of the anal columns mark the anorectal line or junction. Folds of epithelium, called anal valves, connect the inferior ends of the anal columns.

Just superior to the anal valves are the anal sinuses, which release mucus to aid defecation.

The pectinate line is found between the superior and inferior parts of the anal canal. It is the boundary between the columnar epithelium of the superior part and the stratified squamous epithelium of the inferior part.

HINTS AND TIPS

Anal canal structures above the pectinate line have developed from the endodermal hindgut. Structures below the pectinate line have developed from the ectodermal anal pit, or proctodeum. Therefore, the differences in blood, lymphatic and nerve supply above and below the pectinate line are due to embryological development.

Blood supply and lymphatic drainage

The superior and both inferior rectal arteries drain the areas superior and inferior to the pectinate line respectively.

The terminal branches of the superior rectal artery anastomose in the anal valves. The middle rectal arteries anastomose with the superior and inferior rectal arteries.

Venous drainage occurs via the internal rectal venous plexus to the superior and inferior rectal veins respectively.

Clinical Note

The veins in the wall of the anal canal provide a cushion for the passage of faeces and help to close the anus, but they can enlarge to form haemorrhoids.

In the superior part of the anal canal, the lymph drains to the internal iliac lymph nodes and then into the common iliac and lumbar lymph nodes. In the inferior part of the anal canal, lymph drainage is to the superficial inguinal nodes.

Innervation

Superior to the pectinate line, the sympathetic nerve supply is derived from the inferior hypogastric plexus. The parasympathetic supply comes from the pelvic splanchnic nerves.

Inferior to the pectinate line, the nerve supply comes from the inferior rectal nerves, which are branches of the pudendal nerve. This region is sensitive to touch, temperature and pain.

The pelvic splanchnic nerves (parasympathetic) and the aortic and pelvic plexuses (sympathetic) innervate the internal anal sphincter.

The inferior rectal nerve, a branch of the pudendal nerve and the perineal branch of S4 innervate the external anal sphincter.

EMBRYOLOGY AND DEVELOPMENT

This section focuses solely on the development of the large intestine. However, as it develops in tandem with the small intestine, it may be useful to read this section with its counterpart in Chapter 4.

The caecal bud appears on the caudal limb of the primitive gut tube at about week 6 and develops into the caecal swelling, which is the last part of the developing tube to re-enter the abdominal cavity.

The appendix develops from the distal end of the swelling during the descent of the colon and may come to lie in a variety of positions. However, it is usually found posterior to the large intestine.

Clinical Note

Failure of the intestinal loops to return to the abdominal cavity results in exomphalos, the protrusion of abdominal contents through the abdominal wall at the site of insertion of the cord. The contents of this hernia are covered by amnion (which distinguishes them from gastroschisis—see below).

The distal third of the transverse colon and the upper part of the anal canal arise from the hind-gut. They are supplied by the inferior mesenteric artery.

The distal part of the hindgut grows into the cloaca, an endodermal-lined cavity, which is in contact with the surface ectoderm.

During the 9th week of development, the anal membrane ruptures to open up the rectum to the external environment.

In the anal canal, the pectinate line indicates the junction between the endodermal and ectodermal parts. It is also the point at which the columnar epithelium in the upper part of the anal canal changes to stratified squamous epithelium in the lower part.

HISTOLOGY

The tissue layers of the large intestine are essentially the same as those in the rest of the gastrointestinal tract (see Fig. 1.2).

However, the muscle walls are thicker in order to facilitate faecal movement, the lumen is larger and the outer longitudinal muscle layer forms taeniae coli visible on the outside of the intestine.

Mucosa

The mucosa is thrown into folds when not distended. It consists of simple columnar epithelium and contains numerous straight tubular glands that extend throughout its thickness. Unlike the small intestine, there are no villi or plicae circulares. The glands consist of two main types of cells:

* Columnar absorptive cells found at luminal surfaces
* Mucus-secreting goblet cells found at the gland bases.

Paneth cells are present only when young. Isolated nodules of lymphatic tissue are found that extend into the submucosa.

The muscularis mucosae is prominent. Its contractions prevent clogging of the glands by aiding faecal movement.

Anorectal junction

The rectum narrows towards its terminal end when it becomes the anal canal.

The upper portion of the anal canal contains longitudinal folds (anal or rectal columns) separated by depressions (anal sinuses).

The sinuses contain straight, branched tubular glands (anal glands) which produce mucus and extend into the submucosa and sometimes into the muscularis externa.

The ducts of the anal glands open into crypts in the anal mucosa, and may thus become infected or blocked, forming a cyst.

The mucosa of the upper anal canal is similar to that of the large intestine but the lower portion consists of stratified squamous epithelium, continuous with the skin surrounding the anal canal. The middle portion contains stratified columnar epithelium.

Small folds of mucosa (anal valves) are present at the lower end of the anal canal. Above these, the mucosa is folded longitudinally forming the columns of Morgagni.

THE FLORA OF THE LARGE INTESTINE

Most of the flora of the large intestine are anaerobes, e.g. *Bacteroides fragilis*. The large intestine also supports coliforms such as *Escherichia coli* and faecal streptococci, including *Enterococcus faecalis*.

There are at least 400 species of bacteria in the large bowel, with over 10^{10} organisms per gram of stool. Approximately one quarter of the weight of stool is bacteria.

Commensal bacteria keep pathogenic bacteria at bay by competing with them for space and nutrients. The significance of this becomes apparent during antibiotic administration. Antibiotics disrupt the normal flora and predispose to clostridial and other gut infections.

The intestinal flora convert conjugated bilirubin to urobilinogen, some of which is reabsorbed and excreted in the urine. The flora also convert the remainder of the urobilinogen to stercobilinogen which is excreted in the faeces.

Clinical Note

Many patients taking broad-spectrum antibiotics, e.g. cephalosporins and ampicillin develop diarrhoea which normally resolves on stopping the drug. However, in some patients an overgrowth of *Clostridium difficile* may ensue, causing pseudomembranous colitis (see below).

FUNCTIONS AND PHYSIOLOGY

Water absorption

Absorption of water in the colon is similar to the mechanism used to concentrate the contents of the gall bladder described in Chapter 7.

Na^+ and Cl^- are pumped into the paracellular (lateral intercellular) spaces and water follows by osmosis. Water molecules, Na^+ and Cl^- then flow through the lateral intercellular spaces away from the lumen, and across the basement membrane of the epithelial cells of the colon.

Some Cl^- from the colonic lumen also crosses the tight junction into the intercellular space because of the potential difference. It travels in the opposite direction to K^+ and increases the concentration of Cl^- in the intercellular space and, therefore, the passage of water.

The concentration of ions in that part of the intercellular space closest to the lumen is hypertonic, but the fluid at the basement membrane end is isotonic. It is the isotonic fluid that crosses the basement membrane and moves into the intestinal capillaries. Absorbed amino acids and sugars also increase the osmotic absorption of water.

Abnormalities in water absorption in the intestines can result in diarrhoea (see below).

Transport of urea and electrolytes

The main function of the colon is absorption. It absorbs over 90% of the water from the contents passing through it, reducing the volume from 1–2 L to about 200 mL of semi-solid faecal matter.

By the time they reach the end of the gastrointestinal tract, faeces are about 50–75% water. The remainder is solid material, which is partly composed of bacteria and desquamated mucosal cells. Desquamated cells largely account for the fact that a starving person continues to produce stools.

The ion transport processes of the colon are shown in Fig. 7.5. Na^+ in the lumen is exchanged for H^+ (Na^+ is pumped into the epithelial cells and H + pumped out of it). HCO_3^- is exchanged for Cl^- (Cl^- is reabsorbed, bicarbonate pumped out).

In addition, paracellular spaces exist into which Na^+ and Cl^- is pumped, and from which K^+ passes out into the lumen. K^+ is pumped into the cells in exchange for the Na^+ pumped out into the paracellular spaces.

The net result of this is the creation of a potential difference of about -30 mV across the colonic mucosa (a greater difference than that across the jejunal and ileal mucosa). It is this potential difference that allows the passage of K^+ across the tight junctions from the paracellular space into the lumen and accounts for the potassium-rich secretions found in the colon.

Urea synthesis is greater than its excretion by about 20%. The excess is secreted into the colon for metabolism by bacteria. The products are then absorbed.

Metabolism occurs near the mucosa, rather than in the lumen. NH_4^+ and HCO_3^- ions are produced and converted into NH_3, CO_2 and water. These freely diffuse across the mucosal epithelium into the circulation. The NH_3 is transported to the liver for synthesis of amino acids. Electrolyte movement in the colon is shown in Fig. 5.4.

Secretion of mucus

The colonic mucosa has many goblet cells in its crypts and surface epithelium. They secrete mucus in response to mechanical irritation of the mucosa caused by substances passing through it, and as a result of cholinergic stimulation.

Mucus lubricates the colon, preventing trauma from the contents passing through it, which become increasingly solid as water is reabsorbed on the way through. The ratio of mucous to aqueous secretion is greater in the colon than elsewhere in the gastrointestinal tract.

The aqueous component contains bicarbonate, which plays an important role in buffering, and is rich in potassium. Chloride is absorbed in exchange for bicarbonate.

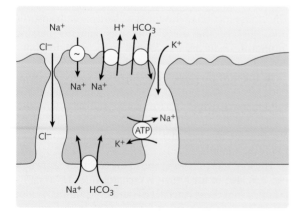

Fig. 5.4 Electrolyte movement in the colon.

Motility of the large intestine

The movement of intestinal contents through the colon is slower than that seen in the rest of the gastrointestinal tract. This is partly due to the nature of the activity and partly due to its absorptive function of water and electrolytes.

The large intestine has three main modes of movement:

- Segmental (or haustral) contractions
- Peristalsis
- Mass movement.

Segmental contractions

Segmental (or haustral) contractions are brought about by the contraction of the taeniae coli. These three bands of longitudinal muscles gather the colon into haustra. The haustra fill with intestinal contents and the distension stimulates contraction.

Contraction of adjacent haustra causes a mixing effect and allows the contents to be in contact with the mucosal surfaces, thus facilitating absorption.

Segmental contractions are initiated by acetylcholine and substance P release.

Peristalsis

Peristalsis is slower in the large intestine than in the small intestine. It provides waves of propulsive contractions, slowly moving the intestinal contents towards the anus. As in the small intestine, distension initiates the contractions and vagal inhibitory and excitatory fibres control the movement.

Mass movement

Mass movement describes the intense contraction that begins halfway along the transverse colon and pushes the intestinal contents towards the rectum. This type of contraction occurs only a few times a day and is responsible for colonic evacuation.

It occurs shortly after a meal and if faeces are present in the rectum, stimulates the urge to defecate. This is called the gastrocolic reflex. It is partly neuronal and partly hormonal (via the action of cholecystokinin).

Control of colonic motility

As in other parts of the gastrointestinal tract, Auerbach's and Meissner's plexuses are present in the walls of the colon (see Fig. 1.2). Their activity is modulated by parasympathetic and sympathetic activity.

Parasympathetic stimulation is via branches of the vagus and pelvic nerves from the sacral spinal cord.

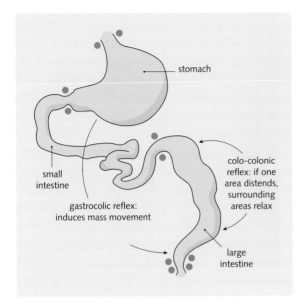

Fig. 5.5 Control of large intestinal motility.

It increases contraction of the proximal colon, allowing greater absorption of salts and water.

Sympathetic innervation is via the superior and inferior mesenteric and hypogastric plexuses. It decreases colonic movements.

Colo-colonic reflexes occur (mediated in part by the sympathetic system) causing one part of the colon to relax if an adjacent part is distended (Fig. 5.5).

Defecation

Control of defecation

The urge to defecate is felt because stretching of the rectum causes impulses in the cholinergic parasympathetic nerves of the pelvis. These are transmitted to a nerve centre in the sacral spinal cord. A pressure of about 18 mmHg in the rectum is needed.

Impulses are then conveyed to higher centres, allowing an individual to decide whether to defecate, i.e. whether to voluntarily relax the external sphincter, or not. In the latter case, the internal sphincter will recontract and the urge to defecate will subside.

As mentioned earlier, the external anal sphincter is made up of striated (voluntary) muscle while the internal sphincter is composed of involuntary smooth muscle. The latter relaxes as a reflex in response to distension of the distal rectum.

Intact Auerbach's and Meissner's plexuses are needed for this reflex relaxation to occur. Thus in Hirschsprung's disease (see later), the internal sphincter does not relax in response to colonic distension as there is

a congenital absence of ganglion cells in these plexuses in the rectum.

If there has been damage to the spinal nerves and therefore to the control of the external sphincter, it will relax when the pressure in the rectum reaches about 55 mmHg.

The anal canal can differentiate between air, liquid and solid contents, and allow the selective release of air as flatus.

Mechanics of defecation

When a person decides to defecate, i.e. when the external sphincter is voluntarily relaxed, an increase in intra-abdominal pressure must be achieved to expel the faeces.

Thus, a breath is taken in and the glottis closes over the trachea. The respiratory muscles contract on lungs filled with air, which increases both the intrathoracic and intra-abdominal pressures.

The pelvic floor muscles relax and the floor 'drops', thus straightening the rectum and preventing rectal prolapse. The faeces are then expelled from the anus.

PHARMACOLOGY OF INTESTINAL MOTILITY

Bowel motility is under autonomic control. Two classes of drugs increase bowel movements: laxatives, which cause purgation and true motility stimulants, which do not. Antidiarrhoeals and antispasmodics decrease bowel movements. The modes of action of these drugs vary (Fig. 5.6).

Drugs which increase movements

Laxatives

Strictly speaking, laxatives (also known as purgatives) do not increase gastrointestinal motility. However, they do increase the speed with which food passes through the intestine, hence the purgation. There are four kinds of laxatives:

- Osmotic laxatives, e.g. lactulose, movicol
- Bulk laxatives, e.g. methylcellulose, fybogel
- Stimulant laxatives, e.g. senna, picolax
- Faecal softeners, e.g. docusate sodium.

Osmotic laxatives

Osmotic laxatives accelerate the transit of food by preserving the higher water contect of residue in the small intestine. An increased (hydrated) volume is thus delivered to the colon, distending it and causing purgation. They are poorly absorbed solutes, which accounts for their osmotic effect.

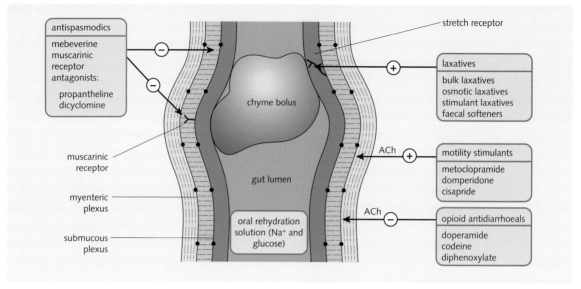

Fig. 5.6 Sites and mechanisms of action of drugs which affect intestinal motility. (ACh = acetylcholine.)

Two most frequently used osmotic laxative is lactulose. Lactulose is a semisynthetic disaccharide of fructose and galactose which is degraded to its component monosaccharides by gut bacteria. These are then fermented, producing lactate and acetate which draw water into the intestine by osmosis. Lactulose takes 2–3 days to have an effect.

The other commonly used osmotic laxative is movicol. Movicol sachets contain macrogel, sodium bicarbonate, sodium chloride and potassium chloride. Macrogel passes through the bowel without being absorbed, and so water is retained in the bowel making the stool softer.

Bulk laxatives

These are polysaccharides which cannot be digested. They act by retaining water and promoting peristalsis. However, they take several days to work but have no major side-effects. Examples include methylcellulose, bran and fybogel (ispaghula).

Stimulant laxatives

As their name suggests, they act possibly by stimulating enteric nerves causing increased mucosal water and electrolyte secretion. Senna is an important example of this class of drug. It is a glycoside of sugars with anthracene derivatives like emodin. In the colon, senna is hydrolysed, releasing free anthracene derivatives which then stimulate the myenteric plexus. As a result, smooth muscle activity is increased and defecation occurs.

Other examples are bisacodyl and sodium picosulphate (Picolax); the latter is commonly used when preparing the bowel for surgery ('bowel prep').

Faecal softeners

An example of a faecal softener is docusate sodium, which acts via a detergent action on the stool in the intestine. It is also a weak stimulant laxative.

Motility stimulants

There are two main drugs in this category: metoclopramide and domperidone. All increase motility but without causing purgation.

The anti-emetic function of metoclopramide has already been mentioned above. In addition to that, however, metoclopramide also acts locally in the stomach to stimulate acetylcholine release. Consequently, gastric motility is stimulated, with an increase in gastric emptying but without a corresponding increase in gastric acid secretion.

Domperidone is another dopamine-receptor antagonist. However, the mechanism by which it enhances gastrointestinal motility is unexplained, although it has been suggested that it acts to facilitate acetylcholine release from the myenteric plexus as well. Its effects are to increase gastric emptying (without increasing gastric acid secretion) and duodenal peristalsis, as well as increasing the pressure of the lower oesophageal sphincter.

Drugs which decrease movements

Antidiarrhoeal drugs

When treating diarrhoea (see later), the maintenance of normal fluid and electrolyte balance must be the first priority. Then, depending on the aetiology, either antimicrobial drugs or non-antimicrobial drugs may be necessary. Antimicrobial drugs are beyond the scope of this book; for more information on them consult the relevant chapter in *Crash Course: Pharmacology*.

If fluid and electrolyte balance is deranged due to excessive loss, it can be restored by means of oral rehydration solutions. These are easy to use; the most common preparation is dioralyte, a powder mix of glucose and sodium chloride which can be dissolved in water. Glucose increases sodium, and thus water absorption as it is absorbed by secondary active transport with sodium. The use of oral rehydration therapy may be sufficient in many cases; in fact, it is the treatment of choice for cholera.

The main non-antimicrobial antidiarrhoeal drugs are opioids. Opioids act on μ-receptors on myenteric neurons. The tone and contractions of the intestinal smooth muscle are increased, but opioids also reduce peristalsis, making a reduction in gastrointestinal motility their overall effect. Additionally, they also increase the tone of the pyloric, ileocolic and anal sphincters.

Loperamide, codeine and diphenoxylate are the main opiates used in the treatment of diarrhoea. Loperamide and codeine also have antisecretory effects besides inhibiting gastrointestinal motility. Note, however, that the opioids used to treat diarrhoea have side-effects such as constipation, drowsiness and abdominal cramps.

Antispasmodics

Antispasmodics are sometimes used in the treatment of irritable bowel syndrome and diverticular disease. Two types exist: muscarinic receptor antagonists and mebeverine. The former decrease muscle tone by inhibiting parasympathetic activity in the alimentary tract. Examples are dicyclomine and propantheline. As would be expected of parasympathetic blockade, side-effects include dry mouth, decreased sweating and blurred vision. Mebeverine acts directly on gastrointestinal smooth muscle causing it to relax.

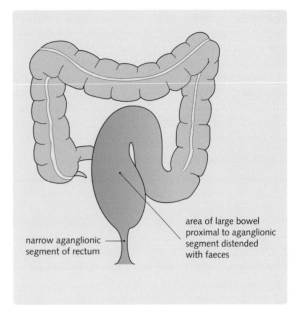

narrow aganglionic segment of rectum

area of large bowel proximal to aganglionic segment distended with faeces

Fig. 5.7 The large intestine in Hirschsprung's disease.

When these parasympathetic plexuses fail to develop, the circular muscle layer of the intestine goes into spasm, resulting in intestinal obstruction. As in other causes of obstruction, dilatation of the intestine occurs proximal to the area in spasm (Fig. 5.7).

Hirschsprung's disease usually affects the rectum and distal colon but, in severe cases, it may also affect the small intestine. The colon may become distended with faeces resulting in megacolon and death from acute enterocolitis.

It is four times more likely to occur in males and severe cases may become apparent shortly after birth with symptoms of obstruction. Less severe cases may simply result in chronic constipation.

DISORDERS OF THE LARGE INTESTINE

The diseases and disorders covered in this section affect primarily the large intestine and/or both the small and large intestine.

Congenital abnormalities

Hirschsprung's disease

Hirschsprung's disease is caused by an absence of ganglion cells in Auerbach's and Meissner's plexuses in the distal bowel as a result of the failure of neuroblasts to migrate during weeks 5–12 of gestation, resulting in congential megacolon.

Clinical Note

Megacolon may also be acquired. Causes of acquired megacolon include Chagas' disease, inflammatory bowel disease, bowel obstruction and chronic constipation in childhood.

Acquired megacolon may be differentiated from Hirschsprung's disease by rectal examination. In patients with Hirschsprung's disease, a narrow empty segment of rectum can be felt, above which the colon is dilated and full of faeces. In patients with acquired megacolon, in contrast, no empty segment of rectum is felt and faeces are present in the distal rectum.

The incidence is 1 in 5000 live births; it is ten times as likely to occur in children with Down's syndrome (trisomy 21) and is often found in association with other congenital abnormalities.

Diagnosis is by barium enema and biopsy showing an absence of ganglion cells. Pressure studies show a failure of relaxation of the internal anal sphincter. Treatment is with surgery.

Gastroschisis and exomphalos

Gastroschisis is a congenital herniation of bowel through the abdominal wall, usually just to the right of the umbilical cord.

The bowel is exposed to fetal urine in utero which causes inflammation and paralytic ileus, and so neonates cannot be fed orally until the bowel recovers. The condition is not associated with other abnormalities and overall mortality is about 5%.

Exomphalos occurs when the gut fails to return to the abdominal cavity after its physiological herniation and development outside the cavity during weeks 7–11 of gestation. Affected children are born with gut and sometimes liver protruding through the umbilicus, covered by amnion and hence protected from fetal urine. This is the key feature distinguishing it from gastroschisis, where the amnion does not cover the herniated intestine. The condition is associated with other congenital abnormalities however, most commonly cardiac, renal or chromosomal. Overall mortality is 25–50%.

Treatment of both conditions is surgical.

Infectious and inflammatory disease

Diarrhoea

Diarrhoea is an increase in frequency of bowel opening associated with looser stools. A more technical definition is passage of more than three unformed stools per 24 hours. It is important to note that a change in bowel habit, not the absolute frequency, is the key abnormality.

More water is reabsorbed in the intestine than is secreted. Clearly, if there is failure of absorption, the faeces will contain abnormal amounts of water and diarrhoea will result.

Dysentery is painful, bloody, but low-volume, diarrhoea.

Reduced absorption may be due to one or more of a number of factors including:

- An increase in the number of osmotic particles in the lumen, resulting in a flow of water into the lumen (osmotic diarrhoea)

Fig. 5.8 Types and causes of diarrhoea.

Osmotic diarrhoea
Disaccharidase deficiencies
Drug-induced
Galactose
Generalized malabsorption

Secretory diarrhoea
Infectious
Defects in intraluminal digestion and absorption
Excess laxative use

Deranged motility
Increased intestinal transit time
Decreased motility

Malabsorption

Exudative diseases
Infectious
Inflammatory bowel disease

- An increase in the rate of flow of intestinal contents, leaving less time for the absorption processes to take place (deranged motility diarrhoea)
- An abnormal increase in secretions of the gastrointestinal tract (secretory diarrhoea).

The main categories and causes of diarrhoea are summarized in Fig. 5.8. The investigation of choice is a stool sample to determine whether an organism is responsible, which can then be treated accordingly. Treatment has been discussed in the pharmacology section, with the initial focus on maintaining fluid and electrolyte balance.

Osmotic diarrhoea

Both electrolytes and absorbed nutrients (such as sugar and amino acids) contribute to osmosis. If the absorption of either of these is reduced, e.g. in a protein-losing enteropathy, osmotic diarrhoea will occur.

Secretory diarrhoea

Mature cells near the tips of the small intestinal villi are responsible for absorption. They are stimulated to increase their rate of secretion by a number of factors such as acetylcholine, substance P, 5-hydroxytryptamine (serotonin) and neurotensin, all of which increase intracellular calcium.

Potentially fatal secretory diarrhoea can also be caused by cholera. The causative organism, *Vibrio cholerae*, is endemic in certain parts of the developing world. Infection is spread by the faecal–oral route and pandemics are by no means unusual.

The organism can survive in the acid conditions of the stomach and multiplies in the small intestine where it produces an enterotoxin that binds to receptors on the immature cells in the crypts.

This causes an increase in adenylate cyclase, elevating cyclic AMP and increasing the secretion of Na^+, Cl^- and water into the lumen. The main symptom is profuse 'rice water' stools.

Treatment with oral rehydration therapy to replace water and electrolytes is curative.

Deranged motility (rapid transit) diarrhoea

Increased gut motility leads to lack of absorption (due to rapid transit), which can result in diarrhoea. Some agents may stimulate secretion as well as motility. Gastrointestinal stasis may also cause diarrhoea by facilitating bacterial overgrowth.

Parasitic causes of diarrhoea

The protozoan organisms *Entamoeba histolytica* and *Giardia lamblia* commonly cause diarrhoea. Both are transmitted by the faecal–oral route and are found most commonly in developing countries.

Infection with the former may be asymptomatic or cause amoebic dysentery (a notifiable disease), which may have a gradual onset accompanied by systemic symptoms, such as anorexia and headache.

Treatment of acute amoebic dysentery is with metronidazole. Diloxanide is given in chronic disease.

Giardiasis causes steatorrhoea and abdominal pain. It may also lead to malabsorption (see Chapter 4). Treatment is with metronidazole.

> **HINTS AND TIPS**
>
> Inflammation, infection or neoplasms can cause bloody diarrhoea. If the diarrhoea is very bloody then it is due to chronic disease, such as a neoplasm or ulcerative colitis. Inflammatory bowel disease can cause chronic exudative diarrhoea.

Infective enterocolitis

Enterocolitis is inflammation of the intestines. It may be caused by a variety of agents. In 40–50% of cases, no specific agent is isolated and an educated guess must be taken according to the age, circumstances and degree of immunocompetence of the patient.

Improved sanitation has led to a decreased prevalence of infective enterocolitis in the developed world, but it still accounts for more than 50% of all deaths before the age of 5 years worldwide and over 12 000 deaths each day among children in developing countries.

Viral gastroenteritis

Gastroenteritis is the inflammation of the stomach and intestines. The illness includes vomiting, fever, abdominal pain and diarrhoea. The rapid loss of water and electrolytes can result in metabolic disturbances which need correcting.

It is transmitted by the faecal–oral route, and causes include rotaviruses, enteric adenoviruses, caliciviruses, astroviruses and noroviruses (Fig. 5.9).

Bacterial enterocolitis

The major causes of bacterial enterocolitis are summarized in Fig. 5.10. In the UK, *Campylobacter* infection, usually acquired by eating contaminated poultry, is the commonest cause.

The principal mechanisms by which bacterial infection may lead to gastroenteritis are:

- The ingestion of a bacterial organism that proliferates in the gut lumen and that is enterotoxic
- Ingestion of a ready-made (preformed) toxin in contaminated food, which is heat stable, e.g. *Staphylococcus aureus*, *Vibrio cholerae* and *Clostridium perfringens*
- The ingestion of an enteroinvasive bacterial organism, which proliferates in the gut and destroys the mucosal epithelial cells.

Fig. 5.9 Common causes of viral gastroenteritis.

Virus	Host age	Transmission method
Rotavirus (group A)	6–24 months	Person-to-person, food, water
Astroviruses	Child	Person-to-person, water, raw shellfish
Norwalk-like viruses	School age, adult	Person-to-person, water, cold foods, raw shellfish
Enteric adenoviruses	Child under 2 years	Person-to-person
Caliciviruses	Child	Person-to-person, water, cold foods, raw shellfish

Fig. 5.10 Common causes of bacterial enterocolitis.

Organism	Source of transmission
Campylobacter	Milk, poultry, animal contact
Clostridium difficile	Nosocomial environment
Clostridium perfringens	Meat, poultry, fish
Escherichia coli	Food, water, undercooked beef products, weaning foods, cheese, person-to-person
Mycobacterium tuberculosis	Contaminated milk, swallowing of coughed-up organisms
Salmonella	Milk, beef, eggs, poultry
Shigella	Person-to-person, low-inoculum
Vibrio cholerae, other vibrios	Water, shellfish, person-to-person
Yersinia enterocolitica	Milk, pork

The incubation period can give clues as to whether the food poisoning was due to bacterial contamination or preformed toxins. Usually, the incubation period of bacterial contamination is longer, as time is required to establish an enterotoxic colony in the gut.

Treatment consists of fluid replacement alongside antibiotics.

Necrotizing enterocolitis

As the name suggests, this is a necrotizing inflammation of the small and large intestines (primarily the terminal ileum and ascending colon) and is the most common acquired gastrointestinal emergency in neonates.

It is most common within the first few days of life (when infants start oral feeding), but it may occur at any time within the first 3 months, especially in premature or low-birth-weight babies being given formula milk rather than breast milk.

Symptoms vary from mild gastrointestinal upset to perforation of necrosed intestine leading to shock and, if untreated, death. Surgical resection of affected intestine may be necessary.

Pseudomembranous colitis

Pseudomembranous colitis is caused by an overgrowth of Clostridium difficile, a bacillus which is carried by 2 % of the population, asymptomatically. It usually occurs post antibiotic therapy which suppresses the normal colonic flora allowing C. difficile to proliferate.

There is loss of epithelial cells and the formation of a whitish pseudomembrane on the bowel surface composed of mucin, polymorphs and fibrin.

While pseudomembranous colitis is associated mainly with broad-spectrum antibiotics, especially cephalosporins, almost any antibiotic may precipitate it. Elderly patients should not be put on cephalosporins for this reason.

Transmission is promoted within the hospital environment, where patients with C. difficile have a mortality of up to 30%.

Treatment is with oral metronidazole, while vancomycin is often used for recurrent infections.

Appendicitis

As mentioned above, acute appendicitis is usually caused when the appendix is obstructed, mostly by faecaliths. Rarely, it can occur when the appendix is not obstructed, e.g. when the lymphoid follicles are infected.

Typically, patients initially present with central abdominal pain, which then becomes localized to the right iliac fossa as the peritoneum adjacent to the appendix is affected. Movement and coughing exacerbate the pain. There may be fever, vomiting, and tachycardia may be present.

Appendicectomy is curative, and needs doing urgently to prevent the appendix from rupturing and causing peritonitis.

Inflammatory bowel disease

There are two major non-specific inflammatory bowel diseases: Crohn's disease and ulcerative colitis. The main differences between them are demonstrated in Figs 5.11 and 5.12.

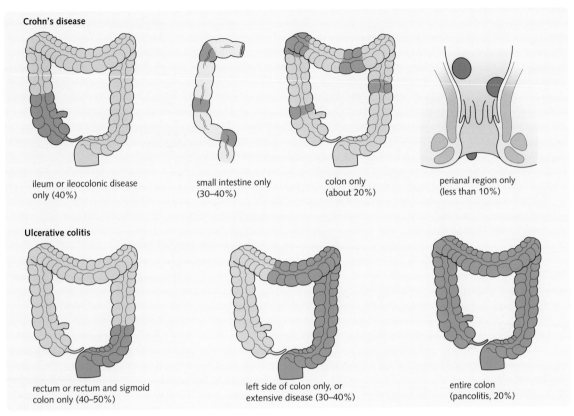

Crohn's disease

ileum or ileocolonic disease only (40%)

small intestine only (30–40%)

colon only (about 20%)

perianal region only (less than 10%)

Ulcerative colitis

rectum or rectum and sigmoid colon only (40–50%)

left side of colon only, or extensive disease (30–40%)

entire colon (pancolitis, 20%)

Fig. 5.11 Distribution patterns of inflammatory bowel disease.

Crohn's disease

Crohn's disease may affect any part of the gastrointestinal tract from the mouth to the anus (Fig. 5.13). It is most common in the terminal ileum and ascending colon.

Crohn's disease is more frequent in the Western world, particularly amongst Caucasians, where the prevalence is approximately 50–100 per 100 000. Its peak onset is between 20 and 40 years of age and both sexes are equally affected.

There is a high rate of concordance in monozygotic twins, which suggests both a genetic and environmental cause. However, the exact aetiology is unknown. There is a 3–4-fold increase in risk with smoking and Crohn's patients generally eat a diet higher in refined sugars and lower in fibre than those without Crohn's.

Macroscopically, the bowel appears bright red and swollen. Later, small, discrete aphthoid ulcers with a haemorrhagic rim form, so named because they look similar to aphthous ulcers in the mouth.

These progress to deeper longitudinal ulcers, which may develop into deep fissures involving the full thickness of the wall of the gastrointestinal tract. Because of this, the mucosa is often described as cobble-stoned (Fig 5.12). Aggregations of inflammatory cells and lymphocytes infiltrate the bowel wall. Mesenteric lymph nodes may be enlarged due to reactive hyperplasia. Granulomas may be present in the lymph nodes.

> **HINTS AND TIPS**
>
> Granulomas are collections of epithelioid macrophages and giant cells surrounded by a cuff of lymphocytes. The non-caseating granulomas in Crohn's disease are different from those found in tuberculosis, which are tubercular granulomas characterized by central caseous (cheese-like) necrosis.

Damage to the gastrointestinal tract in Crohn's disease is often patchy (skip lesions) with normal areas of tissue found in between the patches.

Symptoms include diarrhoea, with or without malabsorption, abdominal cramps, fever, malaise and weight loss. Clinical signs include:

- Abdominal tenderness
- Perianal lesions
- Anaemia
- Aphthous ulcers in the mouth
- Weight loss.

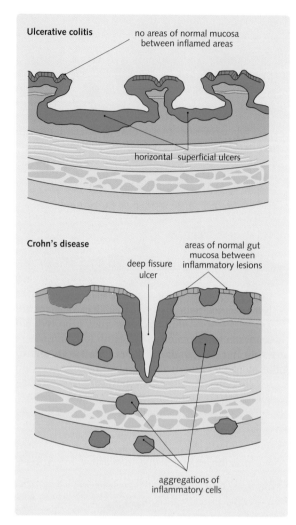

Fig. 5.12 Histopathological features of ulcerative colitis and Crohn's disease. Unlike Crohn's disease, ulcerative colitis is continuous and areas of normal gut are not found between lesions.

Diagnosis involves colonoscopy with biopsy and contrast radiography.

Complications

Complications depend on the site and extent of the lesions.

Malabsorption may occur where large areas of small intestine are affected (short bowel syndrome, following surgical resection). Fistulae may form because of deep fissuring. These may be internal (between loops of gut or from the gut to the bladder), perianal, or, following surgery, open onto the skin.

Crohn's disease may also cause stricture formation, which may lead to obstruction.

Acutely, perforation or haemorrhage may occur.

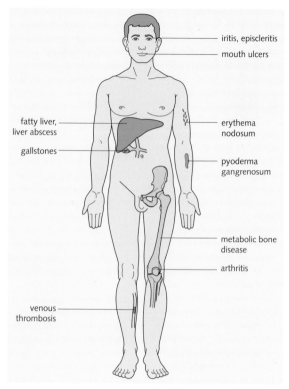

Fig. 5.13 Systemic complications of inflammatory bowel disease.

A variety of lesions may be seen around the anus, most commonly skin tags, fissures and fistulae in 60% of patients.

Treatment

All Crohn's disease patients require symptomatic relief and, for some, this is all the treatment they ever need. Diarrhoea is treated with anti-diarrhoeal drugs, such as loperamide and codeine phosphate. Depending on disease activity, further treatments are often required.

To treat an acute flare up, corticosteroids are the main treatments used to induce remission. In secondary care, immunosuppressive treatments such as ciclosporin or azathioprine are often required. Sulfasalazine (an aminosalicylate) is also used to prevent relapses. Cytokine-modulating drugs such as infliximab induce remission in 70–80% of patients unresponsive to corticosteroids.

Antibiotics, such as metronidazole are useful in severe perianal disease.

However, 80% of patients will require surgery at some point in their life because of:

* Failure to thrive in children
* Complications, e.g. perforation, obstruction, stricture or fistula formation
* Failure or side effects of drug therapy.

Surgery is never curative. Remission is achievable, but most patients have significant relapses.

Ulcerative colitis

Ulcerative colitis only affects the large intestine (Fig. 5.11). Ulcerative colitis affects more patients than Crohn's disease with a prevalence is 100–120 per 100 000. It affects women more than men and is most common between the ages of 20 and 40 years, although it can occur at any age.

It usually starts in the rectum and it may extend proximally, although never beyond the colon. Occasionally, inflammation of the terminal ileum is seen (backwash ileitis) but this is a result of an incompetent ileocaecal valve rather than ulcerative colitis itself. Its aetiology is unknown, although possible causative agents include genetics, infection and immunological factors.

Unlike Crohn's, which commonly shows skip lesions, ulcerative colitis is continuous. Areas of normal gut are not found between lesions.

The disease is a chronic relapsing inflammatory disorder. Inflammation is diffuse but superficial. The mucosa is granular and haemorrhagic (Fig. 5.12), rarely involving the muscle layer.

Both acute and chronic inflammatory cells are found infiltrating the mucosa, and aggregates of polymorphs are seen in the crypts (crypt abscesses). Healing of ulcers leads to periods of remission but, in areas of healing, the normal large bowel epithelium may be replaced by a simple layer of mucus-secreting cells without crypts.

The major symptom in ulcerative colitis is bloody exudative diarrhoea. Often lower abdominal pain, anorexia and malaise accompany this. If the disease is confined to the rectum, urgency and tenesmus accompany the bloody diarrhoea.

Diagnosis requires rectal examination, sigmoidoscopy and biopsy. A barium enema can show fine ulceration.

Complications

The mucosa may haemorrhage, leading to blood loss and anaemia.

Toxic megacolon, where the colonic diameter is greater than 6 cm may occur in acute fulminating cases. It allows passage of bacterial toxins into the systemic circulation and predisposes to perforation.

Extraintestinal complications may also occur in both Crohn's disease and ulcerative colitis (Fig. 5.13). These include:

- Skin involvement: pyoderma gangrenosum and/or erythema nodosum
- Primary sclerosing cholangitis
- Fatty liver and/or liver abscesses
- Iritis and/or episcleritis
- Arthritis and spondylitis.

Treatment

There are two types of treatment for ulcerative colitis, depending on whether acute management or the maintenance of remission is needed. Acute cases are treated with corticosteroids. All ulcerative colitis patients are treated with 5-aminosalicylic acid (5-ASA, e.g. mesalazine) or sulfasalazine (a compound of 5-ASA and sulfapyridine) to maintain remission and reduce the risk of colon cancer.

Azathioprine is an immunosuppressant can induce remission in more resistant cases.

Surgery is curative in ulcerative colitis. Indications include:

- Toxic megacolon (surgical emergency)
- Acute ulcerative colitis not responding to medical treatment
- Chronic colitis leading to poor quality of life.

Prognosis of inflammamtory bowel disease varies greatly depending on the extent of the disease. It is important to distinguish between a diagnosis of Crohn's and ulcerative colitis as the management of each is different (Fig. 5.14).

Inflammatory bowel disease and colon cancer

In patients with ulcerative colitis there is a 5–10-fold increased risk of developing colorectal carcinoma compared to the normal population. This risk is thought to be comparable for patients with Crohn's disease, however there are no accurate figures yet.

Currently all patients with inflammatory bowel disease are offered enrolment into a national surveillance programme where they have episodic colonoscopies and random biopsies taken. Patients are classed as either low risk, intermediate risk or high risk, and then followed up at 5, 3 and 1 years, respectively.

The finding of dysplasia from a biopsy taken at endoscopy is an indication for colectomy.

Irritable bowel syndrome

Irritable bowel syndrome (IBS) is a functional bowel disease. No single cause has been identified, and it is diagnosed on the basis of the presence of particular symptoms and the exclusion of organic diseases.

IBS is very common, affecting 10–20% of the general population, and is more prevalent in young women. It comprises a cluster of symptoms, the most important being abdominal pain, altered bowel habit, abdominal distension, tenesmus and the presence of rectal mucus.

Diagnostic criteria for IBS are:

- Exclusion of structural or metabolic abnormalities, e.g. ulcers, inflammatory bowel disease, lactose intolerance

Fig. 5.14 Comparison of ulcerative colitis and Crohn's disease.

Crohn's disease	Ulcerative colitis
Affects anywhere from mouth to anus	Only affects large bowel (but backwash ileitis occurs in 10%)
Deep ulcers and fissures (rose-thorn ulcers) in mucosa	No fissures, horizontal undermining ulcers
Malignant change less common than ulcerative colitis	Malignant change relatively common
10% have fistulae	Fistulae rare
60% have anal involvement	25% have anal involvement
Fibrous shortening and early strictures of intestine	Muscular shortening of colon but strictures rare and late
Skip lesions	No skip lesions
Fat and vitamin malabsorption (if small intestine affected)	No fat or vitamin malabsorption
Granulomas in 50%	No granulomas
Marked lymphoid reaction	Mild lymphoid reaction
Fibrosis	Mild fibrosis
Serositis	Mild serositis (if any)
No raised ANCA	Raised ANCA
Increased incidence in smokers	Decreased incidence in smokers

- Abdominal pain for 12 weeks or more in a 12-month period
- Presence of two or more accompanying symptoms:
  - Pain relieved by defecation
  - Onset of pain associated with a change in frequency of the stools
  - Onset of pain associated with a change in the form of the stools.

Irritable bowel syndrome is generally referred to as constipation-predominant or diarrhoea-predominant. The course of the disease is often relapsing and remitting. Stress can bring on attacks of IBS.

A management algorithm for IBS is given in Fig. 5.15. Reassurance and explanation is very important, alongside lifestyle and dietary advice.

Bowel obstruction

Bowel obstruction may have mechanical or non-mechanical causes (pseudo-obstruction).

The signs and symptoms are similar, regardless of the cause, and depend primarily on the level of the obstruction. Patients will usually complain of absolute constipation, were they don't pass any flatus. Vomiting is a symptom of high obstruction, but it may be absent (or occur late) in low-level obstruction. Conversely, distension and colic are early symptoms of obstruction lower in the intestine.

Obstruction causes distension of the gut, with a build-up of gas and intestinal secretions above the level of the obstruction. There is progressive depletion of extracellular fluid and the multiplication of bacteria, especially coliforms, Enterococcus faecalis, Clostridium perfringens and Bacteroides.

Diagnosis requires a thorough history and erect and supine radiography. This shows distended, gas-filled loops of bowel with multiple horizontal fluid levels.

Treatment depends on the cause and level of the obstruction, and whether the bowel is strangulated. Strangulated bowel is an emergency and requires urgent surgery.

Simple obstruction, i.e. not due to strangulation may be treated conservatively initially. Conservative treatment consists of 'drip and suck': intravenous fluids and continuous aspiration by nasogastric tube.

HINTS AND TIPS

In general, obstruction high in the gastrointestinal tract presents with vomiting. Obstruction lower down causes distension.

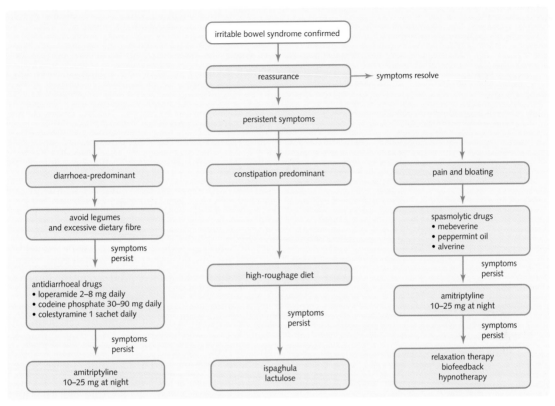

Fig. 5.15 Management of irritable bowel syndrome. (Reproduced with permission from Haslett C et al. Davidson's Principles and Practice of Medicine, 19th edn. Edinburgh: Churchill Livingstone, 2002.)

Causes of bowel obstruction

Mechanical causes of obstruction of a tube like the intestine may be:

- In the wall, e.g. malignancy, inflammatory bowel disease, congenital strictures and diverticular disease
- In the lumen, e.g. foreign material, faecaliths, polypoid tumours and meconium in cystic fibrosis
- Outside the wall, e.g. intussusception, adhesions, hernias, volvulus and intra-abdominal tumours.

Pseudo-obstruction may be due to Hirschsprung's disease, paralytic ileus and bowel infarction.

Paralytc ileus is an obstruction of the intestine caused by partial or complete paralysis of the intestinal muscles, resulting in lack of peristalsis. It occurs transiently after almost every laparotomy. Other major causes include interruption of the autonomic innervation of the gut, peritonitis (which may cause toxin-mediated paralysis of the intrinsic nerve plexuses of the gut) and potassium depletion.

Hernias

A hernia is the protrusion of any organ or tissue through its coverings and outside its normal body cavity.

Hernias are common, occurring in about 1% of the population, and may be congenital or acquired (Fig. 5.16). Within these two groups, they may be reducible, irreducible or strangulated (Fig. 5.17).

Reducible hernias can be pushed back into the compartment from which they came, while irreducible ones cannot and may become strangulated if their blood supply is cut off by the neck of the sac.

Strangulated hernias present with signs and symptoms of obstruction and if untreated, become gangrenous and necrotic. The most common sites of herniation through the abdominal wall are:

- Inguinal (about 90%)
- Femoral
- Umbilical
- Incisional
- Ventral and epigastric.

Inguinal hernias may be:

- Direct (protruding through the posterior wall of the inguinal canal)
- Indirect (passing through the inguinal canal).

Direct inguinal hernias are less common (20% of inguinal hernias) and they lie medial to the inferior epigastric vessels. Indirect hernias are much more common,

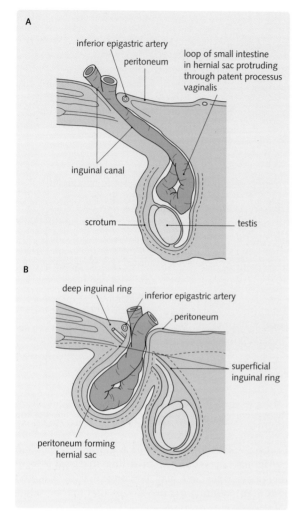

A

inferior epigastric artery

peritoneum

loop of small intestine in hernial sac protruding through patent processus vaginalis

inguinal canal

scrotum

testis

B

deep inguinal ring

inferior epigastric artery

peritoneum

superficial inguinal ring

peritoneum forming hernial sac

Fig. 5.16 (A) Congenital indirect hernia passing into scrotum through patent processus vaginalis. (B) Acquired direct hernia passing through a defect in the abdominal wall. (Redrawn with permission from Hall-Craggs ECB. Anatomy as a Basis for Clinical Medicine. London: Waverly Europe, 1995. http://lww.com)

lie lateral to the inferior epigastric vessels and are more likely to strangulate, as the neck (the internal ring of the inguinal canal) is narrower. See also *Crash Course: Anatomy*.

Treatment depends on the type of hernia. Reducible hernias often require no treatment so long as they remain reducible. Strangulated hernias must be treated surgically.

Synthetic meshes are often used to reinforce closure of hernia orifices.

Adhesions

Adhesions occur where two parts of the body that are normally separate are connected by bands of fibrous tissue.

Some are congenital, but most occur as a result of post-inflammatory scarring, most commonly from scars that form following surgery.

Adhesions may cause external constriction of the bowel, leading to obstruction or strangulation. Urgent surgery is required to relieve the strangulation.

Intussusception

Intussusception occurs when one segment of bowel (the intussusceptum) slides inside the adjacent segment (Fig. 5.18), like a telescope. It is most common in early childhood (95% of all cases) and occurs mainly at the ileocaecal valve (ileocolic intussusception), although it may also occur at other sites. The ratio of males to females affected is 2:1.

The aetiology is unclear, but it may be related to an adenovirus causing enlargement of lymphatic tissue in the intestinal wall. This protrudes into the lumen and is pushed into the adjacent section by peristalsis.

In some cases a polyp (such as Peutz–Jeghers polyps), Meckel's diverticulum or carcinoma may project into the lumen and be pushed along in a similar way.

Patients present aged 5–12 months of age, with periods of screaming, vomiting, blood in the faeces ('redcurrant jelly') and drawing up of the legs. The child is pale and a sausage-shaped mass may be felt on palpation of the abdomen.

Peritonitis and gangrene may occur within 24 hours if untreated. A barium enema may resolve the intussusception by forcing the invaginated segment back with hydrostatic pressure. Alternatively, surgery may be required.

Volvulus

Volvulus occurs when a loop of bowel is twisted 180° about its mesenteric axis. This usually occurs in the sigmoid colon, but it may be found in the caecum, small intestine, gall bladder or stomach. It is rare in the UK.

Risk factors include chronic constipation, adhesions and abnormally mobile loops of intestine.

Twisting of the bowel causes obstruction and occlusion of the vessels supplying the affected section. Potentially fatal gangrene and peritonitis may occur if the volvulus is not treated. Symptoms include the sudden onset of colicky pain in the right iliac fossa and rapid abdominal distension.

Diagnosis is by plain radiography, which shows a dilated section of bowel full of gas and forming a characteristic loop or inverted 'U' (the 'bent inner tube' sign). Treatment depends on the site of the volvulus: surgery is often necessary. Sigmoid volvulus is sometimes resolved by sigmoidoscopy and the passing of a flatus tube.

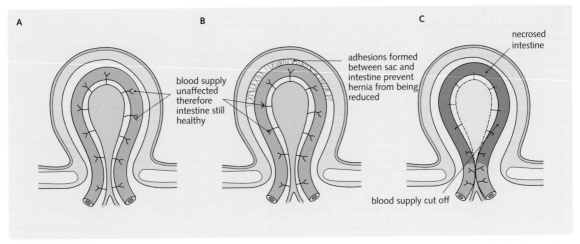

Fig. 5.17 (A) Reducible hernia. (B) Irreducible hernia. (C) Strangulated hernia. Reducible hernias can be pushed back into the compartment from which they came, irreducible ones cannot. Strangulated hernias have had their blood supply cut off.

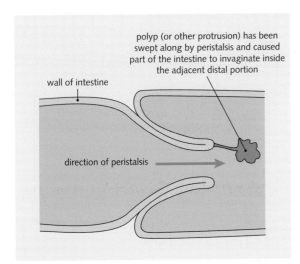

Fig. 5.18 Intussusception. One bowel segment has slipped inside an adjacent one.

Diverticulosis

Some important definitions:

- A diverticulum is an outpouching of the wall of the gut. They occur at weak points in the wall, usually due to increased pressure from within the gut or pulling from outside
- Diverticulosis means that diverticula are present
- Diverticular disease means that diverticula are causing symptoms, such as abdominal pain or change in bowel habit. However, the pain is due to muscle spasm, not inflammation

- Diverticulitis means that one or more diverticula are inflamed. This is usually caused by an infection and leads to inflammatory abdominal pain and diarrhoea, or constipation.

Diverticulosis

Diverticula may be congenital or acquired. They may occur in any part of the gut.

Congenital diverticula are outpouchings of the full thickness of the bowel wall. They are found most commonly in the duodenum and jejunum. They are usually asymptomatic, but they may lead to bacterial overgrowth, steatorrhoea and vitamin B_{12} malabsorption. They may also perforate or bleed.

Acquired colonic diverticula increase in incidence with increasing age. They are predominantly a Western condition, present in about 50% of people aged over 50 years. There is no difference in distribution between the sexes. Low-fibre diets are a risk factor. 95% of diverticulae are found in the sigmoig colon.

They form when the muscle layer of the wall thickens (hypertrophies) and high intraluminal pressures force a pouch of mucosa out through an area of weakness in the muscle layer. Areas of weakness often occur near blood vessels (Fig. 5.19).

Acquired diverticula do not consist of all three layers of the intestinal wall and this differentiates them from congenital ones.

Diagnosis of diverticula is often incidental during other investigations. As over 90% of cases are asymptomatic, in many cases no treatment is required.

Patients should, however, be advised to increase the amount of fibre and liquids in their diet (fibre has no beneficial effect unless there is sufficient liquid in the diet).

Fig. 5.19 Colonic diverticulosis. High intraluminal pressure has forced pouches of mucosa through weak muscle areas. (Redrawn with permission from Ellis H, Calne R, Watson C. Lecture Notes on General Surgery, 10th edn. Oxford: Blackwell Science, 2002.)

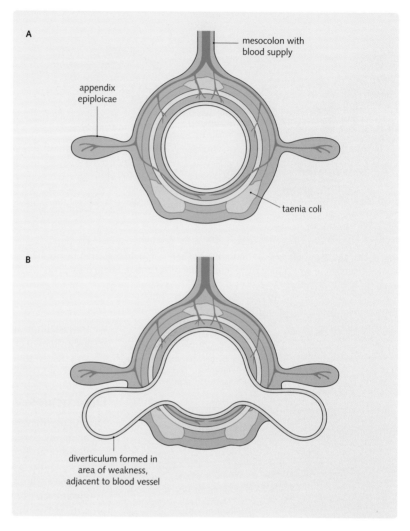

Diverticulitis

Diverticulitis may occur if the neck of the diverticulum becomes obstructed by faeces. Patients with acute diverticulitis often present with severe left iliac fossa pain.

Signs include tenderness and guarding on the left side of the abdomen, pyrexia and tachycardia. Radiographs should be taken to exclude air under the diaphragm (an indication of perforation).

Complications include:

- Haemorrhage if a vessel is eroded
- Perforation, causing peritonitis if it occurs into the peritoneal cavity, abscess formation or fistulae if it occurs into the bladder or vagina
- Chronic infection causing fibrosis and obstruction.

In the absence of complications, acute diverticulitis is treated conservatively with a liquid diet and appropriate antibiotic treatment.

Vascular disorders

Bowel ischaemia

Essentially, the causes of ischaemic bowel disease are the same as ischaemia in other parts of the body. Causes include:

- Stenosis
- Thrombosis
- Emboli
- Strangulation may also cause ischaemia as the blood supply is disrupted.

Ischaemic bowel disease may occur in the small intestine or the colon. The effect depends on the size of the ischaemic area and the length of time ischaemia has persisted. It may be classified as mucosal, mural or transmural.

The blood supply to the wall is 'from outside in' and mucosal or mural infarction often results from

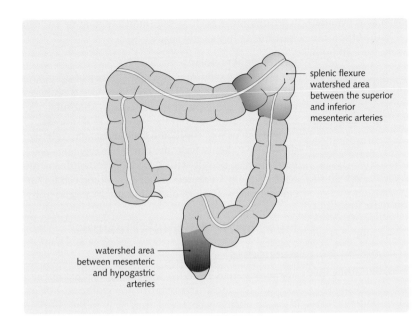

Fig. 5.20 Areas of large bowel particularly prone to ischaemic injury.

splenic flexure watershed area between the superior and inferior mesenteric arteries

watershed area between mesenteric and hypogastric arteries

underperfusion. Transmural infarction is usually due to mechanical compromise of the artery.

The splenic flexure and an area of the rectum are particularly prone to ischaemic damage. These are the 'watershed' areas where the arterial supply switches from the superior to the inferior mesenteric artery, and from the inferior mesenteric and hypogastric arteries, respectively (Fig. 5.20).

Mucosal ischaemia causes release of proteolytic enzymes, which may cause deeper damage to the wall. However, complete regeneration is more common.

After mural ischaemia, ulcers form, the mucosa haemorrhages and granulation tissue forms. This is replaced by fibrotic tissue, which can form a stricture.

Transmural ischaemia leads to gangrene, perforation and, if untreated, death. It should be suspected in any elderly patient with atherosclerosis or atrial fibrillation with a tender abdomen and absent bowel sounds.

Symptoms in acute bowel ischaemia include:

- Acute severe abdominal pain
- No abdominal signs, such as distension
- Shock, due to hypovolaemia
- Increased haemoglobin and white cell count
- Persistent metabolic acidosis
- Gasless abdomen on X-ray.

Diagnosis relies on abdominal X-ray and endoscopy. A sigmoidoscopy shows a normal rectal mucosa, but it also shows blood and mucus coming from further along the bowel. A full colonoscopy is not performed, due to the risk of perforation.

Histological changes in chronic ischaemic bowel disease include fibrosis, haemorrhage, ulceration and granulation. On biopsy, the mucosa has a large infiltration of polymorphonuclear cells. Macrophages laden with haemosiderin are uncommon, but thought to be characteristic of ischaemic bowel disease.

The patient is treated with fluid replacement, heparin and antibiotics. Surgery is absolutely necessary to remove the dead segment of bowel. Revascularization may also be attempted, but note that reperfusion injury caused by free radicals commonly occurs following hypoperfusion.

The prognosis is poor in acute bowel ischaemia, with a less than 20% survival rate.

Angiodysplasia

Angiodysplasia refers to small vascular anomalies, most commonly venous malformations in the mucosa or submucosa. They are usually asymptomatic and their only presentation is bleeding from the large bowel. They occur in the elderly and can be diagnosed by angiography or colonoscopy. The right side of the colon is affected more commonly than the left.

Treatment is by diathermy coagulation or surgical removal.

Haemorrhoids

Haemorrhoids are the enlargement of the normal spongy blood-filled cushions in the wall of the anus. They are the most common cause of rectal bleeding, and patients normally complain of blood on the toilet paper after defecation.

The anal cushions (and hence sites of haemorrhoids) are at 3, 7 and 11 o'clock when viewed in the lithotomy position and attached by elastic tissue and smooth muscle.

However, gravity, increased anal tone and straining on defecation all put stress on the cushions, making them protrude and bleed readily from the underlying capillaries. Pregnancy and portal hypertension (see Chapter 6) can also cause haemorrhoids.

Haemorrhoids are classified as:

- First degree (confined to the anal canal, and which bleed but do not prolapse)
- Second degree (which prolapse on defecation, but spontaneously reduce)
- Third degree (which prolapse on defecation, but require reduction with the fingers).

Patients present with bright red bleeding from the rectum, and they are often very anaemic.Mucus discharge and pruritus ani (anal itching) accompany this. Often internal haemorrhoids are asymptomatic.

Diagnosis involves rectal examination, proctoscopy and exclusion of any abdominal malignancies, which may also cause bleeding.

Haemorrhoids are often self-limiting, however in more troublesome cases injection of a sclerosant or elastic band ligation may be required. Haemorrhoidectomy is usually reserved for irreducible and problematic cases.

Neoplastic disease

Hamartomatous polyps

Some 90% of colonic epithelial polyps are non-neoplastic and therefore benign. Hamartomatous polyps are an example. They are derived from overgrowth of mature tissue and are usually large and pedunculated. They fall into two main categories: juvenile and Peutz–Jeghers polyps.

> **HINTS AND TIPS**
>
> Hamartomas are malformations containing two or more types of mature cell which are normally present in the organ in which they arise. They are always benign.

Juvenile polyps

Juvenile polyps are usually solitary focal hamartomatous malformations of mucosal tissue.

They occur in children and teenagers, but they are most common below the age of 5 years. About 80% of them occur in the rectum.

However, in juvenile polyposis, an autosomal dominant condition presenting with ten or more colonic polyps, the risk of colonic cancer is increased. Children

with this must begin a screening programme to help spot cancer in its early stages.

Peutz–Jeghers polyps

Peutz–Jeghers syndrome is a rare autosomal dominant syndrome characterized by multiple polyps scattered throughout the gastrointestinal tract. Abnormal pigmentation also occurs in the skin and oral mucosa.

The polyps may bleed and cause anaemia. Although the polyps themselves are not premalignant, being hamartomas, people with Peutz–Jeghers syndrome do have a slightly increased risk of developing certain carcinomas, notably in the gastrointestinal tract and ovary.

Neoplastic epithelial lesions

Adenomas

Adenomas are derived from glandular epithelium, and they are the most important of the epithelial polyps. They are relatively common, especially in the elderly.

Of all adenomas, 75% are tubular, 10% villous and the remainder a mixture of the two (tubulovillous).

Villous adenomas are usually sessile and larger (up to several centimetres in diameter) than tubular adenomas, and as the name suggests, have villi lined with dysplastic columnar epithelium protruding from their surface.

Almost all colonic carcinomas originate from an adenomatous polyp. The malignant potential of an adenoma is related to increasing polyp size and the histological type with villous adenomas having a greater tendency to malignant change (Fig. 5.21).

Adenomas and other polyps are usually incidental findings when patients are undergoing endoscopy. They should be removed endoscopically to prevent premalignant transformation.

Familial adenomatous polyposis

People with familial adenomatous polyposis (FAP), a rare autosomal dominant disorder, almost always develop cancer of the intestine by the age of 35 years. FAP is characterized by the development of numerous adenomas in the large and, to a lesser extent, the small intestine during the teens and twenties.

The gene involved in FAP is called APC and is on the long arm of chromosome 5 (between q21 and q22). Non-steroidal anti-inflammatory drugs are thought to be protective.

Hereditary non-polyposis colorectal cancer

Hereditary non-polyposis colorectal cancer (HNPCC) is an autosomal dominant disorder which is similar to FAP in that it greatly predisposes to colorectal cancer, but has an increased prevalence. The carcinomas also

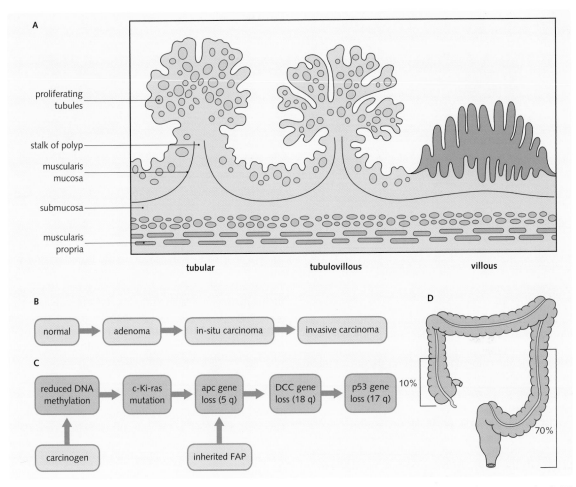

Fig. 5.21 (A) Types of colonic polys. (B) A summary of polyp cancer sequence in the colon. (C) Molecular changes involved. (D) Two-thirds of colon cancers occur within 60 cm of the anal verge and within reach of a flexible sigmoidoscopr. (FAP, familial adenomatous polyposis.) (Reproduced with permission from Fox C, Lombard M. Crash Course: Gastroenterology, 3rd edn. Edinburgh: Mosby, 2008.)

tend to be more aggressive in nature, with a propensity to produce mucin.

Other associated carcinomas include those of the stomach, ovary and endometrium. The cause is a mutation, of which four have been identified, in DNA mismatch genes. The two most important mutations are those in hMSH2 (chromosome 2p) and hMLH1 (chromosome 3p).

Patients with HNPCC or FAP should be offered regular endoscopic screening.

Colorectal cancer

Colorectal cancer is common in the developed world. It is the second biggest cause of cancer death in the UK, coming second only to lung cancer. Incidence increases with age and is more common in males.

As mentioned above the majority of tumours are adenocarcinomas which evolve from polyps. Aetiology is also closely related to diet. Western diets which are high in fat and low in fibre carry a greater risk of colorectal cancer.

Fibre increases the bulk of faeces as long as fluid intake is adequate, which reduces the time taken for the contents of the intestine to pass through and out of the rectum. In a low-fibre diet, faeces remain in the intestine for longer, altering the normal flora. This is thought to predispose to cancer.

The main clinical features are:

- Altered bowel habit for greater than 6 weeks
- Rectal bleeding (more common in left-sided tumours)
- Iron deficient anaemia (often how right-sided tumours present)

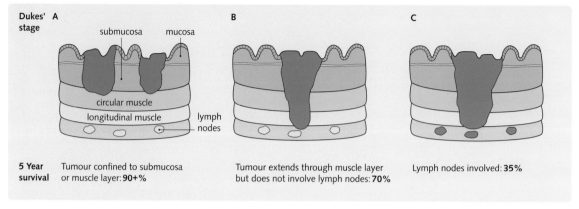

Fig. 5.22 Dukes' staging for colorectal carcinoma.

- Colicky abdominal pain
- Palpable mass (either abdominal or on rectal examination)
- Weight loss.

Colonoscopy is the gold standard investigation as it also allows biopsies to be taken for a histological diagnosis.

Surgery is the mainstay of treatment if the disease is confined to the colon. Depending on the site of the tumour an end-to-end anastomosis or end colostomy will be performed. Chemotherapy is often useful in metastatic disease.

The commonest site for metastases is the liver. Following this, other sites include lung, brain and bone.

Prognosis after diagnosis of colorectal cancer depends on the stage, with an overall survival rate of 30% at 5 years. Dukes' classification is most widely used (Fig. 5.22) and is a common examination question. Dukes' stages are:

- Stage A: invaded submucosa and muscle layer of the bowel, but confined to the wall
- Stage B: breached the muscle layer and bowel wall, but no involvement of lymph nodes
- Stage C1: spread to immediately draining pericolic lymph nodes
- Stage C2: spread to higher mesenteric lymph nodes
- Stage D: distant visceral metastases (5-year survival – 5%).

Colorectal cancer screening

Screening for colorectal cancer has been rolled out across the UK in recent years. Early detection is important as it improves both mortality and morbidity rates. By the time patients present with symptoms of colorectal cancer, the majority of patients are at least Duke's Stage B, so if these patients could be picked up whilst at Duke's stage A it would improve survival rates.

Faecal occult blood screening is offered to all UK residents between the ages of 60–69. Patients are asked to send a stool sample off for analysis, and if they are judged to be at risk then they are offered a colonoscopy. Sensitivity and specificity for the detection of colorectal cancer has still to be confirmed.

Other neoplasms – Carcinoid tumours

These arise from neuroendocrine (APUD) cells (see Chapters 3 and 4) in the gut and elsewhere, e.g. pancreas, biliary tract and lung. They are slow growing and potentially malignant but their malignant potential depends on the site.

Larger tumours in the appendix and ileum tend to spread to regional lymph nodes and the liver. Small tumours (less than 2-cm diameter) near the tip of the appendix rarely do so.

Because of the cells in which they arise, tumours produce hormones that may have local or systemic effects:

- 5-HT produced by midgut carcinoid tumours causes diarrhoea and borborygmi as a result of local stimulation of the contractility of the intestine
- 5-HT may also be produced from metastases in the liver and give rise to the carcinoid syndrome with facial flushing, cyanosis and pulmonary and tricuspid valve stenosis or incompetence
- Adrenocorticotrophic hormone (ACTH) may be secreted and can result in Cushing's syndrome.

Palliative treatment is usually given. Survival can be anything from 3 years to 30 years, even if metastases are present.

After reading this chapter, you should be able to:
- Describe the anatomy of the liver, with regard to its macroscopic structure, relations, arterial supply, venous and lymphatic drainage, and nerve supply
- Outline the embryological development of the liver
- Describe the histological structure of the liver, and understand the function of its different cell types
- Outline the functions of the liver, and the functions of bile
- Define the term 'cirrhosis'
- Outline the clinical features of liver failure
- Define 'jaundice', and explain the pathophysiological mechanisms which cause it
- Describe the effects of alcohol on the liver
- Describe the different types of hepatitis viruses
- Outline the following types of hepatic disorders: congenital abnormalities, infections and inflammatory disease, vascular disease and neoplastic disease

OVERVIEW

The liver is the largest abdominal organ and also the largest gland in the body. It is vital for life, and it has many metabolic, endocrine and detoxifying functions.

ANATOMY

The liver is situated under the diaphragm and weighs about 1.5 kg. It is surrounded by a capsule of strong connective tissue (Glisson's capsule).

It lies in the right upper quadrant and occupies most of the right hypochondriac region, extending into the left hypochondriac and epigastric regions (see Fig. 1.1).

The liver is protected by the rib cage and moves during respiration, owing to its attachment to the diaphragm by the falciform, coronary and triangular ligaments (Fig. 6.1).

The lesser omentum connects the stomach to the liver, and it is continuous with the left triangular ligament.

The liver has diaphragmatic and visceral (posteroinferior) surfaces. The sharp inferior border separates the two surfaces. The visceral surface is related to:

- The abdominal oesophagus
- The fundus and body of the stomach
- The lesser omentum

- The gallbladder
- The superior part of the duodenum
- The transverse colon, including the hepatic flexure
- The right kidney and associated adrenal gland.

Peritoneum covers the visceral surface (except the gall bladder and porta hepatis) and the superior part of the liver, except the posterior part known as the bare area. This area is in direct contact with the diaphragm and is situated between the reflections of the coronary ligament. The inferior vena cava and the right adrenal gland also lie next to the bare area (Fig. 6.2).

Macroscopically and functionally, the liver is comprised of two 'true' lobes, the left and the right, by the plane joining the tip of the gall bladder and the groove of the inferior vena cava. This division is made on the basis of the blood supply (Fig. 6.3) and bile drainage. There are also two minor lobes (used for descriptive purposes) called the caudate and quadrate lobes. The left lobe includes the caudate lobe and most of the quadrate lobe.

In terms of blood supply that can be surgically isolated, the liver has eight segments (of Couinaud) which may be an important consideration when resection for primary or metastatic cancer is being contemplated. The segments can be mapped onto the lobes (Fig. 6.4).

The space between the visceral surface of the right lobe and the right kidney is the hepatorenal recess; the diaphragmatic recess separates the diaphragmatic surface from the diaphragm.

Fig. 6.1 Summary table of ligaments attaching the liver to the diaphragm.

Ligament	Attachments
Falciform ligament (remnant of the ventral mesentery of the abdominal foregut)	Attaches the anterior and superior surfaces of the liver to the anterior abdominal wall and the diaphragm
Coronary ligament	Attaches the posterior surface of the right lobe to the diaphragm
Right triangular ligament	An extension of the coronary ligament
Left triangular ligament	Attaches the posterior surface of the left lobe to the diaphragm

Fig. 6.2 Three different views of the liver, showing the anterior, superior, and inferior sides. The bare area on the posterior part of the liver is not covered with peritoneum.

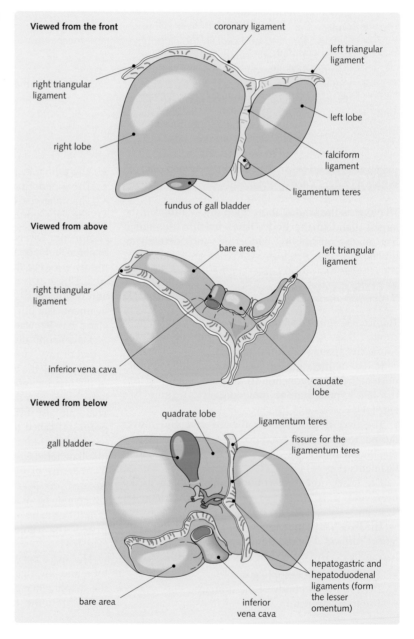

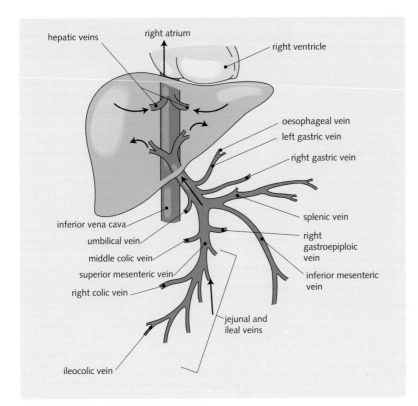

Fig. 6.3 The hepatic portal venous system. (Redrawn with permission from Hall-Craggs ECB. Anatomy as a Basis for Clinical Medicine. London: Waverly Europe, 1995. http://lww.com)

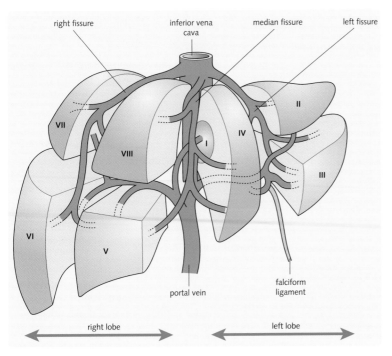

Fig. 6.4 Anterosuperior view of the liver showing the correlation between lobes and vascular segments. Segment I corresponds to the caudate lobe, segments II, III and IV to the left lobe and segments V, VI, VII and VIII to the right lobe. The segments are organized according to the divisions of the hepatic artery and portal vein. (Reproduced with permission from O'Grady J, Lake J, Howdle P. Comprehensive Clinical Hepatology. London: Mosby, 2000.)

Blood supply

The liver has a very rich blood supply from two main sources:

- *The hepatic artery* (a branch of the coeliac trunk), which divides into left and right branches to supply the left and right lobes. This supplies about 30% of the blood to the liver
- *The portal vein*, which carries venous blood rich in products of digestion from the gastrointestinal (GI) tract. It supplies 70% of the blood to the liver, and divides into left and right branches to supply the two functional lobes. An accessory left hepatic artery, often arising from the left gastric artery, may be found.

The main branches of the hepatic artery and portal vein divide each lobe into the vascular segments mentioned earlier. There are eight segments in the whole of the liver.

The hepatic veins drain from the central veins of each lobule into the inferior vena cava.

Lymphatic drainage

The lymphatics of the liver drain to deep and superficial vessels.

The deep vessels come together at the porta hepatis and end in the hepatic lymph nodes scattered along the hepatic vessels, e.g. the cystic lymph node near the neck of the gall bladder. These then drain to the coeliac lymph nodes to enter the thoracic duct.

Some deep lymph vessels follow the hepatic veins through the diaphragm to end in the phrenic lymph nodes.

The superficial lymph vessels follow the same drainage as the deep vessels, but they can also drain to the mediastinal lymph nodes.

Nerve supply

The liver receives both sympathetic and parasympathetic innervation. The nerve fibres reach the liver via the hepatic plexus, which is derived from the coeliac plexus. It also receives parasympathetic innervation from the right phrenic nerve and left and right vagi (Xth cranial nerves).

The hepatic nerves follow the blood supply of the liver and enter at the porta hepatis.

HINTS AND TIPS

The porta hepatis is a deep fissure on the visceral surface of the liver, and it contains the hepatic artery, portal vein, hepatic nerve plexus, hepatic ducts and lymphatic vessels.

EMBRYOLOGY AND DEVELOPMENT

The liver develops from the liver bud (hepatic diverticulum) that appears as an outgrowth of the endodermal epithelium at the distal end of the primitive foregut in the middle of the 3rd week (Fig. 6.5).

The liver bud is composed of rapidly proliferating cells, which penetrate the mesodermal septum transversum. The connection between the liver bud and the foregut (duodenum) narrows and forms the bile duct.

A small ventral outgrowth from the bile duct gives rise to the gallbladder and cystic duct. The structure of the liver is formed by epithelial liver cords that mix with the vitelline and umbilical veins to give rise to hepatic sinusoids.

The liver cords differentiate into the hepatocytes (parenchyma), the bile canaliculi, and the hepatic ducts. The mesoderm of the septum transversum gives rise to:

- Haematopoietic cells
- Kupffer cells
- Connective tissue cells.

The liver is the major haematopoietic organ in the embryo, and by the 4th week, haematopoiesis has already begun.

The lesser omentum and the falciform ligament are both also derived from the mesoderm of the septum transversum, located between the foregut and liver, and the ventral abdominal wall and the liver, respectively.

The rotation of the stomach, liver and spleen occurs between the 6th week and 11th week of embryonic development.

At about the 12th week, the hepatocytes begin to form bile. This is able to enter the duodenum, as the biliary tract and gallbladder are both fully formed.

HINTS AND TIPS

Hepatocytes are highly metabolically active and rich in cytoplasmic organelles, especially mitochondria.

HISTOLOGY

Traditionally, there are three ways of describing the structural units of the liver (Fig. 6.6):

- Classical lobule – each lobule may be thought of as a hexagon with a central vein at its centre and a portal triad at its outer corners. A portal triad consists of a branch of the hepatic artery, a branch of the portal vein and a bile duct

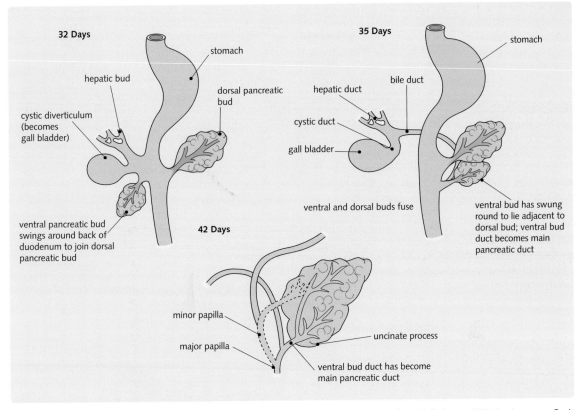

Fig. 6.5 Development of the liver, gall bladder and pancreas. (Redrawn with permission from Hall-Craggs ECB. Anatomy as a Basis for Clinical Medicine. London: Waverly Europe, 1994.)

- Portal lobule – this views the liver as being made up of a series of triangles with a central vein at each corner and a portal triad at the centre, and it emphasizes exocrine function
- Acinus – an elliptical unit with a portal triad at the centre and a central vein at each pole, and it emphasizes endocrine function.

Acinus

This is a more accurate description of the functional unit within the structure of the liver parenchyma. It reflects the gradient of metabolic activity found in the liver, and is divided into three zones for descriptive purposes:

- The periportal zone (zone 1)
- The midzone (zone 2)
- The centrilobular zone (zone 3).

Most oxygenated blood is found in the centre of the acinus around the portal triad (zone 1); this zone is adjacent to the portal canal and receives the most blood from the hepatic artery and portal vein. Therefore, it is most susceptible to damage from toxins carried to the liver in the hepatic portal vein and toxins absorbed from the alimentary tract, e.g. in paracetamol poisoning. Most of the metabolic activity of the liver takes place here.

Conversely, zone 3, being furthest from the portal triad and closest to the central vein, is most susceptible to ischaemic damage, e.g. in heart failure.

Types of cell

Different types of cell make up the architecture of the liver: hepatocytes, Kupffer cells, haematopoietic cells and perisinusoidal cells. The functions of these cells are summarized in Fig. 6.7.

Sinusoids, perisinusoidal spaces and bile canaliculi

The hepatocytes are arranged in 'cords', which radiate out in a spoke-like fashion from the central vein (Fig. 6.8). They are large, eosinophilic cells with round nuclei. An interesting feature is that more than half of the cells are tetraploid, i.e. they have four times the number of normal chromosomes. They have a network of capillaries, or sinusoids, between them, which are lined with discontinuous fenestrated endothelium, stellate cells and phagocytic Kupffer cells. Kupffer cells are

Fig. 6.6 Structural units of the liver.

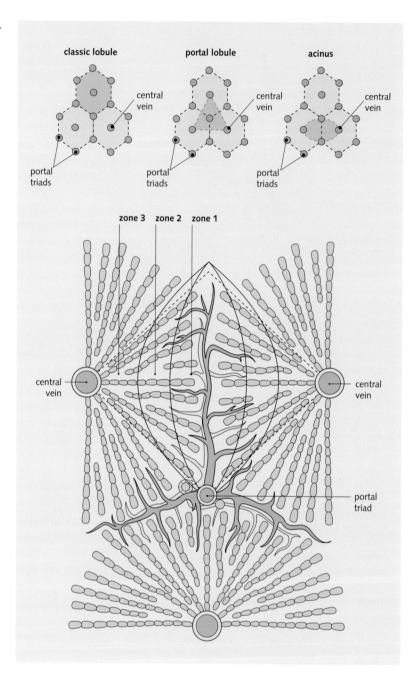

part of the monocyte–macrophage system and phagocytose old erythrocytes and other cellular debris from the circulation.

In between the hepatocytes and the sinusoidal endothelial cells is the perisinusoidal space (of Disse). This contains perisinusoidal cells (stellate, or Ito, cells) which secrete collagen, providing a supportive mesh. It is these cells which contribute to fibrosis in liver damage (see later).

At their sinusoidal surface, the hepatocytes have numerous short microvilli, which extend into the perisinusoidal space. Between the bases of the microvilli lie coated pits that are used for endocytosis.

The microvilli increase the surface area for the transfer of digestive products, nutrients, oxygen, and other substances between the blood in the sinusoids and the hepatocytes.

Cell type	Function
Kupffer cells	Phagocytosis, found in sinusoids
Hepatocytes	Perform most of the functions of the liver (Fig. 6.10)
Ito cells (perisinusoidal cells)	Replace damaged hepatocytes and secrete collagen
Endothelial cells	Scavenger cells for denatured collagen, harmful enzymes, and pathogens: they line the sinusoids
Haemopoietic cells	Haemopoiesis in the fetus, and in adults with chronic anaemia

Fig. 6.7 Cell types of the liver.

Two surfaces of each hepatocyte communicate with a space of Disse and two surfaces communicate with a bile canaliculus (Fig. 6.9).

Bile canaliculi are formed by a groove between surfaces of adjacent hepatocytes and they are sealed by zonulae occludentes, which prevent leakage of bile into the intercellular spaces.

The canaliculi form rings around the hepatocytes and approach the bile ductules in the portal tracts by opening into canals (of Hering). These are short corridors lined with cuboidal cells that drain bile into the ductules of the portal tracts.

Portal canal and limiting plate

The portal canal consists of the portal triad (hepatic portal vein, hepatic artery and bile duct) surrounded by connective tissue.

A small space (the space of Mall) exists between the connective tissue covering and the surrounding hepatocytes. Lymph is thought to originate in the space of Mall.

The limiting plate (the hepatocytes of the periportal zone), which surrounds the portal tract, makes up a protective layer of cells, which are first to be exposed to toxins in the systemic or portal blood. Breaching the plate can lead to liver damage, in particular cirrhosis.

FUNCTIONS AND PHYSIOLOGY

The liver performs many functions vital for life. The main functions of the liver are metabolism of protein, fat and carbohydrate; bile production; storage of vitamins, minerals, and glycogen; biotransformation; and detoxification and protection (by filtration of portal blood). These are summarized in Fig. 6.10.

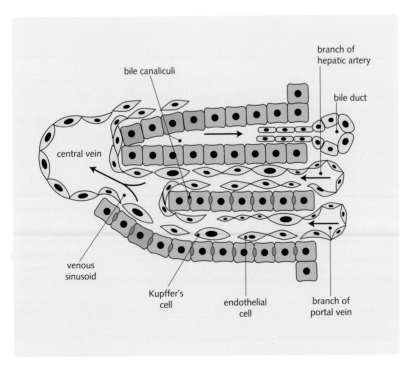

Fig. 6.8 Cords of hepatocytes radiating out from the central vein. The space of Disse (the perisinusoidal space) is located between the hepatocytes and the fenestrated endothelial cells, interspersed with Kupffer cells, that line the sinusoids. Perisinusoidal cells (Ito cells) reside here and secrete collagen. (Redrawn with permission from Marshall W. Clinical Chemistry, 3rd edn. London: Mosby.)

Fig. 6.9 Two sides of each hepatocyte communicate with a sinusoid (via the space of Disse), and bile canaliculi are formed by a groove between adjacent hepatocytes.

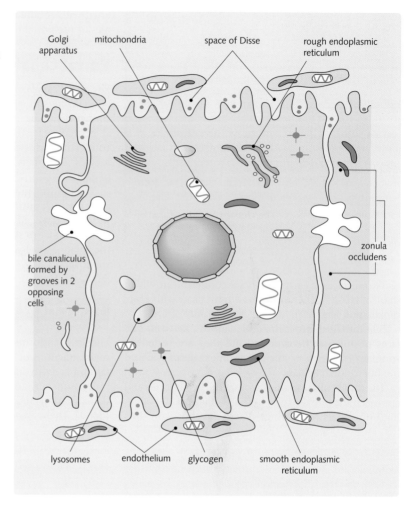

To maintain these functions, the liver must receive 25% of the cardiac output through the portal vein and hepatic artery. Nutrients and other substances are absorbed from the sinusoids into the hepatocytes.

The varied nature of hepatic function requires that the hepatocytes differ functionally from each other. The functional differences correspond to the zones of the liver acinus (see earlier). The cells in each zone differ in ultrastructure, function, and distance from the blood supply, with zone 1 being nearest to the arterial supply and zone 3 the furthest. Functional differences include:

- The periportal hepatocytes take up bile under normal circumstances, but during bile overload, this function is also adopted by the centrilobular (perivenous) hepatocytes
- The centrilobular hepatocytes contain enzymes required in esterification, but the periportal hepatocytes are rich in oxidative enzymes.

Carbohydrate metabolism

In the normal individual, blood glucose levels are carefully regulated. The liver plays an important role in glucose homeostasis.

Blood glucose levels rise transiently after a meal but the liver takes up the glucose and converts it to glycogen.

In the fasting state, glycogen is converted to glucose (glycogenolysis) and released into the bloodstream to keep levels within the range 3.5–5.5 mmol/L.

The liver contains approximately 80 g of glycogen. This is enough to keep blood glucose levels within the normal range for approximately 24 hours at rest, but for less time during heavy exercise.

The peptide hormones insulin and glucagon, both produced by the pancreas, control the levels of plasma glucose. Insulin promotes synthesis of glycogen, protein and fat, while inhibiting gluconeogenesis and lipolysis.

Fig. 6.10 The main functions of the liver and hepatocytes.

Function	Processes involved
Protein metabolism	Synthesis and secretion of albumin Synthesis of plasma proteins Formation of urea from ammonia Deamination of amino acids Synthesis of coagulation factors Metabolism of polypeptide hormone
Fat metabolism	Formation of lipoproteins and fatty acids Synthesis of cholesterol Conversion of cholesterol to bile salts Conversion of carbohydrates and protein to fat Ketogenesis Metabolism and excretion of steroid hormones
Bone metabolism	Hydroxylation Vitamin D
Carbohydrate metabolism	Gluconeogenesis Synthesis and breakdown of glycogen
Bile secretion	Production of bile salts (these emulsify fats for absorption in the intestine: therefore, the liver has a role in fat absorption) Elimination of bilirubin
Absorption	Fat and vitamins A, D, E and K
Storage	Glycogen Vitamins (A and B_{12})
Biotransformation and detoxification	Of drugs and exogenous substances Gonadal hormones Aldosterone Glucocorticoids Nitrogenous gut toxins
Protection	Filtration of portal blood Removal of bacteria/antigens by Kupffer cells (phagocyctosis)
Haematopoiesis	The fetal liver is the major source of blood cell production

Glucagon acts on the liver primarily and has no effect on muscle. It up-regulates gluconeogenesis and ketogenesis.

The liver also contains the hydrolytic enzyme glucose-6-phosphatase, which allows for release of glucose from cells. This enzyme is absent in the brain and muscle so that, in effect, the liver is the only organ which can release glucose into the bloodstream to maintain blood sugar levels.

In diabetes, the utilization of carbohydrates is impaired and ketone bodies are formed in the liver from b-oxidation of fatty acids. Ketones are released from hepatocytes and carried to other tissues where they are metabolized.

In prolonged starvation, ketone bodies and fatty acids are used as alternative sources of fuel, and body tissues (except the brain) adapt to a lower glucose requirement.

Lipid metabolism

Most of the fat (lipids) in the diet is in the form of triglycerides (esters of fatty acid and glycerol). The digestion and absorption of dietary lipids is described in Chapter 5.

Lipids are insoluble in water, and they are assembled into lipoproteins (complexes of lipid and protein) in the liver, for transport in the blood (Fig. 6.11). Depending on their composition, lipoproteins are classified into chylomicrons (the lowest density), very-low-density, intermediate-density, low-density and high-density lipoproteins (Fig. 6.12).

Low-density lipoproteins (LDLs) have been implicated in atheroma and their level in the plasma should be kept low. Conversely, high-density lipoproteins

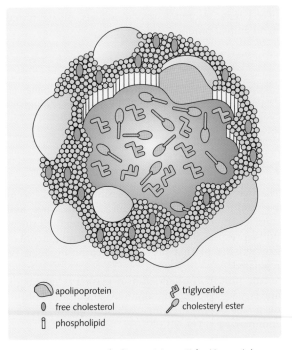

apolipoprotein triglyceride
free cholesterol cholesteryl ester
phospholipid

Fig. 6.11 Structure of a lipoprotein particle. Lipoproteins are complexes of lipids and proteins. They have a triglyceride and cholesterol ester middle and a polar coat, made up of phospholipids, apoproteins and unesterified cholesterol. (Reproduced with permission from Gaw A et al. Clinical Biochemistry: An Illustrated Colour Text, 2nd edn. Edinburgh: Churchill Livingstone, 1999.)

Fig. 6.12 The density classes of plasma lipoproteins.

Class	Abbreviation	Sources	Mean diameter (nm)
Chylomicrons	CHYLO	Intestine	500
Very low density lipoproteins	VLDL	Liver	43
Intermediate density lipoproteins	IDL	Catabolism of very low density lipoproteins and chylomicrons	27
Low-density lipoproteins	LDL	Catabolism of very low density lipoproteins	22
High-density lipoproteins	HDL	Catabolism of chylomicrons and very low density lipoproteins; liver and intestine	8

(HDLs) have a protective function and their levels should be higher.

Cholesterol is needed for the manufacture of steroid hormones and bile acids, and can be synthesized in the liver. It is also a component of most diets, and it is found in all animal products, especially eggs.

> **HINTS AND TIPS**
>
> It is easy to remember the ideal levels of circulating lipoproteins. Low-density ones should be LOW and high-density ones should be HIGH.

Protein metabolism

The liver synthesizes all the plasma proteins except γ-globulins. Amino acids from the intestines and muscles enter the liver and by controlling their metabolism (especially via transamination and gluconeogenesis) the plasma protein concentrations can be regulated.

The protein concentration of plasma is 60–80 g/L and is made up of mainly albumin, globulin and fibrinogen. The plasma proteins synthesized by the liver are summarized in Fig. 6.13.

Urea metabolism

Amino acids are transaminated and deaminated via oxidative pathways in the liver to form ammonia, which is converted to urea via the urea (ornithine) cycle. This occurs mainly in the periportal cells (hepatocytes adjacent to the portal canals).

The cycle occurs partly in the mitochondria and partly in the cytoplasm, so the enzymes are situated in one or the other, according to their function in the cycle.

In liver failure, there is decreased synthesis of urea and increased levels of ammonia—a toxic product. Ammonia can depress cerebral blood flow and cerebral oxygen consumption. Ammonia toxicity is usually due to cirrhosis, but it is also seen in inherited deficiencies of urea cycle enzymes.

Transamination of amino acids is the interconversion of amine ($-NH_2$) groups from amino acids to a-ketoacids, to produce different amino acids. This is catalysed by transaminase in the liver.

Vitamin metabolism

The liver is the main store of the fat-soluble vitamins (A, D, E and K). Vitamin deficiency may occur when there is malabsorption of fat, due to a variety of hepatic and extrahepatic causes.

Vitamin B_{12} is absorbed from the diet in the terminal ileum, provided intrinsic factor is made by the parietal cells of the stomach, and enough is stored in the liver to last 2 or 3 years. Deficiency eventually leads to megaloblastic anaemia (pernicious anaemia).

The liver stores folate and converts it to its active form, tetrahydrofolate. Folate is needed as a coenzyme for the transfer of 1-carbon groups and its deficiency also leads to megaloblastic anaemia, but more quickly than vitamin B_{12} deficiency because body stores of folate are only sufficient for a few months. Folate

Fig. 6.13 Plasma proteins synthesized by the liver.

Protein	Function
Albumin	Maintain colloid osmotic pressure Transport of hydrophobic substances e.g. bilirubin, hormones, fatty acids, drugs
Lipoprotein	Transport of lipids in the blood
Transferrin	Carrier molecule for iron
Caeruloplasmin	Carrier molecule for copper
Globulins (not γ-globulins)	Antibody functions Transport of lipids, Fe, or Cu in the blood
α_1-antitrypsin	Protein inhibitor of the enzyme trypsin
α_1-fetoprotein	Secreted by yolk sac and embryonic liver epithelial cells
	In adults is produced by proliferating liver cells and can be used as an indicator of liver cancer
Fibrinogen	
Prothrombin	Blood clotting factors
Factors V, VII, IX, X, XII	
Complement cascade proteins	Immune function upregulators and coordinators Inflammatory functions

deficiency in early pregnancy may also lead to neural-tube defects in the fetus.

Dietary deficiency of folate is much more common than vitamin B_{12} deficiency, and it is seen in alcoholics and others on a poor diet or suffering from a severe illness where folate utilization is increased, e.g. in cancer.

> **HINTS AND TIPS**
>
> In general, a deficiency of any substance may result from:
> • Increased utilization
> • Increased excretion
> • Decreased manufacture
> • Decreased absorption.

Storage

The liver acts as a store for, among others, glycogen, fat and fat-soluble vitamins, folate, iron and copper. This storage function is important as it enables the body to withstand periods of insufficient intake of the stored nutrients.

Some stores are large enough to sustain the body's needs for a few years, e.g. stores of vitamin B_{12} are sufficient for about 3 years; folate stores can last a few months.

Drug and hormone metabolism

The liver metabolizes drugs and hormones via biotransformation in three stages:

- Phase I (oxidation)
- Phase II (conjugation)
- Phase III (elimination).

These processes are useful, in conjunction with the filtering action of the portal blood supply (see later) in allowing the body to detoxify or degrade toxins or waste products.

Phase I reactions often produce more active metabolites, e.g. they can change prodrugs into the active drugs. Phase II reactions make the substrate more water soluble to facilitate phase III. Phase III occurs via ATPase pumps.

Phase I reactions

Oxidation is carried out mainly by the cytochrome P_{450} enzymes in the hepatocyte smooth endoplastic reticulum. Other enzymes such as xanthine oxidase and

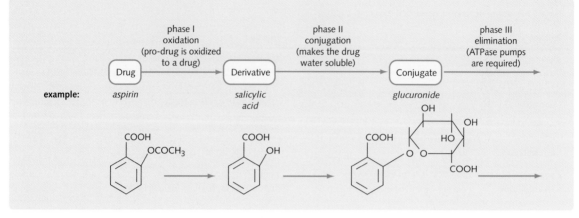

Fig. 6.14 Drug metabolism in the liver. (Adapted from Rang et al. Pharmacology, 5th edn. Edinburgh: Churchill Livingstone, 2003.)

monoamine oxidase, present in other tissues as well as the liver, also assist with oxidation.

A number of drugs induce microsomal enzymes, affecting the metabolism of other drugs taken at the same time, and this should be borne in mind when deciding what dose to prescribe.

Notable examples of enzyme-inducing drugs include phenobarbital, ethanol and phenylbutazone.

Phase II reactions

A number of chemical products are conjugated with drugs or their metabolites in the liver, including glucuronyl, acetyl, methyl, glycyl, sulphate and glutamyl groups, of which glucuronyl is the most common.

Conjugation is important in the metabolism of paracetamol. It is inactivated by conjugation to form a glucuronide or sulphate, but the liver has a limited capacity.

If the normal conjugation pathway is saturated, mixed-function oxidases form a toxic metabolite instead. The toxic metabolite is itself inactivated by conjugation with glutathione, but stores of glutathione are limited.

Phase III reactions

The elimination of conjugated substances is via the blood, which then results in excretion through the kidneys, or via bile through the intestines.

ATPase pumps are required to actively transport the substance out of the hepatocyte. Some pumps are specific for the conjugating molecule, e.g. glutathione.

Some drugs are rapidly inactivated by the liver, e.g. propranolol. The amount of active drug reaching the

circulation is reduced and the drug is said to undergo significant first-pass metabolism. Drug metabolism in the liver is summarized in Fig. 6.14.

Defence

The portal blood supply to the liver allows for toxins and microorganisms to be filtered out before the blood returns to the systemic circulation. This protects the rest of the body from any harmful substances that may have breached the gut defence mechanisms. Kupffer cells in the sinusoids facilitate this via phagocytosis.

Haematopoiesis

In embryonic life, the liver is the main site of haematopoiesis. This occurs from the 2nd to 7th months, but ceases before birth.

By 5 months of gestation, the bone marrow is supplementing the liver in this function.

Between conception and the 2nd month, haematopoiesis takes place in the yolk sac. The liver and spleen can resume their haematopoietic role (extramedullary haematopoiesis) if necessary.

Bile production and function

Bile is an aqueous, alkaline, greenish-yellow liquid produced by the liver to:

- Eliminate endogenous and exogenous substances from the liver
- Emulsify fats in the small intestine and facilitate their digestion and absorption.

Bile consists of bile acids, cholesterol, phospholipids, bile pigments (bilirubin and biliverdin), electrolytes (Na^+, K^+, Ca^{2+}, Cl^-, HCO_3^-) and water.

Waste products found in bile include cholesterol and the bile pigments, bilirubin and biliverdin, which give bile its colour.

Bile passes out of the liver through the bile ducts, and it is concentrated and stored in the gall bladder. During and after a meal, it is excreted from the gall bladder by contraction and passes into the duodenum through the common bile duct.

Most of the bile acids are reabsorbed from the terminal ileum and recycled by the liver (see later). Bile pigments are normally excreted in the faeces, which they colour dark brown.

Bile acids

Bile acids (also called bile salts) are detergents which emulsify lipids. They have a hydrophobic and a hydrophilic end, and they form micelles in aqueous solutions.

Bile acids are synthesized in hepatocytes from cholesterol and excreted into bile. They account for approximately 50% of the dry weight of bile.

The principal primary bile acids are cholic acid and chenodeoxycholic acid. They are made more soluble by conjugation with taurine or glycine.

Of the bile acids excreted into the intestine, 95% are reabsorbed (mostly in the terminal ileum) and recycled by the liver. This is termed enterohepatic recycling (Fig. 6.15). The total pool of bile acids is recirculated six to eight times a day. Reabsorption through enterohepatic recirculation means we only need a small pool of bile acids. Normally about 250–500 mg of bile acids are produced a day, which replaces the amount excreted in the faeces.

The main functions of bile acids are:

- *Triglyceride assimilation* – bile acids emulsify lipids with the aid of lecithin (found in high concentrations in bile) and break them down to 1-mm-diameter droplets. This provides a large surface area for digestive enzymes to act on
- *Lipid transport* – bile acids form mixed micelles with the products of lipid digestion and facilitate transport to the brush border, where they are absorbed
- *Bile flow induction* – bile acids stimulate the flow of bile by osmotically attracting water and electrolytes as they are secreted. It is also thought that some bile acids are secreted in an unconjugated form. They are absorbed without water and electrolytes from the bile ducts to be quickly carried back to the liver for resecretion
- *Regulation of bile acid synthesis* – normal reabsorption of bile acids from the intestines inhibits hepatic synthesis of bile acids. Not all bile acids are equally effective: chenodeoxycholic acid and lithocholic acid significantly reduce cholic acid formation. It is thought that the feedback mechanism acts on the rate-limiting step of bile acid synthesis
- *Water and electrolyte secretion* – if bile acids are present in the colon, they stimulate water and electrolyte secretion. This can result in diarrhoea. A deficiency of bile acids results in malabsorption.

Bilirubin

This yellow pigment, which gives bile its colour, is the principal constituent in bile. Knowledge of bilirubin metabolism is essential to understanding the pathophysiology behind jaundice (see later).

Most bilirubin is formed by the breakdown of haemoglobin from worn-out red cells (Fig. 6.16), but about 15%

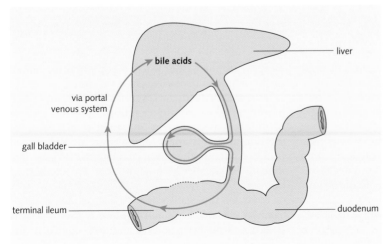

Fig. 6.15 Enterohepatic recycling of bile acids.

Fig. 6.16 Production and fate of bilirubin.

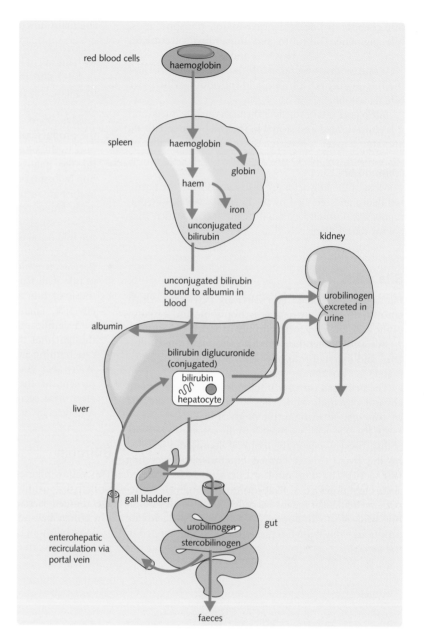

results from the breakdown of other haem-containing proteins such as myoglobin, cytochromes and catalases.

Bilirubin is insoluble and is transported to the liver in the plasma, bound to albumin. There, most of it dissociates from albumin, and is extracted from the blood in the sinusoids by the hepatocytes. It binds to cytoplasmic proteins in the hepatocytes, and is conjugated with glucuronic acid to form bilirubin diglucuronide (a reaction catalysed by glucuronyl transferase, found mainly in smooth endoplasmic reticulum).

Bilirubin diglucuronide is water soluble, unlike bilirubin, and is actively transported against its concentration gradient into the bile canaliculi. A small amount escapes into the blood, where it is transported bound to albumin, and then excreted in the urine.

The intestinal mucosa is permeable to unconjugated bilirubin and to urobilinogen (a colourless derivative of bilirubin produced by intestinal flora); some of the bile pigments and urobilinogens are reabsorbed from the gut into the portal circulation. The intestinal mucosa is relatively impermeable to conjugated bilirubin.

Some of the reabsorbed substances are excreted again by the liver, but small amounts of urobilinogens enter the general circulation and are excreted in the urine.

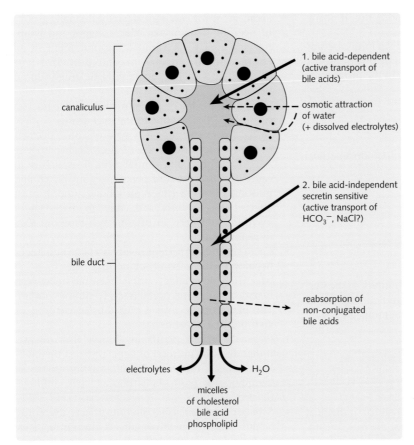

Fig. 6.17 The control of bile acid synthesis and secretion. This involves bile acid-dependent, bile acid-independent and intrahepatic bile duct-dependent control. (From Sanford PA. Digestive System Physiology, 2nd edn. London: Edward Arnold, 1992. Reproduced by permission of Hodder/Arnold Publishers.)

Control of bile production

There are two different mechanisms of control of bile production (Fig. 6.17):

- Bile acid-dependent
- Intrahepatic bile-duct-dependent.

The bile acid-dependent mechanism describes how water and electrolytes passively follow the movement of bile acids, which have been actively transported into the bile canaliculi and ducts. Movement of water and electrolytes is achieved by tight junctions between hepatocytes.

The tight junctions can become more permeable in response to bile acids, vasopressin, epinephrine and angiotensin II. It is thought that bile acids are secreted across the canalicular membrane into bile by protein-mediated facilitated transport, driven partly by the electrochemical difference across the membrane.

The intrahepatic bile duct mechanism describes the aqueous secretion that makes up 50% of the total volume of bile.

The solution is secreted by epithelial cells lining the bile ducts, and is isotonic, with sodium and potassium concentrations similar to those of plasma. It has a higher concentration of bicarbonate and a lower concentration of chloride.

Control of bile acid synthesis and secretion

Cholecystokinin increases the rate of bile acid secretion during the intestinal phase of digestion.

High concentrations of bile acids in the portal blood stimulate bile acid secretion and inhibit its synthesis during the intestinal phase.

Conversely, low levels of bile acids in the portal blood during the interdigestive phase stimulate the synthesis and inhibit the secretion of bile acids.

Secretin stimulates secretion by the bile duct epithelium and this effect is strongly potentiated by cholecystokinin. Secretin alone has no effect on the concentration of bile acids in bile.

PATHOLOGICAL MANIFESTATIONS OF LIVER DAMAGE

The liver is essential to life and has a remarkable capacity to regenerate. Damage from whatever cause (apart from trauma) results in similar pathology but following certain patterns which are dependent on the aetiology. Nevertheless, there is usually an inflammatory reaction, some attempt at regeneration, and, if unsuccessful, cell death.

Because the processes underlying liver injury are similar, the resultant clinical picture will be one of the following types, which represent stages in the progression of liver damage:

- Acute hepatitis
- Chronic hepatitis
- Liver fibrosis
- Cirrhosis, which is the end-point of chronic liver damage
- Complications of the necro-inflammatory or cirrhotic process.

Histopathological patterns of liver injury

These are the different ways in which injury to the liver manifests itself at the tissue level, and should not be confused with the clinical pictures mentioned above.

Necrosis

Hepatic necrosis can be described in a number of ways (Fig. 6.18):

- *Apoptotic necrosis* describes necrosis of individual hepatocytes. It is caused by several diseases, including acute viral hepatitis. Complete recovery with no long-term sequelae is the norm. The dead hepatocytes form eosinophilic Councilman bodies

- *Focal or spotty necrosis* describes small groups of necrotic hepatocytes. Macrophages and lymphocytes tend to accumulate around them in an effort to localize damage or infection. This type of necrosis is seen in acute viral or drug-induced hepatitis
- *Zonal necrosis* describes destruction of hepatocytes within a particular zone of the liver acinus
- *Haemodynamic necrosis* is a type of zonal necrosis because concentric bands of necrotic hepatocytes are seen around the central vein. This occurs in cardiac failure, stasis of hepatic venous blood and poisoning. Zone 3 (the centrilobular zone) is most affected by necrosis, e.g. due to paracetamol overdose, and necrosis of zone 2 is rare, but seen in yellow fever
- *Confluent bridging necrosis* involves a large number of hepatocytes in a 'band' of necrosis stretching between hepatic venules (central to central) or between hepatic venules and portal tracts (central to portal). This pattern of necrosis is caused by severe drug- or viral-induced hepatitis
- *Piecemeal necrosis* occurs in chronic liver disease. It describes the necrosis of hepatocytes at the interface between the parenchyma and fibrous tissue. Lymphocytes, particularly plasma cells, infiltrate the area
- *Submassive or panacinar necrosis* affects the entire acinus. Massive necrosis affects the entire liver. Both are caused by viral- or drug-induced injury. Massive necrosis can result in fulminant hepatic failure.

Fig. 6.18 Patterns of hepatic necrosis. (Redrawn from Underwood JCE. General and Systematic Pathology, 2nd edn. Edinburgh: Churchill Livingstone, 1996.)

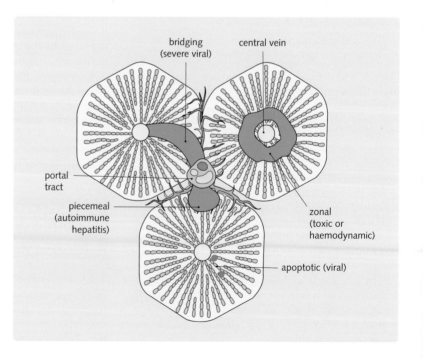

Inflammation

In inflammation of the liver (hepatitis), an influx of acute or chronic inflammatory cells may occur secondary to hepatocellular necrosis.

Regeneration

Regeneration is normal following injury. Hyperplasia and hypertrophy are common after injury. Hepatocyte proliferation results in a thickening of the cords radiating out from the central vein. The architecture may be disturbed unless the connective tissue framework remains intact.

The normal liver can restore its original weight, even if up to two thirds of the liver is removed. This allows for recovery from numerous injuries and even extensive surgical removal of tumours.

Fibrosis

Fibrosis from inflammation or a direct toxic insult may occur around the portal tracts, the central vein or within the spaces of Disse, disrupting the normal architecture and interfering with liver function. In severe cases, cirrhosis results.

Cirrhosis

Cirrhosis is a diffuse and irreversible condition that results from necrosis of hepatocytes followed by the formation of regeneration nodules separated by fibrosis. Cirrhosis has three key characteristics:

- *Chronic hepatocyte necrosis*
- *A chronic inflammatory process* which encourages fibrosis
- *Nodules* caused by *hepatocyte regeneration*.

The process causes architectural disturbances and interferes with normal liver blood flow and function.

The causes of cirrhosis are summarized in Fig. 6.19, and the complications in Fig. 6.20. Many of the complications are similar to those of liver failure, as cirrhosis is a major cause of hepatic failure.

Treatment of cirrhosis

After performing a number of investigations, including liver function tests, liver biopsy, ultrasound and computed tomography (CT) imaging, the severity and type of cirrhosis can be determined.

Treatment depends on the diagnosis and any complications that accompany the cirrhosis. Certain drugs are contraindicated in liver disease, and these should be avoided. Broadly, treatment for cirrhosis may be divided into two categories:

- *Treatment of the underlying cause*, i.e. to stop the pathological process. Depending on the cause, this may include alcohol abstention, antiviral therapy, immunosuppression or withdrawal of drugs

Fig. 6.19 Causes of cirrhosis.

Unknown (10% of cases)
Alcohol (50% of cases)
Hepatitis B (±D) and C
Iron overload (haemochromatosis)
Gall stones
Autoimmune liver disease
Wilson's disease (leading to deposition of copper in the liver)
α_1-antitrypsin deficiency
Type IV glycogenosis
Galactosaemia
Tyrosinaemia
Biliary cholestasis
Budd–Chiari syndrome
Drugs (e.g. methotrexate)
Biliary cirrhosis
Hepatic venous congestion
Cystic fibrosis
Glycogen storage disease

- *Management of complications*, for example ascitic taps and treatment of hepatic encepalopathy (see later).

Patients require 6-monthly checks, involving ultrasound and serum a-fetoprotein measurements. These will enable early detection of hepatocellular carcinoma development.

SYSTEMIC AND ORGANIC MANIFESTATIONS OF LIVER DAMAGE

Portal hypertension

The normal pressure in the hepatic portal vein is about 7 mmHg, but this increases two- to threefold in portal hypertension.

Liver disease is the most common cause, but it is not the only one as many diseases and disorders can result in this condition. Broadly, the causes of portal hypertension may be classified as:

- *Prehepatic* – a blockage of the portal vein before the liver
- *Hepatic* – a disruption or change of the liver architecture
- *Posthepatic* – a blockage in the venous system after the liver.

The causes of these are shown in Fig 6.21.

Fig. 6.20 Consequences of cirrhosis.

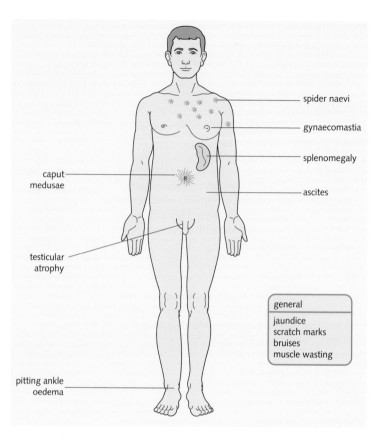

spider naevi

gynaecomastia

splenomegaly

ascites

caput medusae

testicular atrophy

general
jaundice
scratch marks
bruises
muscle wasting

pitting ankle oedema

Fig. 6.21 Causes of portal hypertension.

Prehepatic	Portal vein thrombosis. Arteriovenous fistula. Increased splenic bloodflow, secondary to splenomegaly or arteriovenous fistulae.
Hepatic	Cirrhosis Schistosomiasis. Sarcoidosis. Miliary tuberculosis (granulomata). Massive fatty change. Nodular regenerative hyperplasia. Alcoholic hepatitis.
Posthepatic	Budd–Chiari syndrome (a rare condition caused by hepatic vein obstruction, sometimes associated with the oral contraceptive) (see later). Veno-occlusive disease (see later). Severe right-sided heart failure (very rare with modern cardiac treatment). Constrictive pericarditis (very rare with modern cardiac treatment).

Cirrhosis results in disruption of the normal liver architecture, which increases hepatic vascular resistance and causes intrahepatic arteriovenous shunting. It is the most common cause of portal hypertension in the UK. Worldwide, however, cirrhosis due to viral hepatitis is the main cause of portal hypertension.

Many patients with portal hypertension are asymptomatic, and they are picked up incidentally with low platelet or white cell count related to splenomegaly. Clinical features related to complications include haematemesis or melaena (from ruptured gastro-oesophageal varices), ascites and encephalopathy. The complications of portal hypertension are described below.

Ascites

Ascites is the abnormal collection of fluid in the peritoneal cavity, and is a common complication of portal hypertension secondary to cirrhosis. It may form as a result of:

- Na^+ and water retention, due to peripheral arterial vasodilatation particularly of the splanchnic circulation. This reduces effective blood volume and activates the renin–angiotensin system and sympathetic nervous system (both up-regulate water and salt retention)
- A local hydrostatic pressure increase due to the portal hypertension, resulting in an increased production of lymph in the hepatic and splanchnic

regions. Transudation of the fluid into the peritoneal cavity causes ascites
- Low serum albumin levels (hypoalbuminaemia), due to decreased liver synthesis, causing a low plasma oncotic pressure
- Secondary hyperaldosteronism with reduced catabolism of this salt-retaining hormone.

Clinical Note

The aldosterone antagonist spironolactone is thus often used to treat ascites.

Clinically, ascites may be detected by abdominal swelling, some abdominal pain, a shifting dullness, and a fluid thrill. Many patients also have peripheral oedema, due to hypoalbuminaemia.

It should be managed by reducing sodium intake and increasing renal sodium excretion with diuretics such as spironolactone.

Fluid may be removed by paracentesis (drainage via a needle through the abdominal wall). However, there is a risk that fluid will accumulate again in the peritoneal cavity at the expense of the systemic circulation. This leads to shock, so intravenous albumin should also be given.

A peritoneovenous shunt (a catheter from the peritoneal cavity into the internal jugular vein) may be used to return the fluid to the systemic circulation. This is used in rare cases when diuretic therapy fails.

If the portal pressure rises above 12 mmHg, then dilatation of the venous system causes collateral vessels to form. These are connections between the portal and systemic venous systems, and are found mainly at the gastro-oesophageal junction, rectum, diaphragm, left renal vein, the retroperitoneum and the umbilical region of the anterior abdominal wall and are described further in the next section.

Oesophageal varices can rupture, causing haematemesis and sometimes fatal consequences (oesophageal varices are described in Chapter 2). Enlargement of veins at other sites of portosystemic anastomoses may also occur, forming caput medusae around the umbilicus and rectal varices (see later).

Dilatation of portosystemic anastomoses

These occur at four sites in the body (Fig. 6.22):

- The lower end of the oesophagus, between the left gastric vein (portal) and the azygos vein (systemic): when dilated, they are called *oesophageal varices*

- The lower part of the rectum, between the superior (portal), middle and inferior (systemic) rectal veins: when dilated, they are called *rectal varices*
- The umbilical region of the anterior abdominal wall, between the paraumbilical veins in the falciform ligament of the liver (portal) and the epigastric veins (systemic): when dilated, they are called *caput medusae*
- *The bare areas of the gastrointestinal tract and its related organs*, e.g. veins between the bare area of the liver and the diaphragm
- Additionally, some patients with liver disease who have had intestinal surgery – e.g. colectomy for ulcerative colitis associated with sclerosing cholangitis – can have varices form at the site of the surgical anastomosis or the stoma site and these can subsequently bleed.

HINTS AND TIPS

The locations of the porto-systemic anastomoses is a popular anatomy exam question – make sure you know them. Interestingly, caput medusae at the umbilicus is so-called because it looks like the serpents on the head of Medusa!

These anastomoses may enlarge if the portal vein is obstructed by a thrombus or the venous flow through the liver is impeded by cirrhosis.

Oesophageal varices are clinically the most important cause of bleeding in portal hypertension.

Splenomegaly

Splenomegaly is the term used to describe an enlarged spleen. It can be massive (extending into the right iliac fossa), and has a large number of causes.

Normally the spleen weighs about 200 g; it is oval in shape and found between the 9th and 11th ribs. It plays an important role in immune defence and the removal of expired or abnormal blood cells.

Portal hypertension may cause moderate congestive splenomegaly, as may thrombosis of the extrahepatic portion of the portal vein or of the splenic vein.

A raised pressure in the inferior vena cava may be transmitted to the spleen through the portal vein, and is a cause of posthepatic splenomegaly; other causes include decompensated right-sided heart failure and pulmonary or tricuspid valve disease.

Splenomegaly may cause abdominal discomfort, and an enlarged spleen may occasionally rupture following minor trauma. Additionally, it can cause excess removal of blood cells leading to pancytopenia. This is called hypersplenism.

Fig. 6.22 Diagram showing the sites of portosystemic anastomoses, indicated by a–d.

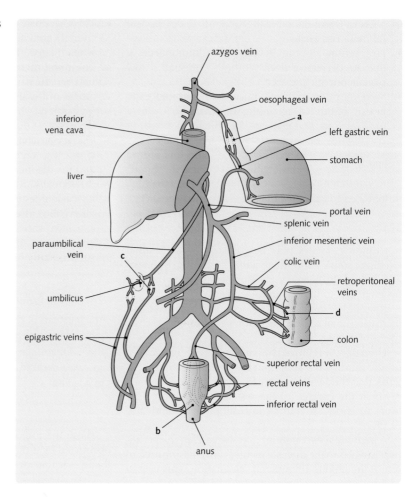

Splenomegaly is easily detected on examination of the abdomen, as it is dull to percussion.

> **Clinical Note**
>
> Do not forget that other non-hepatic causes of splenomegaly include infections and inflammatory and haematological diseases, such as TB, infectious mononucleosis, septic shock, malaria, rheumatoid arthritis and haemolytic anaemia.

Jaundice and cholestasis

Clinical jaundice (icterus) is caused by plasma levels of bilirubin exceeding 50 μmol/L, and it presents as a yellow pigmentation of skin, sclera and mucosa. The colour of the sclera is the best indicator, but it must be examined in good white light. Biochemical jaundice has a much lower threshold, and is simply a plasma bilirubin level above the normal range of 18–24 μmol/L.

Jaundice may be classified by its cause in relation to the hepatocyte as:

- Prehepatic
- Hepatic
- Posthepatic.

Prehepatic jaundice

This describes conditions giving rise to jaundice where the mechanism occurs before the bilirubin gets to the hepatocyte, but its clinical usefulness is extended by considering it as all steps up to conjugation of bilirubin.

Bilirubin is formed from the breakdown of haemoglobin and, normally, is conjugated with glucuronic acid by hepatocytes when it reaches the liver. This makes it more soluble. Unconjugated bilirubin remains in the circulation only when the liver is unable to conjugate all the bilirubin that is delivered to it.

However, increased haemolysis, e.g. in haemolytic anaemias such as sickle-cell disease or haemolytic disease of the newborn, may cause an excess of bilirubin, and this can overcome the liver's capacity to conjugate it. Congenital hyperbilirubinaemias are another cause.

Therefore, haemolytic jaundice results in raised levels of unconjugated bilirubin. This is particularly dangerous in neonates, as the unconjugated bilirubin can cross the blood–brain barrier and cause brain damage (kernicterus).

Because unconjugated bilirubin is not soluble, it does not pass into the urine, so this type of jaundice is often called 'acholuric jaundice'. The urinary urobilinogen is elevated due to increased resorption from the gut, as the total bilirubin load is raised.

The congenital hyperbilirubinaemias are rare, and you do not need to know them in detail at this stage, with the possible exception of Gilbert's syndrome which is relatively more common.

Gilbert's syndrome

This congenital disorder is caused by patients having a reduced amount of the enzyme UDP-glucuronyl transferase (UGT-1), which conjugates bilirubin with glucuronic acid.

This affects between 2% and 7% of the population, and is not a serious disease. The reticulocyte (immature red blood cell) count is normal, and there is only a slight increase in serum bilirubin (unconjugated), often after prolonged starvation or intercurrent illness.

The syndrome is asymptomatic, although some patients complain of fatigue. Treatment is not usually required but carbohydrate loading can help.

Crigler–Najjar syndrome

This is an extremely rare disease due to more severe abnomalities in the translated gene sequence of UGT-1, resulting in total absence of enzyme (type I) or an abnormal but functional enzyme (type II); both types are autosomal recessive and have high serum levels of unconjugated bilirubin.

Type II patients have a decreased level of UDP-glucuronyl transferase and, therefore, they can survive into adulthood. This form is thought to be very similar to Gilbert's syndrome.

Type I patients lack the enzyme altogether, and do not survive, without a liver transplantation.

Hepatic jaundice

This type of jaundice describes mechanisms which occur within the hepatocyte, or more specifically, after the bilirubin conjugation stage. It therefore includes some rare congenital hyperbilirubinaemias and hepatocyte transport 'exporter protein' defects, as well as diseases resulting in hepatocellular damage and cholestasis (loss of bile flow).

Hepatocellular jaundice

Damage to the hepatocytes and the intrahepatic biliary tree leads to an increase in both unconjugated and conjugated serum levels of bilirubin. There is an increase in clotting time, serum alanine aminotransferase and serum aspartate aminotransferase because of the hepatocellular damage.

Clinically, features of a conjugated hyperbilirubinaemia predominate, as excretion, not conjugation is the rate-limiting step in the metabolism of bilirubin, hence this hepatocellular jaundice can be categorized as a form of cholestatic jaundice.

Viruses such as the hepatitis A, B, C and E, and Epstein–Barr viruses, can lead to hepatocellular jaundice, as can leptospirosis (Weil's disease), a bacterial infection spread by infected rat urine.

Autoimmune or drug-induced damage, as well as cirrhosis and tumours, can cause hepatocellular jaundice.

Wilson's disease, an autosomal recessive disorder of copper metabolism, leads to hepatitis and cirrhosis and can manifest as jaundice.

Dubin–Johnson syndrome

This is an autosomal recessive disorder in which the liver fails to excrete conjugated bilirubin (caused by a mutation in the canalicular multispecific organic anion transporter, CMOAT), resulting in jaundice.

Rotor syndrome

This is very similar to Dubin–Johnson syndrome, with a defect in intracellular binding proteins for bilirubin. There is no pigment deposit.

Posthepatic jaundice

Normally, conjugated bilirubin passes from the liver to the gallbladder where it is stored and then released into the duodenum following a fatty meal.

In the terminal ileum, intestinal flora convert it first to urobilinogen (some of which is reabsorbed and excreted in the urine) and then to stercobilinogen, which is excreted in the faeces (giving them their brown colour).

In posthepatic jaundice, the passage of conjugated bilirubin through the biliary tree is blocked, and it leaks into the circulation instead. It is soluble and excreted in the urine, making it dark. However, the faeces are deprived of their stercobilinogen and are pale. These are key symptoms in the history.

There is no problem with the synthesis of any of the bile products in posthepatic obstructive jaundice, only its release into the duodenum. Obstruction also results in cholestasis. Therefore, bile salts, along with conjugated bilirubin, escape into the circulation, and this causes itching (pruritus), another important symptom.

The types of jaundice can be correlated as follows: prehepatic jaundice is where bilirubin is unconjugated, posthepatic jaundice is where bilirubin is conjugated and hepatic jaundice gives a mixed picture.

Causes of posthepatic cholestatic jaundice include gallstones, biliary stricture, congenital biliary atresia (complete blockage from birth), carcinoma of the pancreas or bile ducts and pancreatitis.

One clinical question can be used to separate prehepatic jaundice from the other causes, i.e. whether the patient has pale stools and dark urine. This is a symptom of cholestatic rather than prehepatic jaundice – note that it does not imply obstruction, as obstruction is only one cause of cholestasis. One simple test can be used to identify posthepatic jaundice, i.e. an ultrasound scan.

The symptoms and causes of jaundice are summarized in Fig. 6.23.

Further investigations for jaundice

Investigations other than liver function tests, a full blood count, serum bilirubin levels, virology screening and urinanalysis that can be performed are:

- Ultrasound
- Liver biopsy
- Endoscopic ultrasound (EUS)
- Endoscopic retrograde cholangio-pancreatography (ERCP)
- Magnetic resonance cholangio-pancreatography (MRCP).

Clinical Note

Lack of bile salts and, therefore, a lack of fat absorption, causes the slow clotting time associated with jaundice. Vitamin K (a clotting factor) is a fat-soluble vitamin which requires fat for absorption from the gut. In jaundice: decreased fat absorption = low vitamin K concentrations = slow clotting.

Fig. 6.23 The classification of the different types of jaundice, showing the causes and symptoms or clinical signs. (AST = serum aspartate aminotransferase; ALT = serum alanine amino- transferase; EBV = Epstein–Barr virus; γ-GT = γ-glutamyl transferase; AP = alkaline phosphatase.)

Type of jaundice	Cause	Signs
Prehepatic	Haemolysis Ineffective erythropoiesis	Increased concentrations of unconjugated bilirubin (no bilirubin in the urine because it is insoluble)
Hepatic (congenital and hepatocellular)	• Gilbert's syndrome • Crigler–Najjar syndrome • Rotor syndrome • Dubin–Johnson syndrome • Viral infection, (e.g. Hep. A,B,C,E, and EBV) • Cirrhosis • Drugs • Autoimmune disease • Weil's disease • Wilson's disease	• Increased clotting time • Increased ALT and AST • Hepatocellular damage
Posthepatic (obstructive or cholestatic)	• Pancreatitis • Primary biliary cirrhosis • Gall stones • Drugs • Carcinoma (of head of pancreas or bile duct) • Lymphoma (with enlarged lymph nodes in the porta hepatis) • Biliary stricture • Congenital biliary atresia	• Dark urine (with bilirubin, not urobilinogen) • γ-GT and AP increase (canalicular enzymes raised due to damage to the biliary tree) • Pale stools • Itching

Hepatic failure

Despite its large capacity to regenerate after injury, the liver can sometimes fail due to severe acute liver injury, e.g. in viral hepatitis or drug toxicity, or chronic liver disease, e.g. cirrhosis. Liver failure can therefore be acute or chronic.

The liver has a large number of vital functions, and its failure to perform these can lead to systemic consequences, from neurological problems to decreased coagulation or renal failure.

Acute (fulminant) liver failure

Fulminant means developing suddenly (from the Latin for 'lightning') and fulminant liver failure is the development of hepatic encephalopathy within 2–3 weeks of the first symptoms of hepatic insufficiency. Paracetamol overdose and viral infections are the most common causes.

Clinical features are subtle initially, and are those of hepatic encephalopathy (see below). There is usually jaundice, unless the cause is Reye's syndrome (see later), and the liver is enlarged only in the initial stages, being impalpable after that.

The prognosis depends principally on the cause of liver failure and the health and age of the patient, as in many other diseases.

Clinical Note

In paracetamol overdose, the saturation of liver enzymes and depletion of glutathione lead to liver necrosis and damage to kidney tubules by toxic metabolites. Treatment is with N-acetylcysteine, which increases the formation of glutathione, or with methionine.

Paracetamol has a narrow therapeutic index, i.e. the difference between a beneficial and a toxic dose is small, hence paracetamol overdose is common. Symptoms of liver damage may not be apparent immediately, but when they do occur it is often too late, with fatal consequences.

Hepatic encephalopathy

This is a neurological disorder caused by metabolic failure of the hepatocytes and the shunting of blood around the liver (due to cirrhosis or after portocaval anastomosis).

It may occur in both chronic and acute liver failure, and results in the exposure of the brain to abnormal metabolites, causing oedema and astrocyte changes.

Normally the liver eliminates the toxic nitrogenous products of gut bacteria. In liver failure, their elimination is reduced and some of them act as false transmitters (mimicking the normal neurotransmitters of the central nervous system). This results in central nervous system disturbances.

Other factors may play a part in the pathology, including ammonia and electrolyte disturbances, hypotension, changes in vascular permeability and increased cerebral sensitivity due to the metabolic disturbances.

Symptoms include:

- Disturbances in consciousness (ranging from confusion to coma and death)
- Asterixis (a flapping tremor of outstretched hands)
- Fluctuating neurological signs (muscular rigidity and hyperreflexia).

There is no specific treatment, except to restrict protein intake (to reduce uraemia and endogenous protein breakdown), treat any infection, empty the bowels of nitrogen-containing material and correct the metabolic and coagulation disturbances. Flumazenil, a benzodiazepine receptor antagonist, can improve the encephalopathy in the short term.

Chronic liver failure

This refers to the situation in which the functional capacity of the liver is unable to maintain normal physiological conditions. 'Decompensated liver disease' is a synonymous term.

Clinical features are similar to those of cirrhosis (Fig. 6.20). However, it must be noted that cirrhosis and chronic liver failure are not the same; cirrhosis may cause chronic liver failure but not vice-versa. Infection and hepatic vascular disease may precipitate chronic liver failure, with cirrhosis being a possible step in the pathogenesis.

Management involves treating the underlying cause, treating the symptoms and maintaining normal nutritional status. Liver transplantation (see later) may be an option.

The prognosis is poor, with a 25% 5-year survival rate.

Clinical Note

Cirrhosis and chronic liver failure are very closely related because any condition which may lead to death of hepatocytes and thus predispose to chronic liver failure may also cause cirrhosis. Examples include viral hepatitis, vascular diseases such as the Budd–Chiari syndrome and metabolic diseases affecting the liver. The association with cirrhosis is also why the liver becomes impalpable over the course of the disease, as progressive hepatocyte death and fibrosis cause the liver to shrink.

Hepatorenal syndrome

This is the combination of renal failure in a previously normal kidney and severe liver disease. However, kidney function improves dramatically if the liver failure is reversed.

Renal failure is caused by a drop in renal blood flow and glomerular filtration rate, causing a fall in urine output and increased retention of sodium by the kidney. These mechanisms are brought about by upregulation of the renin–angiotensin–aldosterone system, norepinephrine and vasopressin. It may be fatal.

Treatment includes the use of dopamine to increase renal blood flow, and protein restriction.

Liver transplantation

Liver transplantation is increasingly used in the treatment of:

- Acute and chronic liver disease
- Alcoholic liver disease (provided the patient has given up drinking and is well motivated)
- Primary biliary cirrhosis, when serum bilirubin rises above 100 μmol/L
- Chronic hepatitis B and C when complications ensue
- Primary metabolic disease with end-stage liver disease, e.g. Wilson's disease and α_1-antitrypsin deficiency
- Other conditions, including sclerosing cholangitis or rarely hepatocellular carcinoma.

Clinical Note

For patients with acute liver failure, the King's College Hospital criteria for liver transplantation are:

Paracetamol liver failure

- Arterial pH < 7.3 24 hours after ingestion
Or all of the following:
- INR > 6.5
- Creatinine > 300
- Grade III or IV encephalopathy.

Non-paracetamol liver failure

- INR > 6.5
Or 3 out of 5 of the following:
- Drug-induced liver failure
- Age < 11 or > 40 years old
- 1 week between onset of jaundice and encephalopathy
- INR > 3.5
- Bilirubin > 300.

Absolute contraindications are active sepsis outside the hepatobiliary tree and metastatic malignancy. If the patient lacks psychological commitment, as might occur in alcoholic liver disease, then transplantation is not an option. Complications increase and recovery is impeded with advancing years over 70.

Most organs are taken from beating heart cadavers, but a relative may donate a single lobe to an infant.

The liver is less aggressively rejected than other organs but early (reversible), or late (irreversible) rejection may occur. Acute (cellular), or early rejection occurs within 5–10 days after the transplant. The patient develops pyrexia, general malaise, and abdominal tenderness due to hepatomegaly. This is caused by an inflammatory reaction.

Immunosuppressive therapy is given post-transplant and normally consists of a calcineurin inhibitor, steroids and azathioprine. If further immunosuppression is needed mycophenolate or sirolimus are often used.

Chronic (ductopenic) rejection occurs 6 weeks to 9 months after the transplant. This type of rejection cannot be reversed with immunosuppressive drugs and retransplantation is the only treatment. Graft-versus-host disease is very rare.

DISORDERS OF THE LIVER

As the liver, gallbladder and biliary tract are anatomically and functionally connected, diseases and disorders which affect one part of the hepatobiliary system may therefore have an impact on the other components. It is important to bear this in mind when thinking about the pathological processes that can occur in these organs.

Congenital abnormalities

Polycystic liver disease

In polycystic liver disease, the liver has numerous cysts, lined with flattened or cuboidal biliary epithelium and containing straw-coloured fluid. This is an autosomal dominant condition.

The number of cysts varies from just a few to several hundred, and the cysts themselves vary in diameter from 0.5 cm to 4.0 cm. They may cause discomfort or pain if the patient stoops, and rupture of a cyst may cause acute pain.

Asymptomatic cysts do not need treament; painful ones may require aspiration.

Polycystic liver disease may be associated with polycystic kidney disease, which may lead to renal failure, in which case the prognosis is worse.

Congenital hepatic fibrosis

This is an autosomal recessive disorder. The liver is divided into irregular islands by bands of collagenous tissue that enlarge the portal tracts and form septa. Abnormally shaped bile ducts are scattered throughout the fibrous tissue and the septal margins contain bile duct remnants.

It may present with complications of portal hypertension and, perhaps most importantly, with bleeding varices (a medical emergency).

Associated conditions include polycystic kidneys and medullary sponge kidneys. Diagnosis is by wedge biopsy which allows differentiation between fibrosis and cirrhosis.

Disorders of metabolism

Haemochromatosis and hyperlipidaemias are relatively the most common of these diseases; the others are rare.

Haemochromatosis

Primary haemochromatosis is an autosomal recessive disorder characterized by the absorption of too much iron, which then accumulates (as haemosiderin) in the liver, pancreas, heart, pituitary and joints.

A gene defect near the HLA region on chromosome 6, called the HFE gene, results in a loss of regulation of iron absorption from the small intestine even when the iron-binding protein, transferrin, is fully saturated. Iron stores may be many times greater than normal levels, rising from about 1 g to as much as 20 g.

Heterozygotes have only modest increases in absorption but generally they have normal iron stores. It can take decades for sufficient iron to accumulate to cause organ damage so that most cases present after the age of 40.

Symptoms are rare in women of child-bearing age as menstrual losses and pregnancy compensate for the excess iron absorption. The presenting complaint in men is often loss of libido and hypogonadism, secondary to dysfunction of the pituitary gland, but the commonest presentation now is an incidental finding of abnormal liver enzymes or raised ferritin level.

The clinical features include:

- Liver enlargement
- Fibrosis and cirrhosis
- Bronze discolouration of the skin
- Diabetes mellitus in two-thirds of cases (hence the alternative name, bronze diabetes)
- Cardiac arrythmias, cardiomyopathy and heart failure
- Arthritis in hands and knees.

Untreated, the condition may lead to liver failure and primary hepatocellular carcinoma. Early in the disease, iron is deposited in periportal hepatocytes (as haemosiderin) and then in Kupffer cells, bile duct epithelium and portal tract connective tissue. There is hepatocyte necrosis possibly due to free-radical generation, and cirrhosis occurs as the disease progresses.

Diagnosis is by blood tests (which characteristically show raised ferritin with transferrin saturation of 100%) and liver biopsy showing heavy deposits of iron (as haemosiderin) in hepatocytes.

Treatment is by phlebotomy (venesection) once or twice a week for a year or more until iron levels return to normal, and then three or four times a year.

Chelation therapy (a drug that complexes with a metal ion for its removal) can be used in patients who cannot have venesection due to cardiac disease or anaemia. Desferrioxamine can be given continuously subcutaneously, or as and when required.

Secondary haemochromatosis (haemosiderosis) may result from iron overload, e.g. in thalassaemia patients after repeated blood transfusions or from excess iron absorption, e.g. in congenital haemolytic anaemias.

Hyperlipidaemias

Hyperlipidaemias are a group of metabolic disorders characterized by high levels of lipids (chiefly cholesterol, triglycerides and lipoproteins) in the blood. Several types of hyperlipidaemia have been described, depending on levels of which lipid are raised. Disorders resulting in hyperlipidaemia can stem from:

- Abnormal expression of genes encoding apoproteins
- Lipoprotein lipase deficiency
- Low-density lipoprotein (LDL)-receptor defects.

Hyperlipidaemia is closely associated with atheroma and cardiovascular disease, particularly in the Western world, where diets contain too much fat.

Treatment includes the use of bile acid binding resins such as cholestyramine and colestipol. These prevent the reuptake of bile acids from the terminal ileum and result in a greater de novo synthesis by the liver, using up cholesterol and lowering its circulating levels.

HMG-CoA reductase inhibitors or 'statins', e.g. simvastatin, inhibit the rate-limiting step in cholesterol synthesis and can reduce LDL cholesterol by up to 40%.

Other treatments include fibrates, nicotinic acid and omega-3 marine triglycerides, which limit hepatic triglyceride synthesis, reduce free fatty acid concentrations, and reduce hepatic very low density lipoprotein (VLDL) secretion respectively.

Wilson's disease

Wilson's disease (hepatolenticular degeneration) is a rare, autosomal recessive disorder in which copper accumulates in the liver and the basal ganglia of the brain. The cause is a mutation in a copper transport ATPase gene located on chromosome 13.

Normally copper is secreted into bile, but in Wilson's disease biliary copper excretion is low. In the liver, a chronic hepatitis results, leading to cirrhosis.

Signs and symptoms may appear in patients at any age from about 5 years to 15 years (very occasionally older), and they include hepatic and neurological abnormalities. Faint, brown (Kayser–Fleischer) rings may appear in the eye at the junction of the cornea and sclera in Descemet's membrane. They are diagnostic but usually require slit-lamp examination. Psychiatric symptoms may be seen as a result of copper deposition in the brain.

Diagnosis is by measurement of the copper-binding protein caeruloplasmin in the blood. This is low in Wilson's disease because the non-functioning copper transport protein does not allow copper to stimulate its production. Special staining of liver biopsy tissue will show an excess of copper. Twenty-four-hour urinary copper concentrations are normally raised in Wilson's disease.

Treatment is with penicillamine, a chelating agent that binds to copper and enables it to be excreted.

Prognosis depends on the stage at which treatment is begun. If started early, before significant amounts of copper have been deposited, prognosis is good. Neurological damage may be irreversible, and in hepatic failure or cirrhosis, the only treatment is transplantation. Thus although rare, a high index of suspicion is necessary for Wilson's disease due to the serious consequences.

α_1-Antitrypsin deficiency

α_1-Antitrypsin is a serum protein that is produced in the liver and has anti-protease effects. It is part of the serine protease inhibitors (SERPIN) superfamily of enzymes. One in ten northern Europeans carry a deficiency gene, which is autosomal recessive in inheritance.

The protease inhibitor (Pi) gene controlling its production is located on chromosome 14 and a number of variants exist. The normal variant is M allele, and the most important abnormal one is the Z allele.

Symptoms include emphysema in about 75% of PiZZ homozygotes and liver cirrhosis in approximately 10%. Heterozygotes (e.g. PiSZ) have an increased risk of developing emphysema if they smoke.

In the livers of homozygotes, α_1-antitrypsin accumulates by polymerization in hepatocytes, shown by PAS (periodic acid–Schiff)-positive intracellular globules on liver biopsy. There is a chronic inflammatory picture leading to cirrhosis, but the exact mechanisms causing the cirrhosis are unknown.

Diagnosis is by measurement of serum α_1-antitrypsin and by liver biopsy.

Treatment is symptomatic, and patients should be advised to stop smoking.

Reye's syndrome

Reye's syndrome is a rare disorder affecting children up to 15 years of age. It is characterized by acute encephalopathy and infiltration of fatty microvesicles in the liver (steatosis), and typically occurs during recovery from upper respiratory tract infections, influenza or chickenpox.

The encephalopathy and hepatic microvesicular steatosis are caused by inhibition of β-oxidation and the uncoupling of oxidative phosphorylation in mitochondria.

There is rapid progression to hepatic failure with neurological deterioration and eventual coma.

Treatment is supportive, with corticosteroids and mannitol (to reduce brain swelling) and dialysis or transfusion to correct chemical imbalances resulting from liver damage. Prognosis is poor, with an overall mortality of about 50%, mainly due to cerebral oedema.

Glycogen storage diseases

There are many different types of glycogen storage diseases, each caused by a different enzyme defect. All of these diseases are autosomal recessive, except type IX B, which is X-linked.

Hepatocytes are involved in types I, II, III, IV, VI and VIII, with a different site for glycogen storage in each. Most patients present in childhood with hepatomegaly.

Patients with type I may develop hepatocellular adenoma. Type IV predisposes to cirrhosis and usually results in death by the age of 5 years. The heart and skeletal muscle can be involved, resulting in myopathies and possible cardiac failure.

Liver transplantation is a very successful treatment for glycogen storage diseases.

Lysosomal storage diseases

There are a number of lysosomal storage diseases, all of which have a specific enzyme defect. This results in the abnormal accumulation of the enzyme substrate in lysosomes.

Gaucher's disease (a deficiency of glucocerebrosidase) is the most common type of lysosomal storage disease. This leads to the abnormal storage of glucocerebroside (glycosylceramide) in reticuloendothelial cells (macrophages and monocytes) found in the liver, spleen and bone marrow.

Its incidence is high in Ashkenazi Jews, and it usually presents in childhood with splenomegaly, hepatomegaly, anaemia and elevated levels of serum aminotransferases.

Treatment includes splenectomy, bone marrow transplantation and replacement enzyme therapy (with alglucerase).

Fig. 6.24 Viral hepatitis. (HAV IgM = hepatitis A virus immunoglobulin M; HBsAg = hepatitis B virus surface antigen; HBeAg = hepatitis B virus e antigen; HBc IgM = hepatitis B virus core immunoglobulin M; anti-HCV = anti-hepatitis C virus; PCR = polymerase chain reaction; HDD Ag = hepatitis D virus antigen; HDV IgM = hepatitis virus immunoglobulin; HEV IgG = hepatitis E virus immunoglobulin G; HBIG = hepatitis B immunoglobulin; HNIG = human normal immunoglobulin.) (Data courtesy of Dr Tilzey, St Thomas's Hospital, London.)

Type	Virus	Spread	Incubation period	Carrier state/chronic infection	Diagnosis of acute infection	Specific prevention	Treatment
A	Hepatovirus	Faecal–oral	2–3 weeks	No	HAV IgM	Vaccine HNIG	N/a
B	Hepadnavirus	Contaminated blood and body fluids: • percutaneous • sexual • mother to baby	2–6 months	Yes Adults 5–10% Neonates 70–90%	HBsAg HBeAg HBcIgM	Vaccine, HBIG	α-interferon
C	Pestivirus-like	Contaminated blood and body fluids: • percutaneous • sexual • mother to baby	6–8 weeks	Yes Adults 60–90%	Anti-HCV PCR	N/a	α-interferon
D	Defective RNA virus coated with HBsAG	Contaminated blood and body fluids: • percutaneous • sexual Note: requires HBsAg for propagation and hepatotropism	N/a	Yes	HD Ag HDV IgM (up to 6 wks) HDV IgM (after 6 wks)	Prevent HBV	N/a
E	Calicivirus	Faecal–oral	2–9 weeks	No	HEV IgM	N/a	N/a

Infectious and inflammatory disease

Viral hepatitis

Viral hepatitis is a common cause of liver injury (Fig. 6.24). The most common causes by far are the hepatitis viruses (A, B, C and E). Rarer causes are cytomegalovirus (CMV), Epstein–Barr virus (EBV), hepatitis D and arboviruses, e.g. in yellow fever.

Acute viral hepatitis may be asymptomatic or symptomatic, with or without jaundice and itching. Symptoms are similar, regardless of the infecting virus and present as a non-specific influenza-like illness, or with symptoms of gastroenteritis. Liver function tests are abnormal, with raised serum transaminases indicative of hepatocyte damage. Occasionally, fulminant hepatic failure may occur.

Hepatitis A

This disease is caused by an RNA picornavirus which is found worldwide, especially where thereis poor sanitation and hygiene. It is spread by the faecal–oral route through contaminated food and water, e.g. eating contaminated shellfish or swimming in sewage-polluted water. It may cause outbreaks, and is very resistant to heat and disinfectants.

The incubation period is 2–4 weeks, and infection may be asymptomatic (as in most childhood infections) or cause fever, malaise or a gastroenteritis-like illness followed by jaundice for 1–3 weeks. Diagnosis is by virus-specific IgM. Neither carrier states nor chronic infections occur (Fig. 6.25), but virus is present in the stools of patients about 2 weeks before and up to about a week after jaundice is apparent. Treatment is supportive, and prophylactic vaccines are available.

Hepatitis B

Infection with hepatitis B virus (HBV) may lead to a chronic carrier state, liver cancer or cirrhosis. HBV is a DNA virus.

Transmission is through contaminated blood or blood products, body fluids, sexual contact and vertical

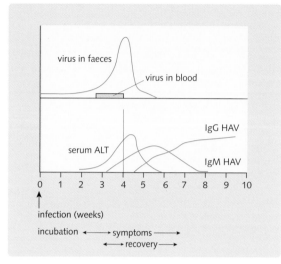

Fig. 6.25 The sequence of events in hepatitis A infection. (ALT = serum alanine aminotransferase; IgG HAV, IgM HAV = antibodies to hepatitis A virus – immunoglobulins G and M.)

transmission from mother to baby during parturition. It is also secreted in breast milk.

HBV is found worldwide, and is especially endemic in Southeast Asia, China and tropical Africa. Areas of low endemicity include Northern Europe, North America and Australia. Infection in these areas is associated with high-risk activities such as intravenous drug use, unprotected male homosexual contact, tattoo and acupuncture practices and the use of blood products by haemophiliacs. In the UK hepatitis B is a notifiable disease.

Incubation is 2–6 months and over 50% of cases are asymptomatic. Hepatitis B infection may lead to arthritis or arthralgia with a rash (caused by immune complexes).

Of infected adults, 90–95% recover completely and become immune, the remaining 5–10% become carriers (either asymptomatic carriers, or suffering from chronic hepatitis which may lead to cirrhosis). Treatment options in this patient group include alpha interferon injections or a number of nucleoside or nucleotide analogues such as entecavir or tenofovir.

About 1% develop fulminant acute hepatitis (a cause of acute liver failure – see above), which has a very high mortality rate. Infants infected perinatally have a worse prognosis: 70–90% become carriers. This may be due to their relatively underdeveloped immune systems.

Complications of chronic carriage include chronic active hepatitis, cirrhosis and hepatocellular carcinoma.

The intact HBV, also called the Dane particle, has a number of antigens. The viral coat contains surface antigen (HBsAg), while the core contains the core antigen (HBcAg) and the e antigen (HBeAg) as well as the viral DNA.

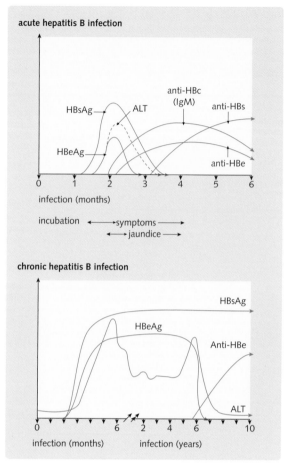

Fig. 6.26 Time-course of infective markers in acute and chronic hepatitis B infection. (ALT = serum alanine aminotransferase; HBc = hepatitis B core; HBs = hepatitis B surface.) (Redrawn with permission from Kumar P, Clarke M. Clinical Medicine, 3rd edn. London: Saunders, 1994.)

All carriers have HBsAg and anti-HBc. A carrier state is defined as one in which HBsAg persists for 6 months or longer (Fig. 6.26). Immune people (those who have recovered from the infection and those vaccinated against it) have anti-HBs and anti-HBc antibodies.

Previously, the e antigen (HBe) used to be a good determinant of infectivity: it is present in highly infectious carriers, carriers without e antigen are intermediately infective, and anti-e antibody means a person has low infectivity. However, HBe-negative but replication-competent mutants have been detected. This means that a patient infected with the mutant virus will, under the old standards, be classified as having low infectivity and a low risk of developing chronic liver disease when this is not the case. Infection with HBe-negative mutants should be suspected if HBV DNA is present in the blood but HBe antigen is negative.

Carriers are defined as people in whom hepatitis B surface antigen has been detected for more than 6 months.

All sexual and household contacts of the infected person with hepatitis B should be vaccinated, if possible. People who are in high-risk groups, and should receive the hepatitis B immunisation vaccine are:

- All healthcare workers
- Members of emergency and rescue teams
- Haemophiliacs
- Homosexual and bisexual men and prostitutes
- Long-term travellers
- Children in high-risk areas
- Morticians/embalmers.

Hepatitis C

Hepatitis C virus (HCV) has been a major cause of post-transfusional hepatitis. It is an RNA flavirus.

HCV may be transmitted parenterally, from mother to baby or through sexual contact, but because blood viral titres are much lower, these routes of transmission are uncommon (unlike hepatitis B). It has a low incidence rate at sexually transmitted disease clinics, suggesting that transmission via sexual contact is uncommon.

HCV shows much genetic diversity, with six genotypes and more than 100 subtypes. However, all are equally pathogenic. It is found worldwide, particularly in Japan, parts of South America, the Mediterranean, Africa and the Middle East.

The UK, Northern Europe and North America are areas of low seroprevalence (< 1% population), and most infection is associated with high-risk activity (mostly intravenous drug use).

The incubation period is 6–8 weeks and infection is asymptomatic in about 90% of cases. However, unlike hepatitis B, only 15% of patients recover fully, with 60–90% of people becoming chronic carriers with a risk of developing chronic active hepatitis, cirrhosis or hepatocellular carcinoma. First-line treatment is pegylated interferon and ribavirin for 24 weeks. Less than 1% will develop fulminant acute hepatitis.

Hepatitis D

Hepatitis D virus (HDV) is a defective RNA virus that can cause infection and replicate only in conjunction with hepatitis B.

It has a worldwide distribution, and is particularly prevalent in the Middle East, parts of Africa and South America.

Infection in Northern Europe is mainly confined to high-risk behaviour (intravenous drug abuse and multiple blood transfusions). Transmission is mainly parenteral. Hepatitis D may infect at the same time as hepatitis B or infect someone already chronically infected with hepatitis B (superinfection).

Infection with HDV rarely resolves and most patients will develop cirrhosis, some within the span of a few years.

Hepatitis E

This is especially common in Asia, Africa and the Middle East, but is seen in some rural parts of the UK particularly associated with pig farming.

It is spread by the faecal–oral route. The incubation period is 2–9 weeks (usually 6 weeks). Clinically, the infection is mild but jaundice is apparent.

High-risk age groups include those aged 15–40 years, and it has a 15–20% mortality rate in pregnant women as it may cause fulminant acute hepatitis in this group. It does not lead to chronic infection.

Liver abscess and non-viral liver infections

Liver abscesses are more common in developing parts of the world.

In the past, they were relatively common complications of appendicitis or perforation of the gastrointestinal tract, but improved management of these conditions has seen a decrease in the formation of abscesses.

They usually result from bacterial infection spread through the biliary tree (ascending cholangitis), carried from the gut in the portal system, from a penetrating injury to the liver, direct extension from a perinephric or other abscess, or infection carried in branches of the hepatic artery.

Amoebic abscesses must be considered in travellers, as *Entamoeba histolytica* causes abscesses as well as amoebic dysentery. Characteristically, the abscesses are filled with necrotic material which looks like anchovy paste.

Symptoms vary from general malaise to febrile jaundice with right upper quadrant pain and tender hepatomegaly.

Diagnosis is by ultrasonography, chest radiography, serological tests and analysis of the aspirated contents of the abscess.

Treatment of large abscesses is by radiologically controlled drainage and the administration of antibiotics. Complications include rupture and septicaemia.

Apart from viral hepatitis and bacterial infections, parasitic infections of the liver also occur, especially in the developing world. The two most important parasitic infections are those caused by helminths (worms) and protozoa.

Malaria (caused by the protozoon *Plasmodium* spp.) and visceral leishmaniasis (caused by *Leishmania donovani*) result in hepatomegaly apart from their other systemic symptoms.

Helminths which infect the liver include *Schistosoma* spp. and *Echinococcus granulosus*, apart from liver flukes. The first causes portal tract fibrosis leading to portal hypertension, while the second is the cause of hydatid cysts containing developing worms.

Clinical Note

Abscesses are collections of pus, caused by an inflammatory reaction, often as a result of bacterial infection. In general, 'if there is pus about, let it out'! Treatment of abscesses in accessible parts of the body is usually by surgical drainage or aspiration.

Autoimmune hepatitis

This form of chronic hepatitis affects predominantly young and middle-aged women, and is associated with the HLA alleles HLA-B8, HLA-DR3 and HLA-DR4. It is also associated with other autoimmune diseases, such as pernicious anaemia and thyroiditis.

The patient may be asymptomatic, or present with symptoms associated with autoimmune disease such as fatigue, fever and arthritis. 25% of patients present with acute hepatitis displaying jaundice. On examination, the patient may have hepatosplenomegaly, bruises, cutaneous striae, acne, hirsutism and possibly ascites. Extrahepatic manifestations may be present, such as glomerulonephritis, fever or pleurisy.

The liver biochemistry shows elevated serum aminotransferases, alkaline phosphatases and bilirubin (to a lesser degree). Serum α-globulins are usually twice the normal titre.

There are two types of autoimmune hepatitis, classified by the autoantibodies detected:

- Type I has antinuclear and anti-smooth muscle autoantibodies
- Type II has anti-liver-kidney-microsomal (LKM) autoantibodies and anti-liver cytosolic autoantibodies.

Type I autoimmune hepatitis affects women, whereas type II mainly affects girls aged 5–20 years, and is generally less common.

Treatment for autoimmune hepatitis involves steroids (prednisolone) and immunosuppressants (azathioprine). The therapy is given indefinitely, and can bring remission to 90% of the cases. Liver transplantation is also an option if drug therapy fails.

Primary biliary cirrhosis (see below) is another form of autoimmune liver disease.

Diseases of the biliary tract associated with cirrhosis

Primary biliary cirrhosis

Primary biliary cirrhosis (PBC) is an autoimmune disorder and thus affects women, especially those 40–50 years of age, more than men. It can occur in conjunction with other autoimmune diseases, e.g. Sjögren's syndrome, rheumatoid arthritis and scleroderma.

The epithelium of the bile ducts (especially that of the smaller intrahepatic ducts) is destroyed by an autoimmune reaction and the damaged areas become surrounded by lymphocytes. The surrounding hepatocytes undergo necrosis, in a pattern resembling piecemeal necrosis. Granulomas may also be present.

All patients with PBC have anti-mitochondrial autoantibodies and this, together with raised serum alkaline phosphatase, is diagnostic for the condition. The presence of antimitochondrial antibodies implies a connection with autoimmunity, although the exact pathogenetic mechanisms are unknown.

An attempt at regeneration then takes place in the form of proliferation of small bile ductules at the edges of the portal tracts, with consequent fibrosis disrupting the normal architecture of the liver.

Eventually, diffuse and irreversible cirrhosis occurs which may be complicated by liver failure, portal hypertension and, rarely, hepatocellular carcinoma.

Clinically, the patient will have pruritus, jaundice and xanthelasma (deposits of cholesterol-laden macrophages around the eyes, easily visible macroscopically).

The course and prognosis of the disease is slow (about 10 years) but variable and there is no effective medical treatment although ursodeoxycholate (a bile acid substitute) is of benefit in some patients, improving liver function and survival.

Treatment is mainly symptomatic, such as cholestyramine for pruritus. Cholestasis results in malabsorption of the fat-soluble vitamins, therefore supplements are given. Treatment of PBC is difficult and often ineffective, so liver transplantation should be considered when the bilirubin levels rise above 100 μmol/L.

Secondary biliary cirrhosis

Secondary biliary cirrhosis is caused by prolonged obstruction of extrahepatic bile ducts, often as a result of gallstones, biliary atresia, strictures caused by previous surgery or carcinoma of the head of the pancreas.

Bile remains in the obstructed ducts and inflammation and periportal fibrosis may result, eventually leading to cirrhosis.

Bile duct proliferation may occur and secondary bacterial infection (ascending cholangitis) may complicate biliary strictures and gallstones.

Diagnosis is by ultrasonography, endoscopic retrograde cholangiopancreatography (ERCP) or percutaneous transhepatic cholangiography.

Primary sclerosing cholangitis

Primary sclerosing cholangitis (PSC) is a chronic inflammatory disease often associated with inflammatory bowel disease. Seventy per cent of cases occur in association with ulcerative colitis.

Male patients outnumber females by 2:1, and they usually present at around 39 years of age.

Intrahepatic, and sometimes extrahepatic, bile ducts become surrounded by a mantle of chronic inflammatory cells.

Eventually onion skin fibrosis occurs (concentric fibrosis around the ducts). The ducts are seen on ERCP as having a 'beaded' appearance. Small ducts near the portal tracts may be totally replaced by fibrous tissue ('vanishing bile ducts').

Patients vary from being asymptomatic to suffering from chronic liver disease, with pruritus, jaundice, fatigue and eventually portal hypertension.

Elevated serum alkaline phosphatase and myeloperoxidase ANCA antibodies in 80% of cases suggest a diagnosis of PSC. However, liver biopsy is the best diagnostic tool. Patients with PSC have a higher risk of developing cholangiocarcinoma. Medical management is based around symptom relief, with liver transplant being the only life-prolonging treatment.

Alcohol, drug and toxin associated disease

Alcoholic liver disease

Alcohol produces a range of liver diseases, from fatty liver (steatosis) to cirrhosis. The pathogenesis of alcoholic liver disease is summarized in Fig. 6.27.

Hepatic steatosis (fatty liver)

Fatty liver is seen in a number of disorders, including alcoholic liver disease and obesity with or without diabetes mellitus.

Normally, lipids from the diet or released from adipose tissue are transported to the liver where they are metabolized.

Alcohol is toxic, and when it is drunk in excess its metabolism becomes a priority (Fig. 6.28). Cellular energy is diverted towards this and away from other essential metabolic pathways, including the metabolism of fat in the liver.

Fat then accumulates in the cytoplasm of liver cells, particularly in zone 3, the area adjacent to the central vein and furthest from the arterial supply.

In chronic ingestion of alcohol, the liver becomes a large greasy organ weighing as much as 5–6 kg.

If alcohol abuse continues, fibrosis and cirrhosis may occur but fatty change is reversible if alcohol intake is stopped.

Alcoholic hepatitis

This is inflammation of the liver caused by alcohol ingestion.

Alcohol is directly cytotoxic at high concentrations and cells swell with granular cytoplasm. Intracytoplasmic aggregates of intermediate filaments (Mallory bodies) appear in the hepatocytes. There is aggregation of neutrophils around damaged liver cells (especially

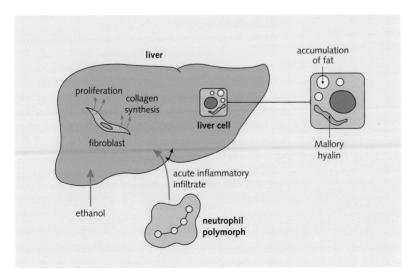

Fig. 6.27 Pathogenesis of alcoholic liver disease.

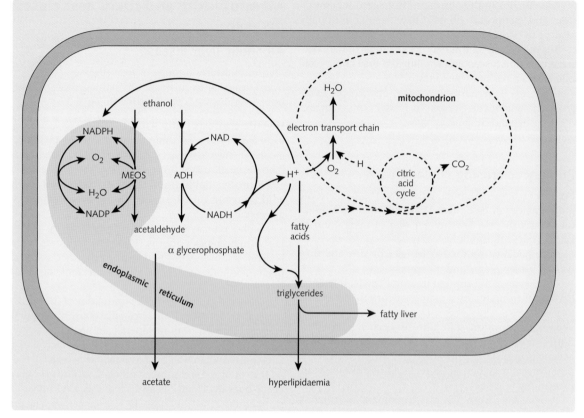

Fig. 6.28 The metabolism of alcohol in hepatocytes. (ADH = alcohol dehydrogenase; MEOS = microsomal ethanol oxidizing system.) (From MacSween RNM, Whaley K. Muir's Textbook of Pathology, 13th edn. London: Edward Arnold, 1992. Reproduced by permission of Hodder/Arnold Publishers.)

those with Mallory bodies), and lymphocytes and macrophages enter the lobule.

Focal necrosis is found in zone 3 (centrilobular zone) aided by damage caused by free radicals. These are produced by phagocytes in response to cytokines, and they are also generated by lipid peroxidation. Ballooning of hepatocytes can occur, due to the retention of proteins and water after injury to organelles.

Collagen deposition almost always ensues, especially with repeated bouts of high alcohol intake, and the risk of cirrhosis is greater than in purely fatty change.

Mallory bodies may also be seen in other conditions including primary biliary cirrhosis, Wilson's disease and hepatocellular carcinoma.

Patients with alcoholic hepatitis have elevated serum levels of alkaline phosphatase, alanine aminotransferase, aspartate aminotransferase, γ-glutamyl transpeptidase, bilirubin and an increased prothrombin time. Often a low serum albumin accompanies these findings.

If the patient stops drinking, the inflammation will resolve of its own accord.

Alcoholic cirrhosis

Cirrhosis is the final and irreversible result of alcohol damage.

It usually develops over a number of years, but it may become apparent in as little as 2–3 years if associated with alcoholic hepatitis.

The underlying pathological mechanisms causing alcoholic cirrhosis are similar to those of cirrhosis due to other causes. The hepatocytes attempt to regenerate but the normal architecture is disturbed and nodules form, separated by fibrous septa. This disrupts the normal blood flow through the liver, and it becomes less efficient at performing its functions. In the early stages, the liver is usually large and fatty but later it shrinks to become small, brown and almost non-fatty.

Remember the major complications of cirrhosis: liver failure, portal hypertension and hepatocellular carcinoma.

Non-alcoholic fatty liver disease

Non-alcoholic fatty liver disease (NAFLD) represents a wide spectrum of liver disease which occurs in individuals who do not consume excess levels of alcohol. This ranges from simple fatty liver (steatosis), to non-alcoholic steatohepatitis (NASH), to irreversible cirrhosis. These are rapidly becoming major contributors to liver disease in the developed world as they are associated with insulin resistance and metabolic syndrome. Risk factors include obesity, diabetes and hyperlipidaemia.

Many patients are asymptomatic, or present with fatigue and malaise. Jaundice is rare. Diagnosis can be difficult and is normally confirmed by raised liver function tests, especially transaminases, for which no other cause can be found; alongside an ultrasound or CT scan which confirms fatty liver. Treatment is usually focused around lifestyle changes such as weight loss and eating a balanced diet, as well as optimizing diabetic control.

Non-alcoholic steatohepatitis

Only a small proportion of patients with NAFLD will develop NASH. This is characterised by hepatic fat accumulation alongside inflammation of the liver, which can ultimately cause hepatic necrosis. Symptoms and investigations are the same as above, with a liver biopsy being the only way to establish a diagnosis of NASH. Treatment is based around exercise, diet and anti-glycaemic drugs. Antioxidants, such as vitamin E are also thought to be effective, and are currently the focus of clinical trials.

Drugs and toxins

The liver is vital in the metabolism and excretion of drugs and toxins. At least 10% of all adverse reactions to drugs affect the liver.

Drug reactions may be predictable (occur in any individual if a sufficient dose is given) or unpredictable (idiosyncratic, or non-dose-related). Predictable drug reactions are also known as intrinsic reactions.

Drugs may cause damage to hepatocytes indistinguishable from viral hepatitis, cholestasis by affecting bile production or excretion, or other liver dysfunction. The mechanisms of drug-induced damage include:

- Direct toxicity to cells
- The conversion of the drug to a toxic metabolite
- Drug-induced autoimmune reaction
- Peroxidation of lipids
- Denaturation of proteins
- Mitochondrial dysfunction
- Free radical generation
- ATP depletion
- Binding or blockage of transfer RNA (tRNA)
- Attachment to membrane receptors
- Disruption of calcium homeostasis
- Disruption of the cytoskeleton in hepatocytes.

Drug-induced autoimmunity usually occurs when the drug, or one of its metabolites, acts as a hapten (a small molecule that is not immunogenic on its own, but which can bind to another molecule and produce an immune response).

A careful drug history should be taken from anyone with signs or symptoms of liver disease, including drugs taken many months before, as there may be a long delay between the administration of the drug and signs of any injury becoming apparent. Injury may also be immediate, depending on the drug or toxin and the type of damage caused.

Diagnosis is made on the history and clinical signs, the fact that improvement should occur if the patient stops taking the offending drug, and by excluding other causes of liver damage.

A summary of hepatotoxins and their effects is given in Fig. 6.29.

Vascular disorders

Liver infarction

Liver infarction is rare because of the dual blood supply of the liver. It may occur if an intrahepatic branch of the hepatic artery is occluded, or the flow of blood through it is interrupted. This is seen in only five situations:

- Trauma to the artery
- Embolization or ligation of the artery, e.g. for therapeutic reasons
- Infective endocarditis
- Eclampsia (seizures during pregnancy)
- Polyarteritis nodosa.

If the main hepatic artery is occluded, blood flow through the portal venous systems is usually sufficient to prevent necrosis, except in the case of a transplanted liver when occlusion usually leads to complete necrosis (in which case another transplant is needed).

Portal vein obstruction and thrombosis

Portal vein obstruction may occur outside the liver (extrahepatic) or inside (intrahepatic). Extrahepatic obstruction is by thrombosis. Intrahepatic obstruction is most commonly caused by cirrhosis, but it can also be caused by congenital hepatic fibrosis and metastases, or primary carcinoma of the liver.

It may lead to portal hypertension (see earlier), with abdominal pain, ascites and oesophageal varices.

Hepatic vein thrombosis (Budd–Chiari syndrome)

Budd–Chiari syndrome is a rare condition in which occlusion (due to thrombosis) of the hepatic vein results in blockage of the flow of venous blood out of the liver.

Fig. 6.29 Hepatotoxins and their effects on the liver. (From Friedman LS, Keefe E. Handbook of Liver Disease. Edinburgh: Churchill Livingstone, 1997.)

Disorder	Hepatotoxic agents
Acute disorders	
Hepatitis-like syndromes (acute necroinflammatory liver disease)	Dapsone, isoniazid, indometacin, phenytoin
Fulminant hepatic failure	Paracetamol, halothane, isoniazid, methyldopa, nicotinic acid, nitrofurantoin, propylthiouracil, valproic acid
Cholestatic syndromes	Amitriptyline, ampicillin, carbamazepine, chlorpromazine, prochlorperazine, cimetidine, ranitidine, captopril, oestrogens, trimethoprim-sulfamethoxazole
Mixed necroinflammatory	Carbimazole, naproxen, phenytoin, thioridazine
Granulomatous hepatitis	Allopurinol, benzylpenicillin, dapsone, diazepam, diltiazem, phenytoin
Macrovesicular steatosis	Alcohol, glucocorticoids, methotrexate, minocycline, nifedipine, total parenteral nutrition
Microvesicular steatosis	Alcohol, amiodarone, aspirin, zidovudine (AZT), piroxicam, sodium valproate, tetracyclines
Budd–Chiari syndrome	Oral oestrogens
Ischaemic necrosis	Cocaine, methylenedioxymethamfetamine
Chronic disorders	
Chronic active hepatitis	Alpha-methyldopa, isoniazid, nitrofurantoin
Fibrosis/cirrhosis	Alcohol, alpha-methyldopa, isoniazid, methotrexate
Peliosis hepatis	Anabolic/androgenic steroids, azathioprine, hydroxyurea, oral contraceptives, tamoxifen
Phospholipidosis	Amiodarone, diltiazem, nifedipine
Primary biliary cirrhosis	Chlorpromazine, haloperidol, prochlorperazine
Sclerosing cholangitis	Floxuridine FUDR via hepatic artery infusion
Steatohepatitis	Amiodarone, total parenteral nutrition
Veno-occlusive disease	Azathioprine, busulfan, cyclophosphamide, daunorubicin, tioguanine, X-irradiation
Oncogenic effects	
Cholangiocarcinoma	Thorotrast
Focal nodular hyperplasia	Oestrogens, oral contraceptives
Hepatic adenoma	Oestrogens, oral contraceptives
Hepatoma	Alcohol, anabolic/androgenic steroids
Hepatoblastoma	Oestrogens
Angiosarcoma	Arsenic, vinyl chloride, Thorotrast

It may be acute or chronic. Acute presentation is usually with sudden onset of abdominal tenderness, epigastric pain, nausea (and vomiting) and shock.

Chronic thrombosis results in hepatomegaly, portal hypertension (and its associated signs and symptoms), jaundice and cirrhosis. Ascites can be found in both acute and chronic forms of the disease.

It may be caused by any condition that predisposes to the formation of thrombi, most notably:

- Polycythaemia
- Pregnancy
- Postpartum states
- Oral contraceptive
- Hepatocellular carcinoma
- Other intra-abdominal cancers.

Surgical treatment, with the creation of a portosystemic anastomosis is required. However, liver transplantation is often the treatment of choice. Mortality is higher in acute cases, with untreated cases resulting in death, but even in its chronic form, 5-year survival is only about 50%.

Veno-occlusive disease

Veno-occlusive disease is similar to Budd–Chiari syndrome in its presentation. It is believed to be caused where damage to the endothelium of the sinusoids allows red blood cells into the space of Disse, which activates the coagulation cascade. The products of coagulation are then swept into the central vein, occluding it.

The incidence is higher in those receiving marrow transplants (25% in allogenic recipients), probably because chemotherapy and radiotherapy, given as part of transplant therapy, damage the endothelium.

Treatment of this disease is aimed at controlling hepatocellular failure and ascites formation.

Neoplastic disease

Hepatocellular carcinoma

Hepatocellular carcinoma (HCC) can develop following hepatitis B and C infections, alcoholic cirrhosis and haemochromatosis. Aflatoxin (a fungal metabolite), androgens and the contraceptive pill are all associated with HCC.

It affects men more than women, and usually presents before 50 years of age. The signs and symptoms include:

- Fever
- Pain in the right hypochondrium
- Hepatomegaly
- Weight loss
- Anorexia
- Ascites.

Diagnosis is made by blood tests and imaging. Liver function tests may be elevated, and alpha-fetoprotein is usually raised in >50% of cases. Ultrasound and CT scan are usually the first line to image tumours.

Treatment usually involves radiological ablation or sometimes surgical resection or liver transplantation. The prognosis is not good. Survival is usually less than 6 months, but up to 30% of cases can be cured if discovered early enough.

The pancreas and biliary tract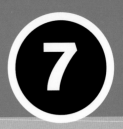

Objectives

After reading this chapter, you should be able to:
- Describe the anatomy of the pancreas, with regard to its macroscopic structure, relations, arterial supply, venous and lymphatic drainage, and nerve supply
- Outline the embryological development of the pancreas
- Outline the histological structure of the pancreas
- Describe the control of pancreatic secretion and the function of the enzymes released
- Outline the following pancreatic disorders: pancreatitis, pseudocysts, pancreatic insufficiency, carcinoma and congenital abnormalities
- Describe the anatomy of the gallbladder and biliary tract, with regard to its structure, relations, arterial supply, venous and lymphatic drainage, and nerve supply
- Outline the functions and physiology of the biliary system
- Outline the following disorders of the biliary system: gallstones, primary and secondary biliary cirrhosis, primary sclerosing cholangitis, malignant neoplasms and congenital abnormalities

THE PANCREAS

The pancreas is both an endocrine and an exocrine gland.

Most of the pancreas consists of exocrine tissue, in which are embedded islands of endocrine cells (islets of Langerhans). The exocrine cells produce enzymes that play an important role in digestion. The hormones produced by the islets are essential for the regulation of blood glucose.

Anatomy

The pancreas is a soft, elongated digestive gland which is grey–pink and 'feather-like' in appearance. It is approximately 15 cm in length, lobular and weighs about 80 g.

It is retroperitoneal and extends transversely across the posterior abdominal wall from the curve of the duodenum to the hilum of the spleen.

The right side lies across the vertebral bodies of L1–L3. It is posterior to the stomach and the transverse mesocolon is attached to its anterior margin. It is located in the left hypochondriac and epigastric regions.

The pancreas has four parts: a head with an uncinate process (from the Latin meaning 'hook'), a neck, a body and a tail (Fig. 7.1):

- The *head* is the expanded right portion. It nestles in the curve of the duodenum, anterior to the inferior vena cava and the left renal vein. In a groove on the posterior surface of the head lies the common bile duct

- The *uncinate process* is a small portion of the head extending superiorly and to the left, 'hooked' around the superior mesenteric vessels
- The *neck* joins the body to the head, overlying the superior mesenteric vessels and the portal vein. The anterior surface of the neck is covered with peritoneum and is adjacent to the pylorus
- The *body* is triangular in cross-section and extends as far as the hilum of the left kidney. It overlies the aorta, the left renal vein, the splenic vessels and the termination of the inferior mesenteric vein. It is crossed anteriorly by the attachment of the transverse mesocolon. Note that where the body crosses the aorta, superior mesenteric artery, left adrenal gland and left kidney, its posterior surface is not covered by peritoneum
- The *tail* lies in the lienorenal ligament and ends at the hilum of the spleen.

The main pancreatic duct traverses the gland from left to right, i.e. from the tail to the head and together with the bile duct, opens into the second part of the duodenum at the hepatopancreatic ampulla (of Vater). This opens into the duodenum at the major duodenal papilla.

There are two important sphincters in this region: the pancreatic duct sphincter at the termination of the pancreatic duct, and the hepatopancreatic sphincter (of Oddi) at the ampulla of Vater. They control the flow of pancreatic juice (as well as bile, in the case of the latter) into the duodenum.

Fig. 7.1 The relations of the pancreas.

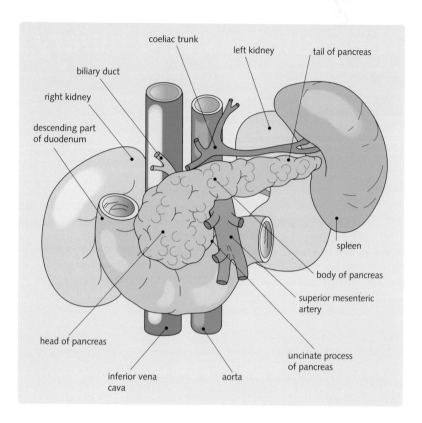

An accessory duct, if present, may drain the inferior part of the head as well as the uncinate process. It has a separate opening into the duodenum at the minor duodenal papilla above the ampulla of Vater.

Blood supply and venous drainage

Because the pancreas has an endocrine function, it has a rich blood supply.

The arteries supplying the pancreas arise from the splenic and pancreaticoduodenal arteries. The anterior and posterior superior and inferior pancreaticoduodenal arteries supply the head, while up to 10 branches of the splenic artery supply the remainder of the pancreas (Fig. 7.2).

Venous drainage is to the portal, splenic and superior mesenteric veins, with most going into the splenic vein.

Lymphatic drainage and innervation

The course of lymphatic vessels draining the pancreas follows that of the blood vessels. Lymphatic drainage is to pancreaticosplenic or suprapancreatic nodes alongside the splenic artery and to preaortic nodes around the coeliac and superior mesenteric arteries. Some vessels also terminate in nodes near the gastric pylorus.

The innervation of the pancreas is from the splanchnic nerves and the vagi through the coeliac and superior mesenteric plexuses.

Embryology and development

The pancreas develops between the mesenteric layers from two buds (the dorsal and ventral pancreatic buds) that originate from the endodermal lining of the caudal foregut (which goes on to form the proximal duodenum) in weeks 4–6 (Fig. 7.3). Most of the pancreas is formed from the dorsal bud, which is larger and appears before the ventral bud.

As the duodenum rotates to form a C-shape, the ventral pancreatic bud, which originates near the ampulla of Vater, migrates 270° around the back of the duodenum to lie below and behind the dorsal pancreatic bud, trapping the mesenteric vessels between them. This allows fusion of the ventral and dorsal pancreatic buds. Ultimately, part of the head as well as the uncinate process is derived from the ventral bud.

The distal part of the dorsal pancreatic duct normally joins with the duct of the ventral pancreatic

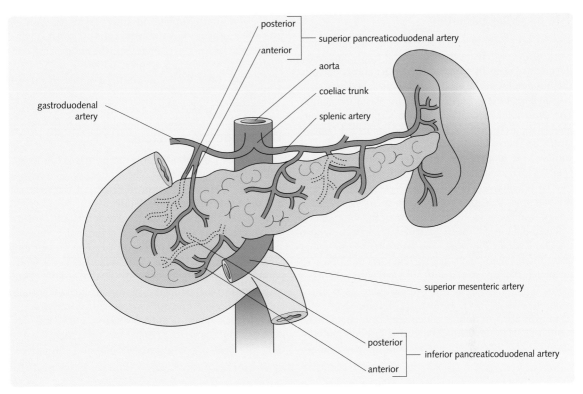

Fig. 7.2 The arterial supply of the pancreas.

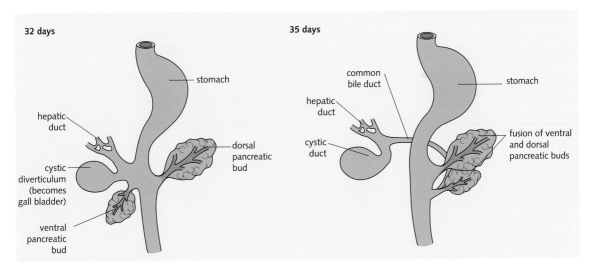

Fig. 7.3 The development of the pancreas.

bud, to become the main pancreatic duct. The proximal part of the dorsal pancreatic duct either regresses and disappears, or becomes an accessory pancreatic duct (of Santorini). The pancreatic islets of Langerhans develop from pancreatic parenchymal tissue in the 3rd month, and are scattered throughout the gland.

Insulin secretion begins during the 5th month of embryonic development and fetal levels of insulin are independent of those of the mother. Note that insulin does not cross the placenta.

Histology

The pancreas is covered with a thin capsule of fibrocollagenous connective tissue, from which septa extend into the gland, dividing it into lobules. Nerves and larger blood vessels travel within the septa.

The exocrine pancreas

The exocrine cells secrete digestive enzymes into a network of ducts that meet to form the main pancreatic duct, which joins the common bile duct and opens into the duodenum at the ampulla of Vater (see Fig. 4.2).

The basic unit of the exocrine pancreas is the acinus. The acini are tubuloacinar glands similar to salivary glands in their organization. They are called 'acinar' (Latin for 'berry-like') because the secretory portion is similar to a grape, with the duct resembling a stalk (Fig. 7.4). The acini consist principally of pyramidal epithelial cells, which produce the digestive enzymes of the pancreas. The apices of the cells surround a central lumen, which marks the termination of the duct system.

From the lumen, the intercalated ducts begin within the acini where the duct cells are called centroacinar cells. Intercalated ducts are the smallest members of the pancreatic duct system and are lined with squamous epithelium. They drain into intralobular ducts lined with cuboidal or low columnar epithelium.

In turn, the intralobular ducts lead into larger interlobular ducts in the fibro-collagenous interlobular connective tissue. These are lined by columnar epithelium and also contain goblet and enteroendocrine (amine precursor uptake and decarboxylation, APUD) cells. As the size of the ducts increases, the supporting connective tissue becomes denser, with the wall of the main pancreatic duct containing a layer of smooth muscle.

The endocrine pancreas

The islets of Langerhans form the primary component of the endocrine pancreas. These clusters of endocrine cells (Fig. 7.5) can be found throughout the pancreas but are most prevalent in the tail.

Pancreatic islet cells can be differentiated from the exocrine cells as they are smaller and paler. There is an extensive network of blood vessels surrounding the islets – each islet has its own capillary network which is in contact with every cell in that islet – into which the hormones insulin, glucagon and somatostatin are secreted. Their functions are described in Fig. 7.6.

Other cell types include vasoactive intestinal polypeptide (VIP)-secreting cells and enterochromaffin cells, which secrete serotonin, motilin and substance P.

Fig. 7.4 A pancreatic acinus. The secretion of alkaline fluid and proenzymes is regulated separately, and pancreatic fluid rich in one or the other can be produced depending on the stimulus. Secretin initiates production of alkaline-rich fluid while cholecystokinin initiates production of an enzyme-rich fluid.

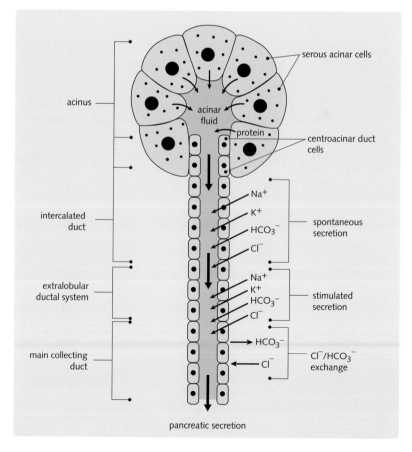

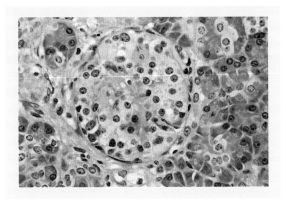

Fig. 7.5 High-power micrograph showing the α and β cells in the islets of Langerhans (in the endocrine pancreas). α cells produce glucagon and β cells produce insulin. Note that each cell is in contact with the capillary network. (Reproduced with permission from Stevens A, Lowe J. Human Histology, 2nd edn. Edinburgh: Mosby, 1997.)

Fig. 7.6 Functions of endocrine hormones.

Insulin	Produced by pancreatic β (or B) cells, which constitute 70% of pancreatic endocrine cells. It acts on all cells in the body to increase the uptake of glucose from the blood into the cells.
Glucagon	Produced by pancreatic α (or A) cells (20%) and it acts mainly on the liver. It increases glycogenolysis and gluconeogenesis to raise blood glucose concentration.
Somatostatin	Secreted from δ (or D) cells (5–10%). It acts locally as a paracrine agent, inhibiting the production of insulin and glucagon. It also inhibits the gut peptides secretin, cholecystokinin (CCK), gastrin and motilin.
Pancreatic polypeptide	Produced by PP or F cells (1–2%). It self-regulates the pancreas secretion activities, both exocrine and endocrine.

A more detailed account of the endocrine function of the pancreas can be found in *Crash Course: Endocrine and Reproductive Systems*.

Pancreatic exocrine functions and physiology

The pancreas secretes about 1.5 L of fluid a day (over ten times its own weight). This fluid contains cations, anions, albumin, globulin and digestive enzymes.

The bulk of the fluid is the sodium- and bicarbonate-rich juice secreted by cells of the small ducts, which neutralizes acid entering the duodenum from the stomach.

The acinar cells secrete a small volume of fluid rich in digestive enzymes, which break down carbohydrates, fats, proteins and nucleic acids.

Most of these enzymes are secreted in an inactive form to protect the pancreas from autodigestion, and are activated in the duodenum (see later).

Alkaline secretion

The pancreas secretes a fluid rich in bicarbonate, which, together with secretions from the gallbladder and the intestinal juices, neutralizes gastric acid in the duodenum, raising the pH to 6 or 7.

Secretion in the pancreas takes place in a similar way to that in the salivary glands. The acini secrete a slightly hypertonic fluid, rich in bicarbonate, which is modified as it travels through the ducts (Fig. 7.4). Chloride is actively exchanged for bicarbonate by the epithelial cells of the extralobular ducts as the fluid travels through the ducts (Fig. 7.7) and concentrations of bicarbonate and chloride are reciprocal.

When the pancreas is stimulated to increase its rate of secretion, there is less time for chloride and bicarbonate to be exchanged and the fluid is richer in bicarbonate. When the rate of secretion is low, the fluid is produced mainly by the intralobular ducts. However, when secretin stimulates an increased rate of production, most of the additional fluid is produced by the extralobular ducts.

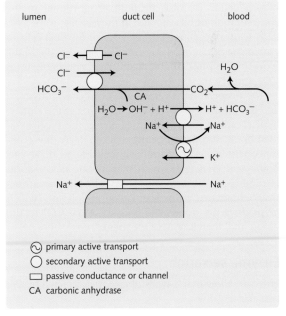

Fig. 7.7 The mechanism by which bicarbonate is taken up by the epithelial cells of the pancreas. (Redrawn with permission from Johnson LR. Physiology of the Gastrointestinal Tract, 4th edn. New York: Raven Press, 2000.)

Fig. 7.8 Pancreatic enzymes.

Enzyme	Activator	Substrate
Trypsin	Secreted as trypsinogen, activated by entero-peptidase (and by trypsin)	Proteins and polypeptides
Pancreatic lipase		Triglycerides
Pancreatic α-amylase	Activated by Cl⁻	Starch
Ribonuclease		RNA
Deoxyribonuclease		DNA
Elastase	Activated by trypsin	Elastin and some other proteins
Phospholipase A₂	Activated by trypsin	Phospholipids
Chymotrypsins	Secreted as chymotrypsinogen, activated by trypsin	Proteins and polypeptides
Carboxypeptidase A and B	Activated by trypsin	Proteins and polypeptides
Colipase	Activated by trypsin	Fat droplets

The bicarbonate in pancreatic juice is derived from the blood and its concentration in the juice and the rate of production of juice are both proportional to the concentration of bicarbonate in the blood.

$H+$ ions, which are pumped out of the duct cells in exchange for K^+ and Na^+, neutralize bicarbonate in the blood by forming carbonic acid. This dissociates to form CO_2 and H_2O.

The dissociation is catalysed by carbonic anhydrase and is a similar reaction to that occurring in the kidney.

The carbon dioxide diffuses across the basolateral membrane into the duct epithelial cell. Here, it is combined with water by carbonic anhydrase, to make carbonic acid (H_2CO_3), which then dissociates to form H^+ and HCO_3^- (bicarbonate) ions. The $H+$ ions are actively eliminated at the basolateral membrane (which helps drive the reaction to produce more CO_2 in the blood and, therefore, HCO_3^- ions).

Enzyme secretion

There are three major types of enzymes secreted by the pancreas:

- Proteolytic enzymes (trypsin, chymotrypsin and carboxypeptidase)
- Amylase
- Lipase.

Additionally, the pancreas also secretes ribonuclease and deoxyribonuclease. These are summarized in Fig. 7.8.

Proteolytic enzymes

The proteolytic enzymes play an important role in protein digestion. It follows that these enzymes are capable of damaging the tissues of the pancreas and so they are secreted as proenzymes, which are activated by substances in the duodenum.

Enterokinase (enteropeptidase) in the brush border of the duodenum secreted in response to cholecystokinin, converts trypsinogen to trypsin. Trypsinogen is therefore not activated until it reaches the duodenum where it is needed.

Trypsin then activates the other proteolytic proenzymes, including its own proenzyme trypsinogen, resulting in an autocatalytic chain reaction.

To protect the pancreas from the chain reaction and autodigestion (that would result from even a small amount of trypsin in the pancreas), the pancreas contains a trypsin inhibitor called the kazal inhibitor. This forms a complex with trypsin and prevents it acting.

Also, the maintenance of an acid pH in the zymogen granules prevents the proenzymes being exposed to their optimal pH. In acute pancreatitis, phospholipase A2 is activated by trypsin in the pancreatic duct. It then acts on lecithin (a normal constituent of bile) to form lysolecithin, which damages cell membranes and causes disruption of pancreatic tissue and necrosis of surrounding fat. Circulating levels of pancreatic α-amylase also increase in acute pancreatitis and measurement of levels in the blood is used as a diagnostic tool.

Amylase
Like salivary amylase, pancreatic amylase hydrolyses polysaccharides into disaccharides, and therefore is involved in carbohydrate digestion in the duodenum. It is secreted in its active form as it does not damage pancreatic tissue.

Lipase
This is the most important enzyme in terms of fat digestion. It hydrolyses triglycerides into glycerol and fatty acids, therefore in pancreatic insufficiency where enzyme secretion is deficient, fats cannot be digested and a malabsorption syndrome occurs (see section on 'Pancreatic insufficiency').

The fate of pancreatic enzymes in the duodenum
The digestive enzymes survive for differing periods of time once they enter the intestines.

Measurements have shown that around 75% of amylase and 20% of trypsin were present in the distal ileum, but only 1% of lipase secreted actually reached this part of the small intestines. Different mechanisms are thought to be involved, and the small intestine is thought to be permeable to several digestive enzymes.

It has been found that chymotrypsinogen and amylase are capable of crossing the basolateral membranes of pancreatic cells.

Some foods contain inhibitors of the digestive enzymes. For example, soybeans contain the Bowman–Birk inhibitor, which stops trypsin and chymotrypsin activities.

Control of pancreatic secretion

Pancreatic exocrine secretion is controlled by neuroendocrine signals, which are hormones and substances released from nerve terminals (Fig. 7.9).

Vagal (parasympathetic) stimulation enhances the rate of secretion of both enzyme and aqueous components of pancreatic juice.

Sympathetic stimulation inhibits secretion, probably by decreasing blood flow.

Secretin and *cholecystokinin* (released from the duodenal mucosa) stimulate secretion of the aqueous component of pancreatic fluid.

Separate control of the aqueous and enzymatic components explains the variation in composition of pancreatic juice.

The control of secretion can be split up into the *cephalic, gastric* and *intestinal (duodenal)* phases, like the control of gastric secretions.

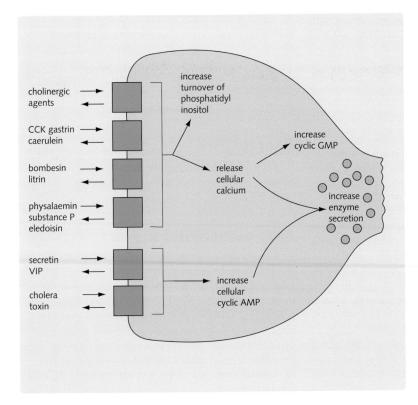

Fig. 7.9 Summary diagram of all the stimulating substances of pancreatic secretion. (CCK = cholecystokinin; VIP = vasoactive intestinal peptide; AMP = adenosine monophosphate; GMP = guanosine monophosphate.)

Cephalic phase

This is very minor in humans. Gastrin is released from the mucosa of the antrum in response to vagal stimulation (via acetylcholine and VIP). This causes the release of a small amount of pancreatic juice with a high protein content.

Gastric phase

Gastrin is released in response to gastric distension (via the vago-vagal reflex) and the presence of amino acids and peptides in the antrum. This continues to stimulate release of pancreatic juice.

Vago-vagal reflexes elicited by distension of the fundus or antrum also cause the release of small amounts of pancreatic juice with a high enzyme content (by acting on receptors on the acinar cells in the pancreas).

Intestinal phase

This is the longest and most important phase. It involves the secretion of two hormones, secretin and cholecystokinin. Chyme in the duodenum and upper jejunum stimulates pancreatic secretion.

Secretin is released from the duodenal and upper jejunal mucosal cells in response to acid in the lumen. Secretin acts on the pancreatic ducts to stimulate the secretion of a large volume of HCO_3^- rich fluid (but with low levels of pancreatic enzymes). It also stimulates bile production in the liver.

Cholecystokinin (CCK, also called pancreozymin) is secreted from duodenal and upper jejunal mucosal cells in response to peptides, amino acids and fatty acids in the lumen. It has two actions:

- It acts on pancreatic acinar cells to stimulate enzyme synthesis and release
- It acts on the gallbladder by stimulating its contraction and the relaxation of the sphincter of Oddi. This allows release of bile into the duodenum.

Therefore, CCK induces the secretion of a pancreatic juice that is rich in enzymes and which is accompanied by concentrated bile for fat absorption. The substances that stimulate pancreatic secretion are summarized in Fig. 7.9.

CCK has little direct effect on ductular epithelium but potentiates the effect of secretin, which is a weak agonist of acinar cells.

Vagal stimulation is important and vagotomy reduces the response to chyme in the duodenum by 50%.

Somatostatin has the opposite effect and by inhibiting adenylate cyclase and decreasing cyclic AMP, it inhibits the secretion of acinar and duct cells.

Insulin, insulin-like growth factors and epidermal growth factor potentiate enzyme synthesis and secretion, through the activation of receptor-associated tyrosine kinase.

DISORDERS OF THE EXOCRINE PANCREAS

Congenital abnormalities

Agenesis and hypoplasia

Congenital abnormalities of the pancreas are rare. However, as with other organs, the pancreas may fail to develop at all (agenesis) or develop incompletely (hypoplasia).

Annular pancreas and pancreas divisum

In normal development, the duodenum rotates and the ventral pancreatic bud migrates around the back of the duodenum to lie caudal and dorsal to the dorsal bud. This allows fusion of the ventral and dorsal pancreatic buds (Fig. 7.3).

Sometimes, migration of the ventral bud is incomplete, or it migrates in both directions, so that a ring of pancreatic tissue surrounds the duodenum. This is called an annular pancreas, and it may cause constriction or complete obstruction of the duodenum.

Pancreas divisum, either partial or complete, may occur where fusion of the two pancreatic buds does not take place. It is found in 5% of patients.

Ectopic pancreatic tissue

Heterotopic pancreatic tissue is sometimes found in the mucosa of the stomach, the duodenum and in Meckel's diverticula.

The pancreatic tissue is normal (although in an abnormal place), and so may produce substances normally made by the pancreas.

Pancreatitis

Pancreatitis (inflammation of the pancreas) is classified as acute or chronic, but it is sometimes difficult to separate the two.

Acute pancreatitis

Acute pancreatitis is relatively common, affecting 1% of the UK population. It can be severe and complicated with a mortality of 5–10% but mild and moderate forms present with variable degrees of pain. The Glasgow criteria (Fig. 7.10) are used to assess severity, although it is difficult to differentiate mild from severe pancreatitis in the first 24 hours. The presence of three or more items on either scoring system implies severe pancreatitis; if more than seven (out of 11) items are present, mortality approaches 100%.

Fig. 7.10 The Glasgow criteria for assessment of the severity of pancreatitis. Three or more signs indicate a severe presentation.

Age > 5 years
Blood glucose >10 mmol/L with no history of diabetes
White cell count > 15 x 10⁹/L
Lactate degydrogenase (LDH) > 600 iu/L
Aspartate transaminase (AST) > 200 u/L
Corrected calcium < 2.0 mmol/L
Blood urea > 16 mmol/L and no improvement with intravenous fluids
Arterial pO₂ < 8 kPa (60 mmHg)
Serum albumin < 32 g/L
Metabolic acidosis

Aetiology

The main cause in the UK, accounting for 50% of cases, is gallstones. The majority of non-gallstone pancreatitis is due to alcohol. Other causes include infection, trauma, drugs, e.g. azathioprine, sodium valproate and diuretics, hypothermia, hypercalcaemia, hyperlipidaemia, post-ERCP (endoscopic retrograde cholangiopancreatography) and post-operative states. Carcinoma of the pancreas may also cause acute pancreatitis. Rarely, it is hereditary (see below).

HINTS AND TIPS

It is easy to remember the causes of acute pancreatitis using the mnemonic 'I GET SMASHED': Idiopathic, Gallstones, Ethanol, Trauma, Steroids, Mumps, Autoimmune, Scorpion bites, Hyperlipidaemia/Hypothermia, ERCP and Drugs (especially azathioprine and diuretics).

Pathology and clinical features

Different agents cause acute pancreatitis by different mechanisms. Fig. 7.11 summarizes the pathogenetic mechanisms of the major causes. Whatever the cause, they all lead to the release of lytic enzymes, which are then activated and cause damage. Pancreatic enzymes, in particular trypsin, lipase and phospholipase A2, digest pancreatic tissue, in particular causing fat necrosis. Blood vessel walls are also damaged causing extravasation of blood or ecchymoses, which may be extensive enough to discolour the skin of the flanks (Grey Turner's sign) or around the umbilicus (Cullen's sign).

The typical presentation is with severe abdominal pain of sudden onset that may radiate into the back, together with nausea and vomiting. The upper abdomen is usually tender to palpation. In severe cases tachycardia, tachypnoea and fever may be present.

Diagnosis

Diagnosis is by measurement of serum amylase. It is normally greatly elevated (five times or more) in acute pancreatitis. It is important to be aware that many other conditions, e.g. perforated peptic ulcer, intestinal obstruction and trauma can cause moderate increases in serum amylase, and only a marked elevation is characteristic of pancreatitis.

Clinical Note

Remember that not every patient with an elevated serum amylase has pancreatitis – there are numerous causes for a raised serum amylase. Only when levels are elevated fivefold or more should pancreatitis be diagnosed. Even then, be sure to correlate the findings on investigation with your clinical findings!

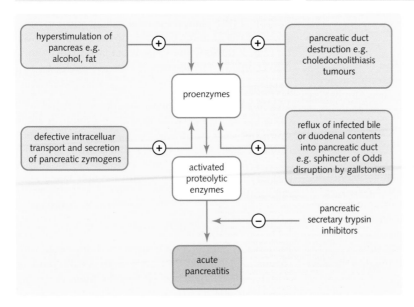

Fig. 7.11 Pathogenesis of acute pancreatitis. (Reproduced with permission from Haslett C et al. Davidson's Principles and Practice of Medicine, 19th edn. Edinburgh: Churchill Livingstone, 2002.)

Radiography shows characteristic findings in the abdomen. The psoas shadow can be absent because of retroperitoneal fluid and an air-filled dilatation of the proximal jejunum will be seen, i.e. a 'sentinel' loop.

An abdominal ultrasound will show whether gallstones are the cause or not.

Treatment

Patients with acute pancreatitis should be treated conservatively and kept 'nil by mouth', along with aggressive intravenous water and electrolyte replacement with opiate analgesia (not morphine). This allows the pancreas to 'rest' by removing secretory stimuli. If the patient is hypoxic then need inspired oxygen.

Complications of acute pancreatitis include formation of an abscess or a pseudocyst (see later), renal failure due to shock, DIC, relapses and diabetes mellitus if the inflammation is severe and necrosis ensues. In severe cases an intensive care bed is often required to manage these systemic complications.

If the pancreatitis is severe, the patient must receive intravenous nutrition. Patients with cholangitis or jaundice and biliary pancreatitis may benefit from gallstone removal via ERCP from the bile duct.

Severe pancreatitis occasionally results in significant necrosis and surgical or laparoscopic necrosectomy may be required.

Chronic pancreatitis

Chronic pancreatitis is an on-going inflammation of the pancreas accompanied by irreversible architectural changes. It causes a great deal of pain and often permanent loss of pancreatic function, and may or may not be preceded by acute pancreatitis.

Aetiology

Alcohol consumption causes more than 85% of cases, and is the most common cause of pancreatitis in developed countries. High-fat and -protein diets amplify the damage done by alcohol. Other causes include:

- Idiopathic chronic pancreatitis: this condition occurs in older people and is associated with peripheral vascular disease
- Trauma and scar formation, leading to the obstruction of the main pancreatic duct
- Previous episodes of acute pancreatitis predispose to others although they may oftenbe subclinical
- Hypercalcaemia causing the formation of calcified plugs, which obstruct the pancreatic duct
- Cystic fibrosis resulting in protein plugs in the duct system
- Hereditary forms of pancreatitis.

Hereditary pancreatitis accounts for 5–15% of causes overall. It should be suspected in an individual with acute or chronic pancreatitis when detailed history either indicates a positive family history or the patient's history began in childhood or early adulthood. It can be confirmed by detection of an increasing number of identifiable genetic mutations, most commonly in the trypsinogen gene, the trypsin inactivator cascade or the cystic fibrosis genes.

Pathology

Chronic pancreatitis has four key pathological features:

- Continuous chronic inflammation
- Fibrous scarring
- Loss of pancreatic tissue
- Duct strictures with formation of calculi.

Clinical features

Patients normally present with a history of prolonged ill-health with chronic epigastric pain, usually radiating through to the back. Steatorrhoea (lipase deficiency prevents complete breakdown and absorption of fat in the diet and weight loss from malabsorption occur due to reduced pancreatic enzyme activity. Secondary diabetes mellitus is caused by destruction of pancreatic islet cells.

Diagnosis

Serum amylase will be normal, in contrast to acute pancreatitis. Diagnosis is by CT scan complemented by endoscopic ultrasound (EUS) or magnetic resonance imaging (MRI); plain abdominal radiography can show speckled calcification of the pancreas (caused by the binding of calcium ions to necrosed fat). Diabetes mellitus should be excluded.

Treatment

Treatment involves stopping drinking alcohol and judicious use of analgesia. Surgery is an option in some cases, but only in those who are committed to stop drinking. Pancreatic enzyme supplements and a low-fat diet help the steatorrhoea, and diabetes mellitus is treated with insulin or diet control and oral hypoglycaemic agents.

Pseudocysts

Pseudocysts are a complication of both acute and chronic pancreatitis. They are localized collections of serosanguinous fluid found 6 weeks after the onset of an acute attack of pancreatitis.

They are usually solitary, 5–10 cm in diameter and lie in the lesser sac. Typically, they are characterized by chronic pain and persistently raised serum amylase levels.

Pseudocysts may produce abdominal pain and, more rarely, haemorrhage, infection and peritonitis. As they usually present as an epigastric mass, they may be mistaken for a tumour in the pancreas.

They differ from true cysts in that true cysts have an epithelial lining and are often congenital, while pseudocysts are surrounded by granulation tissue. Those smaller than 6 cm may resolve of their own accord.

Pancreatic insufficiency

In pancreatic insufficiency, pancreatic enzymes are absent or secreted in lower amounts than normal. Consequently, fat malabsorption occurs, with associated steatorrhoea. A deficiency in the fat-soluble vitamins A, D, E and K may also be found. The patient may be malnourished.

Cystic fibrosis is a major cause of pancreatic insufficiency. It is an autosomal recessive disorder (with a carrier rate of 1 in 25 among Caucasians but the disease incidence is 1:2500 live births), and its other major clinical feature is a tendency to chronic lung infections. The underlying defect is an abnormality in the chloride ion transporter.

Pancreatic insufficiency also occurs in chronic pancreatitis.

Treatment is with high-dose oral pancreatic enzymes. Additionally, a proton-pump inhibitor may help as it produces a pH in the duodenum which is optimal for fat digestion.

Carcinoma of the pancreas

Aetiology

Carcinoma of the pancreas accounts for about 5% of all cancer deaths in the USA and the UK.

It is particularly common in diabetic females, being most common over the age of 60 years. It is associated with smoking. Of all pancreatic carcinomas, 60% occur in the head, 15–20% in the body and 5–10% in the tail. Twenty percent of cases involve the pancreas diffusely.

Clinical features

Those arising in the head are likely to produce symptoms earlier than those arising elsewhere. They may obstruct the ampulla of Vater or common bile duct causing obstructive jaundice; in fact the classical presentation is with painless progressive jaundice. Other presenting symptoms include pain (50% of cases), intermittent jaundice, diabetes mellitus and the general features of malignancy, e.g. weight loss.

Clinical Note

Carcinoma of the head of the pancreas causes jaundice which develops over a few weeks. The jaundice is of the obstructive type, as the tumour compresses the common bile duct at the ampulla of Vater. The obstruction results in accumulation of bile in the proximal biliary tree, and so the gallbladder becomes enlarged. As inflammation is not usually involved, the jaundice is painless. Interestingly, even though the jaundice is due to a conjugated hyperbilirubinaemia, itching is uncommon; although you still get the other symptoms of obstructive jaundice such as pale stools and dark urine.

The gallbladder may be dilated and easily palpable (Courvoisier's sign).

HINTS AND TIPS

If a gallbladder is palpable in the presence of jaundice, Courvoisier's law states that the cause is unlikely to be gallstones.

Carcinomas arising in other parts of the pancreas are less likely to produce symptoms and so are discovered late. Consequently, they have a worse prognosis, often having metastasized before diagnosis.

Most are adenocarcinomas and almost all begin in the ductal epithelium. Less than 1% begin in the acinar cells.

Weight loss usually occurs and some individuals develop thrombophlebitis migrans (flitting venous thromboses).

Diagnosis

An abdominal CT is the first line imaging when there is a suspicion of pancreatic cancer.

EUS is also used to visualize the head of the pancreas and take biopsies. ERCP is used in patients with jaundice to relieve biliary obstruction and acquire cytology samples for diagnosis.

Treatment

The optimal treatment for carcinoma of the pancreas is surgical, but less than 30% of patients are suitable. Survival of up to 30% at 5 years with a surgical mortality of < 5% can be achieved in sub-groups.

The operation is called Whipple's procedure. It is a major operation consisting of a partial gastrectomy, duodenectomy and a partial pancreatectomy. It may or may not include the removal of the gallbladder and distal common bile duct. For small tumours, a modified Whipple's prodecure preserves the duodenum and bile duct. Palliative surgical or endoscopic procedures can be used to relieve jaundice or gastric outlet obstruction.

The overall prognosis is very poor, with a 5-year survival rate of < 5%. This is due to its late presentation.

THE BILIARY SYSTEM

The biliary system comprises the gallbladder and bile ducts. It serves to remove waste products from the liver and carries bile salts to the intestine where they aid digestion. The biliary system is closely related both anatomically and functionally to the liver and pancreas.

The gallbladder

The gallbladder is a pear-shaped sac that concentrates and stores bile secreted from the liver. It can hold between 30 and 60 mL of bile and, when stimulated, it releases its contents into the duodenum, through the cystic and biliary ducts.

It lies on the right edge of the hepatic quadrate lobe, in the gallbladder fossa on the visceral surface, partly covered by peritoneum on its posterior and inferior surfaces. The anterior surface contacts the hepatic visceral surface.

The gallbladder comprises three parts: the fundus, body and neck (see Fig. 5.12), which tapers and makes an S-shaped bend to join with the cystic duct. The cystic duct is 2–4 cm long and joins the common hepatic duct to form the bile duct. This travels anterior to the portal vein and courses through the head of pancreas to open into the second part of the duodenum through the sphincter of Oddi (hepatopancreatic sphincter) at the ampulla of Vater (duodenal papilla).

The neck, as well as the cystic duct, has a spiral folding of its mucus membrane, forming a spiral valve (of Heister). This keeps the cystic duct open constantly for two purposes:

- To allow bile to pass into the gallbladder from the liver when the bile duct is closed (by the sphincter of Oddi and the choledochal sphincter)
- To allow bile to be secreted into the duodenum when the gallbladder contracts.

Blood supply

The blood supply to the gallbladder is from the cystic artery (a branch of the right hepatic artery).

Venous drainage occurs via the cystic vein which drains the neck and ducts, and the veins draining the fundus and body. These terminate in three ways:

- Draining directly into the hepatic visceral surface
- Joining the portal vein
- Joining the gastric, duodenal and pancreatic veins (which then join the portal vein).

Lymphatic drainage

Lymph from the gallbladder passes to the hepatic nodes via the cystic nodes, near the neck of the gallbladder. These drain to the coeliac lymph nodes.

Nerve supply

The innervation to the gallbladder is from the coeliac plexus (sympathetic), the vagus nerve (parasympathetic), the right phrenic nerve (sensory) and the hepatic plexus. The nerves follow the cystic artery.

The biliary tract

The biliary tract, comprising the bile ducts, conveys bile from the liver to the duodenum. The left and right hepatic ducts join to form the common hepatic duct, which descends in the free edge of the lesser omentum and joins the cystic duct to form the common bile duct.

The common bile duct descends in the free edge of the lesser omentum with the hepatic artery and portal vein. It continues its descent behind the superior part of the duodenum and head of the pancreas.

The termination of the bile duct, together with that of the pancreatic duct forms the ampulla of Vater (hepatopancreatic ampulla) in the superior part of the duodenum.

There are two sphincters involved in the movement of bile:

- The *choledochal sphincter* at the distal end of the common bile duct. Contraction of this prevents bile entering the ampulla and duodenum, thus causing its storage in the gallbladder
- The *sphincter of Oddi* around the ampulla of Vater, This controls the secretion of both bile and pancreatic juice into the duodenum.

Embryology and development

The embryology of the biliary system is intimately connected with that of the liver, hence it is worth reading this section together with that of its counterpart in Chapter 6. See also Fig. 7.3.

Important to the development of the biliary tract is the liver bud. The connection between this and the foregut (duodenum) narrows and forms the bile duct.

A small ventral outgrowth from the bile duct gives rise to the gallbladder and cystic duct.

When bile begins to be produced around the 12th week, the biliary tract and gallbladder are fully formed. This allows the bile to enter the duodenum.

Histology of the gallbladder

The wall of the gallbladder consists of a mucous membrane, muscular layer, adventitia and a serous membrane.

The *mucous membrane* is made up of simple columnar epithelium and a lamina propria of loose connective tissue. The columnar epithelial cells have a brush border of many microvilli on their apical surfaces. The mucosa is thrown into folds when the gallbladder is empty. This allows it to distend when needed.

The *muscular layer* consists of smooth muscle oriented longitudinally, transversely and obliquely with associated collagenous elastic fibres.

The *adventitia* is made up of collagen and elastic fibres, and contains a rich blood vessel and lymphatic network.

The intrahepatic bile ducts are lined by cuboidal or low columnar epithelial cells. Increasing amounts of fibroelastic connective tissue surround the epithelium as the ducts become larger near the porta hepatis. The largest ducts have smooth muscle in their walls.

Gallbladder functions and physiology

The primary functions of the gallbladder are the concentration and storage of bile.

In the fasting state, the sphincter of Oddi (Fig. 7.12) is contracted. However, in response to stimulation during and after meals to aid digestion (Fig. 7.13) it relaxes, allowing the gallbladder to release its contents. Nevertheless, it is not essential for life.

> **Clinical Note**
>
> Cholecystectomy is a common operation, following which bile is discharged into the duodenum at a constant, slow rate which allows the digestion of moderate amounts of fat in the diet.

Concentration of bile

The gallbladder stores bile secreted by the liver and has a capacity of about 35 mL.

The stored bile is 5–20 times more concentrated than that secreted by the liver, principally because of the active transport of Na^+ from the gallbladder

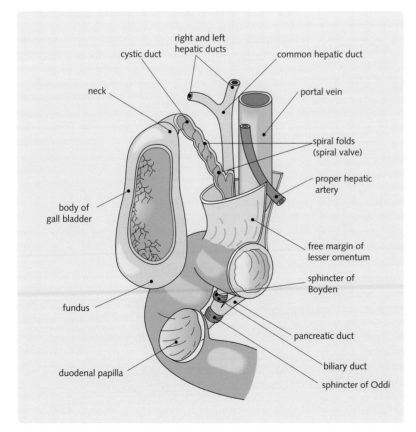

Fig. 7.12 The gall bladder and biliary tract. (Redrawn with permission from Hall-Craggs ECB. Anatomy as a Basis for Clinical Medicine. London: Waverly Europe, 1995. http://lww.com)

cystic duct

right and left hepatic ducts

common hepatic duct

neck

portal vein

spiral folds (spiral valve)

proper hepatic artery

body of gall bladder

free margin of lesser omentum

sphincter of Boyden

fundus

pancreatic duct

duodenal papilla

biliary duct

sphincter of Oddi

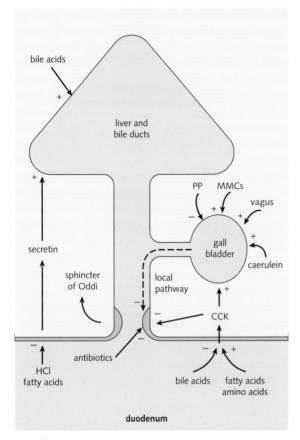

Fig. 7.13 Mechanisms controlling the secretion of bile into the duodenum. (PP=pancreatic polypeptide; MMCs=migrating motor complexes; CCK=cholecystokinin.) (From Sanford PA. Digestive System Physiology, 2nd edn. London: Edward Arnold, 1992. Reproduced by permission of Hodder/Arnold Publishers.)

epithelium into the lateral intracellular spaces (Fig. 7.14). Water passively follows the active transport of Na$^+$ ions.

> ### HINTS AND TIPS
>
> The gallbladder epithelial cells are highly specialized for absorption. They have a brush border of microvilli; they are rich in mitochondria; and they have numerous Na$^+$/K$^+$ ATPase transporters at their lateral surfaces.

Gallbladder contraction

Gallbladder emptying begins several minutes after the start of a meal.

During the cephalic phase, the taste and smell of food and the presence of food in the mouth and pharynx cause impulses in branches of the vagus nerve that increase emptying of the gallbladder.

The highest rate of emptying of the gallbladder occurs during the intestinal phase, mostly in response to cholecystokinin released from the duodenal mucosa as a result of the presence of the products of fat digestion and essential amino acids in the duodenum.

Cholecystokinin enters the circulation and reaches the gallbladder, where it causes strong contractions of the smooth muscle of the wall and relaxation of the sphincter of Oddi.

Gastrin, which has the same sequence of amino acid residues as cholecystokinin at its C-terminal, may also cause contractions of the gallbladder during the cephalic and gastric phases.

Fig. 7.14 The mechanism by which bile is concentrated in the gall bladder. The epithelial cells in the gall bladder mucosa have large lateral intercellular spaces near the basement membrane and tight junctions at the apices. Na$^+$ ions are coupled with Cl$^-$ ions and actively transported into the intercellular spaces. Water passively diffuses into the spaces as it follows the osmotic gradient set up by the active transport of ions.

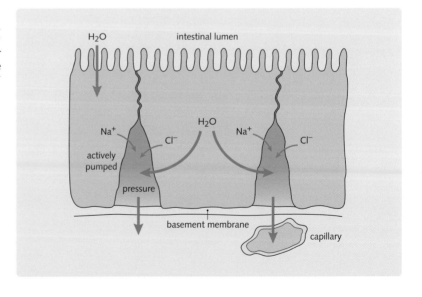

DISORDERS OF THE GALLBLADDER AND BILIARY TRACT

Congenital abnormalities

Anomalies of the biliary tree are characterized by changes in the architecture of the biliary tree within the liver.

In normal development, embryonic bile ducts involute (spiral and roll inwards at the edges). Anomalies of the biliary tree are thus thought to be caused by remnants that have not involuted completely.

Anomalies vary in severity. They may be clinically insignificant or be severe enough to cause hepatosplenomegaly and portal hypertension. They are often inherited.

Gallstones

Gallstones (cholelithiasis) are a common complaint in the West. They affect the gallbladder and extrahepatic bile ducts.

The incidence of gallstones is twice as high in women as in men overall. However, it increases with age in both sexes. Obese people and those with diabetes or haemolysis are also at higher risk of getting gallstones.

Aetiology

Eighty percent of gallstones are composed predominantly of cholesterol. The rest are composed mainly of bile pigment and calcium (pigment stones). Most stones contain all three constituents.

A predisposition to cholesterol stones arises in two situations:

- Increased cholesterol in bile, e.g. due to obesity or diet
- Decreased amount of bile acids in bile, e.g. due to malabsorption in cystic fibrosis patients.

Typically, cholesterol stones are large and can be either single or multiple. In cross-section, cholesterol crystals are seen radiating from the centre.

Pigment stones are seen when levels of unconjugated bilirubin are abnormally high, e.g. in haemolytic anaemias such as hereditary spherocytosis or when enterohepatic recycling of bile is impaired, e.g. in patients who have undergone ileal resections. Another risk factor is chronic infections of the biliary tract, as the bacteria act as foci for the formation of pigment stones. Pigment stones are usually small, black and fragile.

Clinical features

Eighty per cent of patients with gallstones are asymptomatic. These remain in the gallbladder, but stones which impact in the neck of the cystic duct can cause biliary pain and acute cholecystitis.

If gallstones impact in the common bile duct, this can lead to obstruction of bile and cause pain and cholestatic jaundice. This sometimes gives rise to bacterial infections resulting in cholangitis.

If they impact in the gallbladder, either at the neck or in the cystic duct, the bile which is unable to escape becomes concentrated and produces a chemical cholecystitis. The bile may also become infected, resulting in acute cholecystitis. However, if the gallbladder is empty, it will secrete mucus, so that a mucocele results.

The clinical presentations are summarized in Fig. 7.15.

Clinical Note

The cardinal feature of acute cholecystitis is pain in the right upper quadrant, but pain may also be felt at the epigastric or interscapular regions. This is because of the innervation of the gallbladder, which is derived from T5–T9, hence the referral to the corresponding dermatomes. Additionally, visceral pain from the gallbladder may also be referred to the right shoulder tip via C3–C5 if the inflammation irritates the diaphragm.

Treatment

Treatment varies according to the location of the gallstones and how they present, e.g. whether inflammation or a bacterial infection (cholecystitis or ascending cholangitis) is present.

If infection is present, patients should have blood cultures taken, and then broad-spectrum antibiotics. Intravenous fluids, analgesia and antiemetics are often required.

Fig. 7.15 Clinical presentation and causes of gall stones.

Clinical presentations	Cause
Biliary pain (in epigastrium and right hypochondrium)	Impacted in the cystic duct
Biliary pain, cholestatic jaundice, and cholangitis	Impacted in the common bile duct
Asymptomatic	Located in the gall bladder

Cholecystectomy (surgical removal of the gallbladder) is often performed laparoscopically, with good effect. If gallstones are only present in the common bile duct then they can be removed via ERCP.

Cholesterol stones may be dissolved or disrupted by giving bile acids to increase their solubility in bile. Dissolution of gallstones can take up to 2 years and 50% of the stones recur. This treatment is rarely used.

The compications are summarized in Fig 7.16.

Disorders associated with biliary cirrhosis

There are three main diseases in this category: primary and secondary biliary cirrhosis, and primary sclerosing cholangitis. These are disorders affecting the intrahepatic bile ducts which lead to cirrhosis of the liver. They are normally considered as hepatic diseases and so are covered in Chapter 6.

Fig. 7.16 Complications of gall stones.
Acute cholecystitis
Pancreatitis
Gall stone ileus
Biliary enteric fistula
Ileum obstruction
Carcinoma of the gall bladder

Neoplastic disease

Cholangiocarcinoma

Cholangiocarcinomas (carcinomas of the bile ducts) are relatively uncommon, accounting for approximately 10% of all liver tumours.

These mucus-secreting adenocarcinomas cause jaundice and are not associated with the hepatitis B or C viruses, or cirrhosis. They are, however, associated with inflammatory bowel disease, especially if primary sclerosing cholangitis is present as well.

The prognosis is poor. There is usually no curative treatment but palliation can be effective for a couple of years.

Primary adenocarcinoma of the gallbladder

This occurs mostly in patients over 70 years of age, and more frequently affects women. It presents with right hypochondrial pain and nausea, and it is usually palpable. Obstructive jaundice occurs as the disease progresses.

Cholecystectomy is a possible treatment, but again, prognosis is poor due to late presentation.

Ampullary tumours

An adenocarcinoma of the ampulla of Vater is relatively rare. It presents much earlier than the previous cancers mentioned, mainly with obstructive jaundice. It can be diagnosed by ERCP or EUS. The prognosis is good with a 5-year survival rate of 60% after surgical resection.

Clinical assessment of gastrointestinal disease

8

After reading this chapter you should be able to outline the following presentations of GI disease:
- Dysphagia
- Dyspepsia
- Vomiting
- Abdominal pain
- Weight loss
- Gastrointestinal bleeding
- Diarrhoea
- Constipation

You should also be able to:
- Describe the process of taking a history focusing on the gastrointestinal system
- Describe the process of a complete abdominal examination
- Outline biochemical, haematological and microbiological tests
- Outline endoscopic investigations
- Outline radiological investigations

COMMON PRESENTATIONS OF GASTROINTESTINAL DISEASE

DYSPHAGIA

Dysphagia means having difficulty in swallowing. This can be caused by simple reflux oesophagitis, but is a symptom of several conditions, principally obstruction, stricture, neurological problems or uncoordinated peristalsis as in achalasia (Fig. 8.1). Note it is different from globus, where a 'lump in the throat' is felt in anxiety states, or odynophagia, which is pain on swallowing.

Important questions to ask in the history include duration of symptoms; is it difficult to make the swallowing movement? Is it difficult to swallow fluids as well as solids? Is it painful? Does the neck bulge or gurgle when drinking? Any recent weight loss? Has there been a history of GORD?

Difficulty making the swallowing movement is likely to be caused by a neurological problem such as a stroke. The ability to drink liquids, but not to swallow food suggests a stricture, Failure to swallow both fluids and solids is seen in achalasia. Constant, painful dysphagia with weight loss is suggestive of a malignancy. Bulging or gurgling is a symptom of pharyngeal pouch.

DYSPEPSIA

Dyspepsia is a general term encompassing several symptoms which originate in the gastrointestinal tract. These include heartburn, indigestion and peptic symptoms.

Although most of the time no abnormality is found, if a patient has 'alarm symptoms' they require a rapid referral for further investigations to exclude serious gastrointestinal disease. This should be unusual in patients <55 years.

HINTS AND TIPS

The ALARM Symptoms in dyspepsia are:
- Anaemia
- Loss of weight
- Anorexia or vomiting
- Refractory to antisecretory medications
- Melaena
- Swallowing difficulties.

Heartburn is common, especially in developed countries. Pain is felt behind the sternum (retrosternal pain) that may radiate up towards the throat. It is worse on lying flat, and can also be exacerbated after drinking alcohol or eating a fatty or spicy meal (Fig. 8.2). It is

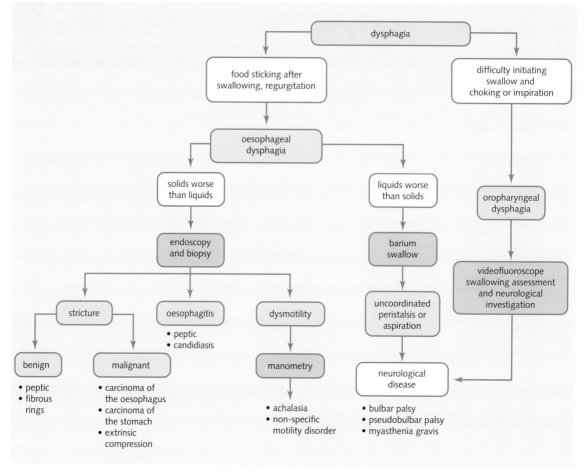

Fig. 8.1 Investigation of dysphagia. (Reproduced with permission from Haslett C et al. Davidson's Principles and Practice of Medicine, 19th edn. Edinburgh: Churchill Livingstone, 2002.)

important to distinguish this from the retrosternal pain of a myocardial infarction (typically a central crushing pain which may radiate to the neck or arm).

Indigestion is used to describe any discomfort experienced after eating or drinking. People will interpret this differently so it is import to establish exactly what the patient means by the word (Fig 8.3).

NAUSEA AND VOMITING

Nausea is a feeling that one is about to vomit. It is often accompanied by hypersalivation, which protects the mouth against the acid contents of the stomach. A differential diagnosis is shown in Fig 8.4.

Vomiting is the reflex act of ejecting the contents of the stomach through the mouth. Note it is important to differentiate true vomiting from regurgitation of gastric contents.

The content of the vomit (either blood or bile), the frequency and amount all give important diagnostic information. The presence of bile suggests that the lesion is below the ampulla of Vater.

A thorough history needs to be taken as nausea and vomiting are non-specific symptoms. You should enquire about associated symptoms, including abdominal pain, onset relative to food consumption, headache, fever, weight loss, and also take a drug history.

ABDOMINAL DISTENSION

Abdominal distension may be caused by one of the five Fs (flatus, fluid, fetus, fat or faeces). It is typically caused by obstruction low in the gastrointestinal tract.

Aetiologies can be split into gaseous causes such as functional gas, gastric outlet obstruction, small bowel obstruction, pseudo obstruction and ileus; solid causes

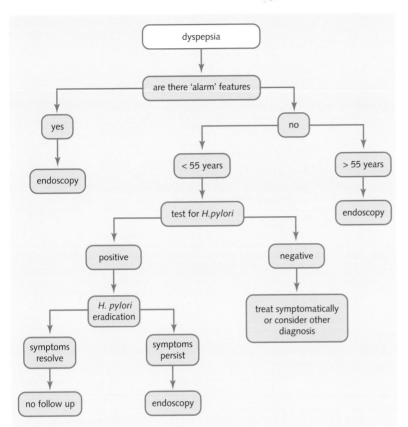

Fig. 8.2 Investigation of dyspepsia. (Reproduced with permission from Haslett C et al. Davidson's Principles and Practice of Medicine, 19th edn. Edinburgh: Churchill Livingstone, 2002.)

Fig. 8.3 Differential diagnosis of indigestion. (From Greene HL et al. Clinical Medicine, 2nd edn. St Louis, USA: Mosby, 1995.)

Peptic disease
Gastro-oesophageal reflux
Oesophagitis
Gall bladder disease
Pancreatitis
Ischaemic heart disease
Malabsorptive diseases
Irritable bowel syndrome
Motility disorders
Inflammatory bowel disease
Abdominal angina

ABDOMINAL PAIN

There are several causes of abdominal pain (Fig. 8.6). Broadly abdominal pain may be classified as one of the following types: visceral (from organs), parietal (from the parietal peritoneum), referred or psycogenic. Accompanying symptoms will give clues to the mechanisms behind the pain.

HINTS AND TIPS

Because of the embryological development of the gut, pain in a structure that develops from the foregut may be referred to the epigastric region, that from midgut structures to the umbilical area and hindgut structures to the suprapubic area.

including hepatomegaly, splenomegaly, tumour and constipation with faecal retention; and finally fluid causes such as ascites, abdominal haemorrhage, cysts and abscesses. A diagnostic algorithm is given in Fig 8.5.

In the history it is important to ask about the rate of onset. A neoplasm, for example will not produce distension as quickly as gas.

Abdominal pain can also be divided into acute and chronic pain. Diagnostic algorithms are shown in Figs 8.7 and 8.8.

Fig. 8.4 Differential diagnosis of nausea and vomiting. (From Greene HL et al. Clinical Medicine, 2nd edn. St. Louis, USA: Mosby, 1995.)

| Associated abdominal pain | Associated neurological signs | Predominant symptoms | |
		Acute	Recurrent or chronic
Viral gastroenteritis	Increased intracranial pressure	Digitalis toxicity	Psychogenic vomiting
Acute gastritis	Midline cerebellar haemorrhage	Ketoacidosis	Metabolic disturbances
Food poisoning	Vestibular disturbances	Opiate use	Gastric retention
Peptic ulcer disease	Migraine headaches	Cancer chemotherapeutic agents	Bile reflux after gastric surgery
Acute pancreatitis		Early pregnancy	Pregnancy
Small bowel obstruction		Inferior myocardial infarction	
Acute appendicitis		Drug withdrawal	
Acute cholecystitis		Binge drinking	
Acute cholangitis		Hepatitis	
Acute pyelonephritis			
Inferior myocardial infarction			

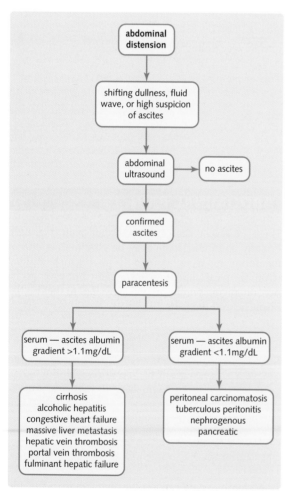

Fig. 8.5 Investigation of abdominal distension. (From Greene HL et al. Clinical Medicine, 2nd edn. St Louis, USA: Mosby, 1995.)

Fig. 8.6 Mechanisms of abdominal pain. (From Greene HL et al. Clinical Medicine, 2nd edn. St Louis, USA: Mosby, 1995.)

Obstruction

Gastric outlet
Small bowel
Large bowel
Biliary tract
Urinary tract

Peritoneal irritation

Infection
Chemical irritation (blood, bile, gastric acid)
Systemic inflammatory process
Spread from a local inflammatory process

Vascular insufficiency

Embolization
Atherosclerotic narrowing
Hypotension
Aortic aneurysm dissection

Mucosal injury

Peptic ulcer disease
Gastric cancer

Altered motility

Gastroenteritis
Inflammatory bowel disease
Irritable colon
Diverticular disease

Metabolic disturbance

Diabetic ketoacidosis
Porphyria
Lead poisoning

Nerve injury

Herpes zoster
Root compression

Muscle wall disease

Trauma
Myositis
Haematoma

Referred pain

Pneumonia (lower lobes)
Inferior myocardial infarction
Pulmonary infarction

Psychological stress

Depression
Situational stress
Intrapsychic conflict

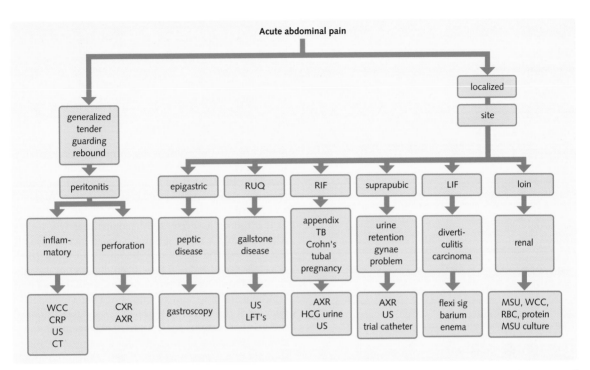

Fig 8.7 Algorithm for the investigation of acute abdominal pain. (AXR, abdominal X-ray; CRP, C-reactive protein; CT, computed tomography; CXR, chest X-ray; HCG, human chorionic gonadotrophin (pregnancy test); LFTs, liver function tests; LIF, left iliac fossa; MSU, midstream urine; RBC, red blood cells; RIF, right iliac fossa; RUQ, right upper quadrant; US, ultrasound; WCC, white cell count). (Reproduced with permission from Fox C, Lombard M. Crash Course: Gastroenterology, 3rd edn. Edinburgh: Mosby, 2008.)

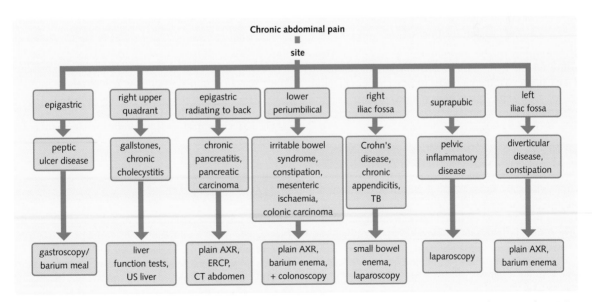

Fig. 8.8 Algorithm for the investigation of chronic abdominal pain. (AXR, abdominal X-ray; CT, computed tomography; ERCP, endoscopic retrograde cholangiopancreatography; US, ultrasound;). (Reproduced with permission from Fox C, Lombard M. Crash Course: Gastroenterology, 3rd edn. Edinburgh: Mosby, 2008.)

Fig. 8.9 Causes of the acute abdomen.

Inflammation
Acute appendicitis
Cholecystitis
Pancreatitis
Diverticulitis
Abscess
Pelvic inflammatory disease

Perforation
Peptic ulcer
Aortic aneurysm
Diverticula

Obstruction
Intestinal
Biliary

Other causes
Torted ovarian cyst
Ectopic pregnancy

The acute abdomen

This accounts for about half of urgent general surgical admissions. Many of the causes are serious and require prompt intervention, although relatively simple conditions such as constipation are also admitted (Fig 8.9). Generally the causes of acute abdomen are:

- Inflammation – the pain develops gradually and is exacerbated by movement
- Obstruction – the pain is colicky as the bowel goes into spasm trying to move the obstruction
- Perforation of a viscus – severe sudden-onset pain which needs urgent treatment.

Examination of the abdomen is necessary to determine whether the patient shows signs of peritonitis (see Chapter 5). If so it needs to be treated as an emergency case with resuscitation and prompt surgical treatment.

WEIGHT LOSS

Any significant, unintentional weight loss within a 6-month period needs to be investigated. Gastrointestinal causes that need to excluded include malignancy, malabsorption, inflammatory bowel disease, dysphagia and obstruction.

It is important to take a detailed history as there are many other medical problems associated with weight loss, These include systemic causes such as malignancy and tuberculosis, psychiatric causes such as anorexia nervosa, and endocrine diseases including diabetes mellitus and hyperthyroidism.

GASTROINTESTINAL (GI) BLEEDING

Generally bright red blood signifies fresh bleeds, and dark black blood is from an old bleed.

Upper GI bleeding

Acute upper GI bleeding is the commonest gastrointestinal emergency. Approximately half of all cases are caused by bleeding from peptic ulcers. Other important causes are bleeding oesophageal varices, oesophagitis and gastric erosions.

If bleeding is severe, the haematemesis will be red with clots; black 'coffee ground' haematemesis is usually less serious. The stools may be tarry and black (melaena), as the blood will have been digested in the gut.

A patient suffering from an acute upper GI bleed may rapidly deteriorate and go into shock with fatal consequences if the bleeding is severe, hence assessment of the circulatory status is a key part of management. Intravenous access and fluid resuscitation is a priority. Blood should be cross-matched for either transfusion or if surgical treatment is needed.

Once the patient is sufficiently resuscitated, endoscopy may be carried out. This is diagnostic in about 80% of cases.

Lower GI bleeding

This is caused by bleeding from the intestine or anus, and may be acute, subacute or chronic. Patients typically complain of blood on the toilet paper when they open their bowels.

Subacute or chronic lower GI bleeding is very common. Usually this is due to haemorrhoids or anal fissures. Nevertheless, in patients over 50 years of age, colonoscopy may be required to rule out colorectal carcinoma.

Severe, acute lower GI bleeding is uncommon. Diverticular disease is the most likely cause.

Fig 8.10 gives an algorithm for the management of GI bleeding.

ANAEMIA

Anaemia is a decreased number of red blood cells in the blood, when the haemoglobin level drops below normal values. It can be classified by the size of the red bloods as either microcytic, normocytic or macrocytic.

This can often be picked up on routine blood tests, or the patent may look pale and feel short of breath.

Anyone over the age of 50 who has iron-deficient anaemia (microcytic), should be investigated with an OGD and colonoscopy to exclude colorectal malignancy.

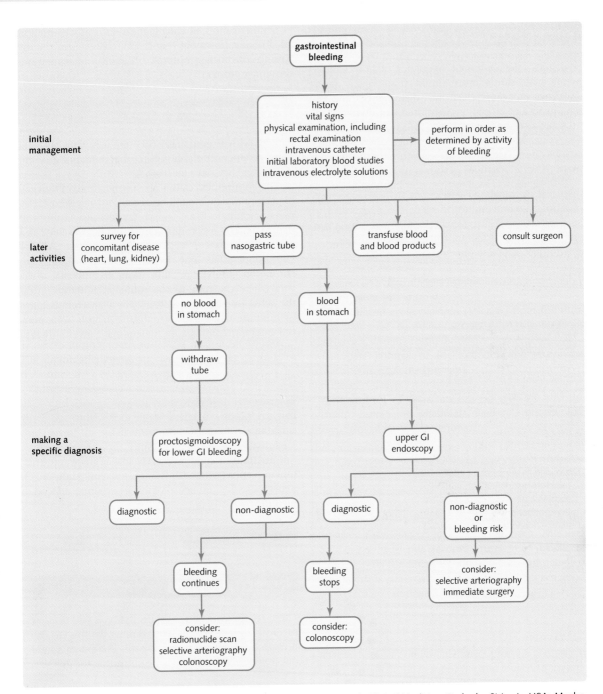

Fig. 8.10 Management of gastrointestinal bleeding. (From Greene HL et al. Clinical Medicine, 2nd edn. St Louis, USA: Mosby, 1995.)

JAUNDICE

Jaundice is characterized by yellow skin and yellow sclerae, and is caused when plasma bilirubin levels exceed 50 μmol/L. An important question is whether the urine is dark coloured as this would distinguish acholuric jaundice (pre-hepatic causes) from conjugated hyperbilirubinaemias (hepatic and post-hepatic causes).

The mechanisms by which the levels may become elevated, and the classification of jaundice are described in Chapter 6.

DIARRHOEA AND CONSTIPATION

Diarrhoea refers to excess frequency of bowel movements with stools more liquid than usual. Severe diarrhoea can cause electrolyte disturbances and is a major cause of mortality in children worldwide.

Acute cases are usually due to infections or dietary indiscretion, whereas chronic diarrhoea often has more serious causes (Fig. 8.11). An algorithm for the management of acute diarrhoea is shown in Fig. 8.12.

Constipation is a subjective complaint. Some people believe they must open their bowels at least once a day, but in fact anything from once every three days, to three times daily is within the normal range. Consequently it is important to ask in the history, 'What frequency is normal for you?'

Fig. 8.11 Aetiology of diarrhoea. (From Greene HL et al. Clinical Medicine, 2nd edn. St Louis, USA: Mosby, 1995.)

Viral	Norwalk agent
	Rotavirus
	Enteric adenovirus
Bacterial toxin	*Staphylococcus*
	Clostridium perfringens
	Clostridium difficile
	Clostridium botulinum
	Bacillus cereus
	Toxigenic *Escherichia coli*
	Vibrio cholerae
Bacterial invasion	Shigella
	Invasive *E. coli*
	Salmonella
	Gonorrhoea
	Yersinia enterocolitica
	Vibrio parahaemolyticus
	Campylobacter fetus and *jejuni*
Parasites	*Giardia lamblia*
	Cryptosporidium
	Entamoeba histolytica
After infection	Lactase deficiency
	Bacterial overgrowth
Drugs	Laxatives
	Antacids with magnesium
Food toxins	Ciguatoxin, scombroid, pufferfish
Metabolic	Hyperthyroidism
	Adrenal insufficiency
	Hyperparathyroidism
	Diabetes mellitus
Chronic illness	Inflammatory bowel disease
	Ischaemic colitis
	Malabsorption
	Irritable bowel syndrome

Serious causes of constipation such as obstruction need urgent treatment (Fig. 8.13); however, in the the absence of other symptoms a high-fibre diet may improve symptoms.

ANAL MASS

Patients with an anal mass will often complain of tenesmus (an uncomfortable feeling that something is still there after they have defecated).

The commonest causes are haemorrhoids (varices), hypertrophied anal papillae, rectal prolapsed, condylomata acuminata (anal warts), faecal impaction and neoplasia. The most important thing is to exclude is a malignancy.

Anal papillae may hypertrophy in response to chronic irritation or inflammation. Rectal prolapse occurs where the tone of the sphincter is reduced and the pelvic floor weakened. It may be a late complication of multiple childbirth. Neoplasms include squamous cell carcinoma, malignant melanoma, Bowen's disease and basal cell carcinoma.

A rectal examination is essential to investigate an anal mass, followed by proctoscopy.

FAECAL INCONTINENCE

This may be of faeces or of flatus.

Structural changes such as the loss of angle at the rectum and anus (which contributes to faecal continence), neuromuscular and neurological lesions may all lead to incontinence.

HISTORY AND EXAMINATION

INTRODUCTION

These are the core clinical skills that you will need as a medical student, so it is worth taking the time to learn how to do them properly. Use this section as a guide, but remember that there is no substitute for practice!

HISTORY-TAKING

Most diagnoses are made on the history alone – if not, it should allow you to come up with a list of differential diagnoses. In most cases, the examination and investigations should confirm the diagnosis or exclude the differentials.

Remember, the patient has far more information about his or her condition than you do. Introduce yourself, be polite, listen carefully and look interested. Give

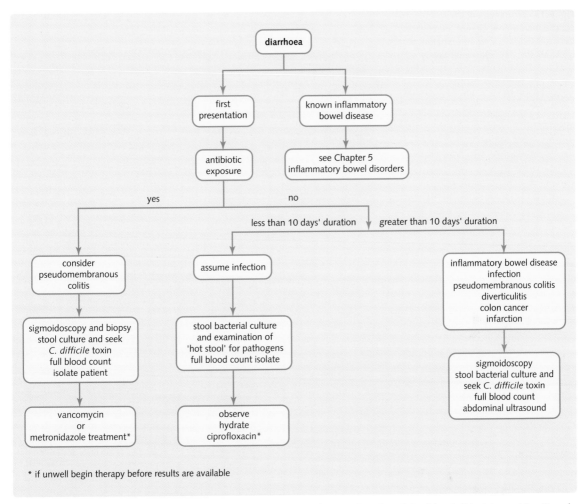

Fig. 8.12 Management of diarrhoea. (Reproduced with permission from Haslett C et al. Davidson's Principles and Practice of Medicine, 18th edn. Edinburgh: Churchill Livingstone, 1999.)

the patient the time and opportunity to tell you what you need to know, and put him or her at ease. Many symptoms are embarrassing.

Watch the patient carefully. How ill does the patient look? Are they agitated or distressed? Is he or she in pain? Can you notice any tremors? Has the patient lost a lot of weight (cachexia)? Look around the bedside for clues, such as inhalers, oxygen, a walking stick or frame, sputum pots, special food preparations etc.

THE STRUCTURE OF A HISTORY

When recording a history, use the headings below. You are less likely to leave things out if your history is structured. It is also easier for others to find the information they need quickly when looking at your notes.

Remember, patients notes are a legal document. They should have the patients name on it, along with other identification such as hospital number or date of birth. Make sure that you include all the details discussed, date the entry, and sign your name legibly.

The presenting complaint (PC)

This should be brief - a sentence stating the symptoms, not the diagnosis. For example write 'abdominal pain', not 'appendicitis'. Ideally you should use the patient's own words.

If the patient has a number of problems (not uncommon in the elderly) ask them to state the main ones first.

The history of the presenting complaint (HPC)

This is essentially a complete description of the presenting complaint.

Fig. 8.13 *Management of constipation. (From Greene HL et al. Clinical Medicine, 2nd edn. St Louis, USA: Mosby, 1995.)*

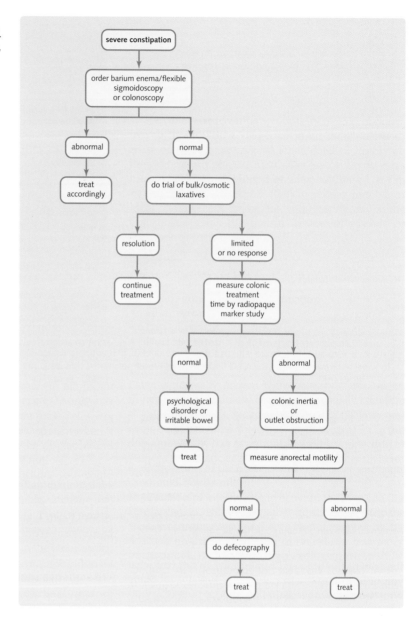

It is usually good to start off with:

- How and when the symptoms started
- The speed of onset: was it rapid, or slow and insidious?
- The pattern of symptoms, their duration and frequency. Are they continuous or intermittent? How often do they appear?

If the complaint appears to be gastrointestinal, you should always ask about the following:

- Weight loss or gain, and appetite
- Dysphagia
- Nausea and vomiting
- 'Indigestion' or 'heartburn'
- Abdominal pain (see the following section)

- Change in bowel habit – a deviation from what is normal for the patient is the key point, not the absolute number of times they open their bowels
- Change in the nature of stools: ask about stool colour and consistency, pressure of mucus or blood. If blood is present, was it fresh blood?

Pain

If pain is present, use the mnemonic SOCRATES as a guide to the questions which need to be asked:

- Site: where about is the pain?
- Onset: you should ask what the patient was doing at the time, and whether the onset was acute or

gradual. Ask whether there is any relationship to food
- Character: sharp, dull, shooting, crushing (like a band around the chest), stabbing, colicky, etc.
- Radiation
- Associated factors: nausea, vomiting, sweating, diarrhoea, migraine, etc.
- Timing: duration, number of episodes
- Exacerbating and relieving factors: lying down, sitting up, food, movement etc.
- If movement exacerbates the pain, peritoneum is likely to be involved; if the patient is rolling around, the pain is likely to be visceral colic, e.g. intestinal spasm
- Severity: this should be graded out of 10, with 10 being the most severe.

Additionally you should ask:

- If the patient has had it before. If yes, is it the same kind of pain?
- What happened last time? Did he or she have any treatment or investigations, or did it go away by itself? If treatment was given, was it effective?

Past medical history (PMH)

Has the patient had any other medical problems? This question often needs persistence. It is amazing how many people forget operations, spells in hospital, or visits to the GP! Ask what previous investigations have been carried out and their results.

It is also good practice to ask whether the patient has had any of the following: myocardial infarct, thyroid disease, asthma, tuberculosis, rheumatic fever, diabetes mellitus and epilepsy.

Drug history (DH)

Ask about all drugs, including over-the-counter medicines and the contraceptive pill, as well as medications which have been prescribed. If the patient is an in-patient you should check their drug chart. If appropriate, you could ask whether the patient actually took the prescribed medication, if non-compliance is suspected.

You should always ask about allergies (i.e. type 1 hypersensitivity reactions which may result in anaphylaxis) in this section. It is important to ask what the allergic reaction was, as sometimes patients have just experienced a normal side effect, e.g. diarrhoea after taking penicillin. It is important to establish whether they are really allergic, as you may be denying them the best treatment, but do not give them anything they say they are allergic to unless you are absolutely sure they are not.

Family history (FH)

Ask whether any diseases run in the family, specifically if first-degree relatives (parents and siblings) are affected.

If any first-degree relatives are deceased, also ask about the cause of death, and at what age they died. Practise drawing quick sketches of family trees. Make a note on the family tree of any diseases that relatives may have had, to help you notice trends.

Social history (SH)

This is to useful to gain some insight into the patient's life; how their illness is affecting the patient, what support they have or need at home, and whether he or she can reduce any health risks.

It should include information about the patient's:

- Marital or cohabitation status
- Children and other dependants
- Occupational history: this is especially relevant with regard to toxin/chemical exposure and musculoskeletal disorders
- Accommodation: assess whether the patient will be able to cope at home, e.g. getting upstairs
- Activities of daily living: can they manage cooking, cleaning, washing themselves and other essential tasks? If not, do they get any help?
- Smoking: is it cigarettes, cigars or a pipe that the patient smokes? How many cigarettes do they smoke per day, and for how long have they been smoking?
- Alcohol: what type of alcoholic beverages do they drink, and how much per week? You should calculate weekly consumption using units (Fig. 8.14), but remember that patients often underestimate their drinking
- Diet: Is it adequate? High cholesterol? Vegetarian?
- Exercise.

Review of systems (RoS)

Briefly go through all the systems of the body (Fig. 8.15) and ask specifically whether the patient has experienced any symptoms relating to them.

Presenting the history

You may be asked to present your history, for example on a ward round. This should be a short concise summary recapping the most important features. For example:

'Reginald Smith, a 69-year-old male presented with dysphagia. This started about 3 months ago and has become progressively worse, initially only with solids but now with liquids and he has lost 2 kg in weight. He is otherwise fit and well. His father died of cancer of the stomach at the age of 50. He has smoked 30 cigarettes a day since his early 20s, but does not drink.'

Fig. 8.14 Calculating alcohol consumption using the unit system. (Reproduced with permission from Cameron AD. Crash Course: Psychiatry, 2nd edn. Edinburgh: Mosby, 2004.)

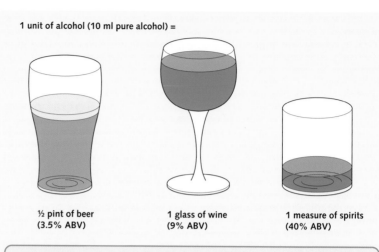

1 unit of alcohol (10 ml pure alcohol) =

½ pint of beer (3.5% ABV)

1 glass of wine (9% ABV)

1 measure of spirits (40% ABV)

Note: this is an approximate guide only, as many beers contain 4–5% ABV and many wines 11–12% ABV
ABV, alcohol content by volume

Safe daily alcohol limits
Men: 3–4 units/day (<21 units/week)
Women: 2–3 units/day (<14 units/week)

Note: Alcohol can confer health benefit mainly by giving protection from coronary heart disease but this only applies to men over 40 and postmenopausal women: The maximum health advantages are obtained by drinking 1–2 units per day

---

Fig. 8.15 The systems enquiry.

Cardiovascular system

- Chest pain (site, referral, precipitating and relieving factors)
- Palpitations

- Ankle oedema
- Shortness of breath/orthopnoea/ paroxysmal nocturnal dyspnoea

Respiratory system

- Chest pain
- Cough
- Sputum production

- Haemoptysis
- Shortness of breath and/or wheeze

Gastrointestinal system (also see section on Presenting Complaint above)

- Abdominal pain
- Nausea/vomiting

- Diarrhoea/constipation
- Chest pain (non-cardiac)

Nervous system

- Headache
- Fits
- Dizziness
- Numbness/tingling/loss of sensation

- Weakness
- Alteration or loss of vision
- Hearing loss
- Weakness

Endocrine system

- Polyuria/polydipsia
- Heat/cold intolerance
- Weight loss or gain

- Skin changes
- Mood changes

Continued

Fig. 8.15 The systems enquiry—cont'd

Musculoskeletal system and skin

- Pain
- Swelling

- Stiffness
- Rash

Genito-urinary system

- Frequency/oliguria/polyuria/nocturia
- Dysuria
- Haematuria

- Menstrual history in females
- Prostate symptoms in males

GASTROINTESTINAL SYSTEM EXAMINATION

Most clinical examinations comprise inspection, palpation, percussion and auscultation. Not all examinations will require all four components but it is useful to keep to this sequence so you do not leave any part undone. Before zooming in on the abdomen, there are a few other steps to the gastrointestinal system examination.

General inspection

The main purpose of a general inspection is to determine how unwell the patient is (Fig. 8.16). It may also enable you to pick up some clues.

Look at the patient's facial expression. Is he or she comfortable; or in obvious distress? If the patient is very ill, do not waste valuable time asking questions that can wait until later.

Many diseases and conditions do not have a direct effect on the gastrointestinal system. However, always

Fig. 8.16 Possible signs on general inspection.

Test performed	Sign observed	Diagnostic inference
Inspection of skin colour	Pallor	Anaemia, shock, myxoedema
Inspection	Yellow skin (and sclerae)	Jaundice
	Pink nodules and/or areas of baldness on scalp (alopecia neoplastica)	Metastases from internal carcinoma, usually from gastrointestinal tract, breast, kidney, ovary or bronchus
	Dark pigmented flexures, especially armpits and under breasts (acanthosis nigricans)	Obesity, endocrine disease, genetic, adenocarcinoma of gastrointestinal tract or other internal malignancy
	Vellus hair over face and body (hypertrichosis lanuginosa)	Anorexia, neoplasm
	Patient sitting forward on edge of bed using accessory muscles of respiration (respiratory distress)	Airway obstruction, anaemia, heart failure, pulmonary embolism, obesity
	Abdominal distension	Fluid, fat, faeces, fetus, flatus
	Large masses	Neoplasm, cysts, congenital abnormalities
	Telangiectasia (abnormal dilatation of blood vessels)	Cirrhosis, outdoor occupation
	Severe muscle wasting and loss of body fat (cachexia)	Severe illness
Inspection and questioning	Itchy tissue-paper skin (ichthyosis)	Lymphoma, drugs, malabsorption, malnutrition
	Generalized itching	Jaundice, systemic malignancy
	Painful tender veins in different sites at different times (thrombophlebitis migrans)	Carcinoma of pancreas

Fig. 8.17 Clinical signs in the hands indicative of disease. (Reproduced with permission from Fox C, Lombard M. Crash Course: Gastroenterology, 3rd edn. Edinburgh: Mosby, 2008.)

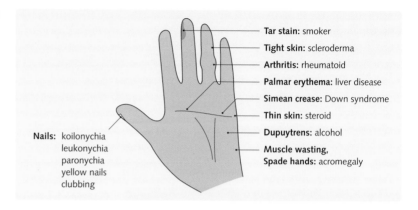

Tar stain: smoker

Tight skin: scleroderma

Arthritis: rheumatoid

Palmar erythema: liver disease

Simean crease: Down syndrome

Thin skin: steroid

Dupuytrens: alcohol

Muscle wasting, Spade hands: acromegaly

Nails: koilonychia
leukonychia
paronychia
yellow nails
clubbing

Fig. 8.18 Nail changes and their causes.

Nail changes	Diagnostic inference
Koilonychia (spoon shaped nails)	Iron deficiency, syphilis
Leukonychia (white nails)	Hypoalbuminaemia
Paronychia (inflammation of nail fold)	Bacteria or fungal infection
Clubbing	Cirrhosis, inflammatory bowel disease, coeliac disease, endocarditis, congenital heart disease, fibrosis alveolitis, bronchial carcinoma

Fig 8.19 Possible signs on examination of the limbs.

Test performed	Sign observed	Diagnostic inference
Palpation	Pulses	Information about cardiovascular system
Inspection	Central dilated arteriole with small red vessels radiating out from it, like a spider (spider naevus)	If more than five or six: pregnancy, cirrhosis or chronic liver disease
	Scratches	Pruritus
	Muscle wasting	Damage to innervation of muscles, malnutrition, chronic illness
	Thinning of skin	Steroid use

remember that the patient may be receiving medication for a pre-existing condition, which may affect the dose of drug you are intending to give for his or her gut condition, e.g. he or she may already be receiving enzyme-inducing drugs for another condition. Current medication might even be producing his or her gut symptoms, e.g. diarrhoea caused by antibiotic therapy.

Inspection of the hands and limbs

Physical examination of the patient should start with an inspection of the hands. This is relatively non-invasive and allows the patient to get used to your touch. It also gives you a lot of information (Figs 8.17 and 8.18).

When examining a patient, be methodical. Examine the hands and then work your way up the arm to the head and neck. Possible signs on limb examination are listed in Fig. 8.19.

Examination of the head and neck

Face, scalp and eyes

You need to pull down the lower eyelid to take a look at the sclerae for pallor (do not say anaemia— this is a

haematological finding) or jaundice. This may be uncomfortable, so always warn a patient beforehand. Remember, however, that jaundice is not clinically detectable unless serum bilirubin levels reach 50 μmol/L (twice the normal value).

Examination of the head and face is covered in Fig. 8.20.

Mouth

Use a pen torch to inspect the inside of the mouth. Ask the patient to stick their tongue out and then let you look under it. This will tell you if the patient is dehydrated or cyanotic (Fig. 8.21). Also inspect carefully for any mouth ulcers.

Wear gloves if you need to feel anything in the mouth and ask the patient to remove any false teeth.

Fig 8.20 Possible signs on examination of the head and face.

Test performed	Sign observed	Diagnostic inference
Inspection of colour of sclera	Yellow	Jaundice
Inspection of colour of conjunctiva	Pale	Anaemia
Inspection	Red eye from subconjunctival haemorrhage	Bleeding disorder from liver disease or other Cause, diabetes, vomiting
	Inflamed connective tissue beneath conjunctiva (episcleritis)	Reiter's syndrome (may follow dysentery)
	Red eye from conjunctivitis	Stevens–Johnson syndrome
	Chronic red eye	Cirrhosis, renal failure, hereditary Haemorrhagic telangiectasia (Osler-Weber-Rendu syndrome), iron deficiency anaemia
	Acute swelling of eyelids	Adverse reaction to penicillin, bee sting or other allergen, infection
	Firm, chronic swelling of eyelids	Lymphoma, sarcoidosis
	Yellow swelling in periorbital area (xanthelasma)	Hypercholesterolaemia, age
	Erythematous, swollen eyelids	Dermatomyositis
	Malar flush	Mitral stenosis
	White ring around edge of iris (arcus)	Hypercholesterolaemia, ageing
	Protruding eye with sclera visible above iris	Graves' disease
	Constricted pupils	Ageing, drugs (opiates, glaucoma treatment), Damage to sympathetic innervation
	Swollen, purple nose and ears (lupus pernio), prominent scars, orange–brown papules, nodules and plaques	Sarcoidosis
	Patches of hair loss on scalp (alopecia neoplastica)	Metastases from internal carcinoma (usually gastrointestinal tract, kidney, ovary, bronchus or breast)
	Flushing	Carcinoid syndrome
	Periorbital oedema, erythema of face and neck	Dermatomyositis
Inspection of cornea	Brown rings (Kayser–Fleischerrings) at periphery	Wilson's disease
Pupil reaction	Pupils constrict to accommodation but not to light (Argyll–Robertson pupil)	Syphilis

HINTS AND TIPS

Stomatitis simply means ulceration of the mucosal surface of the mouth – it can occur in the mouth or at the edges, where the upper and lower lips meet.

Neck

Inspect both the front and back of the neck, then stand behind the patient and palpate for enlarged nodes in the back, front and sides of the neck (Fig. 8.22).

Always palpate for the supraclavicular lymph nodes carefully, especially in the left supraclavicular

Fig. 8.21 Possible signs on examination of the mouth.

Test performed	Sign observed	Diagnostic inference
Inspection	Puckered mouth	Scleroderma
	Swollen gums	Pregnancy, acute leukaemia, puberty, phenytoin, infection
	Fissuring at edges of mouth (angular cheilosis or stomatitis)	Iron-deficiency anaemia, malabsorption, candidal or other infection
	Vesicles on lips and in perioral area	Herpes simplex infection
	Blue spots on mucosa	Hereditary haemorrhagic telangiectasia (Osler–Weber–Rendu syndrome)
	Small pigmented areas on lips and on mucosa (lentigines)	Peutz–Jeghers syndrome
	Bleeding and necrosis of gums	Acute leukaemia
	Bleeding gums	Vitamin C deficiency
	Beefy, raw, red tongue	Pernicious anaemia, malabsorption, pellagra
	Dry discoloured tongue	Gastrointestinal or other infection
	Ulcer	Carcinoma, lymphoma, trauma, infection (tuberculosis, herpes, Vincent's angina, diphtheria, measles), Stevens–Johnson syndrome, Behçet's syndrome, drugs, pemphigus, bullous pemphigoid
	Swellings	Cysts, stones in salivary glands, infection
	High-arched palate	Marfan's syndrome
	Black tongue	Antibiotic treatment
	Blue tongue and lips	Cyanosis
Inspection and touch with spatula	White patches that cannot be brushed off (leucoplakia)	Trauma, infection (including HIV)
	White patches that can be brushed off	Candidal infection (thrush)
Smell	Halitosis	Infection, poor hygiene, hepatic coma, uraemia, Diabetic coma

Fig. 8.22 Possible signs on examination of the neck.

Test performed	Sign observed	Diagnostic inference
Inspection of JVP (jugular venous pressure)	JVP raised (vertical height of column of blood in internal jugular vein exceeds 3 cm, measured from the sternal angle with the patient lying at 45°)	Superior mediastinal obstruction, e.g. carcinoma of bronchus (if JVP non-pulsatile), right heart failure, fluid overload, tricuspid incompetence, cardiac tamponade (if JVP pulsatile)
Palpation	Swellings	Infection, carcinoma, bronchial cyst, thyroglossal or other cyst, goitre (iodine deficiency or thyroid disorder)
	Enlarged lymph nodes (lymphadenopathy)	Infection, carcinoma
	Enlarged supraclavicular lymph node on the left (Virchow's node)	Carcinoma of stomach
Palpation of trachea	Deviation, not central	Superior mediastinal mass, collapse one lung, fibrosis
Palpation of carotid pulse	Character of pulse	Information about cardiovascular system

fossa, as this is a common site for gastrointestinal metastases. An enlarged node is indicative of gastric carcinoma (Virchow's node, or Troisier's sign – see Chapter 3).

Examination of the abdomen

As mentioned earlier, follow the sequence inspection, palpation, percussion and auscultation.

Inspection

The abdomen should be examined from the nipples to the knees, but not all at once. Respect the patient's dignity and only uncover as much as you need to at any one time.

Ask the patient to remove their clothes and lie flat on the bed or the couch, with the head on one pillow and arms by the sides. Cover the patient with a folded sheet or blanket. It is easy to move this up or down, exposing or revealing different parts, as you complete your examination.

Stand at the end of the bed to look at the abdomen as a whole before going nearer and taking a closer look. Look out for the following:

- Asymmetry
- Distension
- Dilated veins – obstruction of inferior vena cava

- Caput medusa – veins radiating out from umbilicus. Suggestive of portal hypertension.
- Spider naevi – these are found in the distribution of the superior vena cava, i.e. chest and upper back. More than five or six are significant in chronic liver disease
- Bruising – may imply acute pancreatitis
- Visible peristalsis – suggestive of bowel obstruction
- Visible pulsation – aortic aneurysm
- Masses
- Scars (Fig. 8.23)
- Striae.

Palpation

Make sure your hands are warm and tell the patient that you are about to feel their abdomen.

Before you do so, ask whether the abdomen is tender anywhere. If it is, then start your palpation as far away from the tender area as possible. Start with light palpation before pressing more deeply and always ask the patient to tell you if he or she feels anything. Most people will understandably tense their abdominal muscles if they think you are about to cause them pain.

Additionally, never take your eyes off the patient's face while you are palpating. You are looking for any

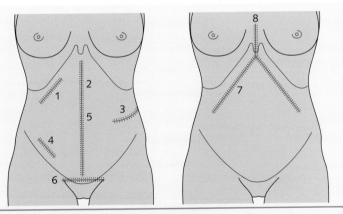

Fig. 8.23 Illustrations of common abdominal surgical scars, and their possible significance. (DU, duodenal ulcer; IVC, inferior vena cava.) (Reproduced with permission from Fox C, Lombard M. Crash Course: Gastroenterology, 3rd edn. Edinburgh: Mosby, 2008.)

1. Kocher's incision commonly for cholecystectomy
2. Upper midline incision commonly for peptic ulcer surgery: vagotomy, pyloroplasty, oversewn DU, gastrectomy
3. Lateral loin scar often for nephrectomy
4. Short scar in right iliac fossa for appendicectomy
5. Lower midline scar for colonic resection, laparotomy, caesarean section
6. Pfannensteil's incision for caesarean section
7. 'Rooftop' scar common for pancreatectomy or liver resection
8. 'Mercedes' scar is an upper extension of 'rooftop' to enable access to the IVC required in liver resection or transplantation

signs of pain or discomfort. Do not hurt the patient — you will fail exams if you do.

Light palpation of all four quadrants or nine regions will alert you to any obvious tenderness or peritonism— this is all you want to gain from it.

Patients with a tender abdomen are naturally apprehensive about having them palpated. However, when you have been around the quadrants once without hurting them they will often relax the abdominal muscles enough to let you palpate more deeply.

During deep palpation, you should be looking for:

- Tenderness on deep palpation only
- Guarding (tensing of the abdominal muscles)
- Rovsing's sign (more pain in the right iliac fossa than in the left iliac fossa, when palpated)
- Obvious masses.

HINTS AND TIPS

To describe any lump in the body, remember the six Ss – site, size, shape, surface, smoothness (as well as consistency and fluctuance) and surroundings, i.e. whether it is tethered or not.

Following general deep palpation, you will need to palpate for any enlarged abdominal organs (organomegaly). You should attempt to feel the liver, spleen and kidneys.

Palpating the liver

To examine the liver, start at the right iliac fossa and move your hand up, using the long, flat edge of your index finger to feel for the liver edge. The normal position of the liver is shown in Fig. 8.24.

Its edge can usually be felt just below the edge of the costal margin. You need to palpate quite deeply to feel it. Ask the patient to take deep breaths in and out; the edge should be felt moving against your fingers with respiration.

If you can feel the liver edge, make a note of what it feels like and how many centimetres you can feel. Is it smooth (possible hepatitis) or hard and craggy (tumours)? Remember that cirrhotic livers may not be felt as they often shrink. Some patients may have a palpable extension (Riedel's lobe) to the right lobe which is entirely normal.

Palpating the spleen

To examine the spleen, start in the right iliac fossa and move up diagonally to the left costal margin. A grossly enlarged spleen can extend into the right iliac fossa. A normal spleen cannot be felt.

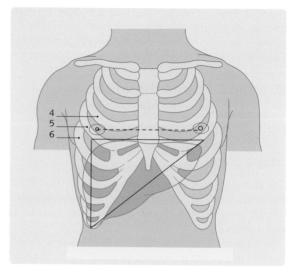

Fig. 8.24 The position of the normal liver in relation to the nipple line and to the 4th, 5th and 6th ribs.

A distinguishing feature of the spleen is its notch, which may be palpable in splenomegaly. Additionally, if you can feel an upper margin, you are not feeling the spleen, as you cannot get 'above' it.

Palpating the kidneys

The kidneys should be 'balloted', using two hands. This is the procedure of bouncing the kidney between the hand at the renal angle and the hand positioned anteriorly to this.

Normally they should not be able to be felt. Enlarged, tender kidneys may indicate infection. Fig. 8.25 lists the signs elicitable on abdominal palpation.

Percussion

The abdomen is not routinely percussed. It is usually done if there is a suspicion of ascites or when confirmation of hepato- or splenomegaly is needed.

The liver and spleen are dull to percussion. You can trace their margins (and confirm organomegaly) by percussing in the directions you palpated when examining them both. Always percuss for the upper border of the liver as well as the lower one. The liver may be pushed down by a hyperinflated chest or other respiratory pathology. Hepatomegaly may be wrongly diagnosed if the upper border has not been located.

If a patient has ascites, there will be shifting dullness. This is when a patient lies on their back, and on percussion the flanks are dull, and the midline is resonant. Get the patient to roll on their side, and this time on percussion the

Fig. 8.25 Possible signs on palpation of the abdomen.

Test performed	Sign observed	Diagnostic inference
Palpation	Enlarged liver (hepatomegaly)	Malignancy, infection (especially glandular fever and malaria), hepatitis, sickle-cell disease, porphyria, haemolytic anaemia, connective-tissue disease, portal hypertension, lymphoma, leukaemia, glycogen storage disorders, myelofibrosis
	Pulsatile liver	Tricuspid incompetence
Palpation of right iliac fossa	The right iliac fossa is more painful than the left (Rovsing's sign)	Acute appendicitis
Press on abdomen	Pain occurs when you press in and also when you remove your hand (rebound tenderness)	Peritonitis
Place fingers over right upper, quadrant, ask patient to breathe in	Pain on inspiration (Murphy's sign)	Inflamed gall bladder
Palpation	Sausage-shaped mass	Pyloric stenosis, intussusception
	Mass	Carcinoma, obstruction, hernia, faeces

upper flank is resonant, and the lower flank is dull. Note that it takes a minute or two for the fluid to drain.

Auscultation

You should listen for bowel sounds. There should be some and they should not be too loud. Absent bowel sounds suggest paralytic ileus, while tinkling bowel sounds suggest intestinal obstruction. Listen also for bruits (evidence of disturbed blood flow).

Examination of the rectum and external genitalia

These are considered part of a complete abdominal examination, although for obvious reasons you will not be asked to do them in examination situations. You should always finish by saying you would perform them.

Rectal examination

Many patients find rectal examinations distressing and embarrassing. It is therefore essential to take the time to explain what the examination entails, why it is being done and gain verbal consent. Ensure you have a chaperone present and always wear gloves, ensuring your examining finger is well lubricated.

To perform a rectal examination, ask the patient to lie on his or her left side with the knees drawn up. Inspect the anus for redness, bleeding, external haemorrhoids, skin lesions or fistulae. Before you begin, ask the patient if there is any tenderness and ask them to tell you if they feel any pain during the examination.

Gently insert a well-lubricated index finger into the anal canal and rectum. Note the tone of the anal sphincter. Gently sweep your finger around the walls to check for any masses or abnormalities. You should be able to feel the prostate in the male and cervix in the female through the anterior wall of the rectum. The prostate has a shallow central groove.

Withdraw your finger: there should be faecal matter on it but no blood or mucus. Take your glove off cuff-first, pulling the glove off inside out, and dispose of it in a clinical waste bag. Possible abnormal findings are listed in Fig. 8.26.

Genital examination

You should be looking for any signs of infection, gross abnormality and hernias.

It is best to look for hernias with the patient standing and you crouching down so that you are at the same level as the area you are examining. Many hernias disappear if the patient lies down. Hernias are common. About 1 in 100 people will have a hernia at some time in their life. About 70% of hernias are inguinal, 20% are femoral and 10% are umbilical.

Palpate over the external and internal rings (above and medial to the pubic tubercle) to detect an inguinal hernia and ask the patient to cough. You may feel a lump when he or she does. Repeat this procedure below and lateral to the pubic tubercle to check for a femoral hernia, and above and below the umbilicus for an umbilical hernia.

Try to reduce any swelling. The femoral pulse and lymph nodes in the groin should be palpated.

In the male, inspect the penis and scrotum, carefully palpating the testes, epididymis and spermatic cords. Note any scrotal swelling.

Fig. 8.26 Possible signs on rectal examination.

Test performed	Sign elicited	Diagnostic inference
Rectal examination and inspection of glove after rectal examination	Bloody mucus	Chronic inflammatory bowel disease, ulcerating tumour
	Watery mucus	
	Pale faecal material	Villous adenoma
	Bright red blood and slime	Obstructive jaundice
	Nodular prostate	Intussusception, colitis
	Tender prostate	Carcinoma, calcification
		Prostatitis
	Enlarged, smooth prostate	Age-related benign prostatic hyperplasia
	Narrow empty rectum and a gush of faeces and flatus on withdrawing finger	Hirschsprung's disease

Vaginal examination is not routine and is only performed when indicated.

Concluding the examination

An examination should also ideally include checking the feet and legs for pitting oedema. This can give clues about respiratory, cardiac or hepatic function.

Urinalysis should also be performed.

INVESTIGATIONS AND IMAGING

OVERVIEW

Investigations are part of patient management, and so a good working knowledge of common tests is essential. However, it is worthwhile remembering that 80% of the diagnosis comes from the history and the remainder from the examination and investigations, so investigations cannot replace clinical skill!

Before requesting investigations, a list of differential diagnoses should have been made. The tests ordered should be relevant to the possible diagnoses, as unnecessary or inappropriate tests waste time and resources.

HINTS AND TIPS

Clinical history taking and examination should always take precedence over investigations. Remember the main function of tests is to confirm or exclude a provisional diagnosis.

ROUTINE HAEMOTOLOGICAL AND BIOCHEMICAL INVESTIGATIONS

A number of simple blood tests are available to confirm (or disprove) diagnoses arrived at from the history and examination.

The results below are particularly relevant to gastrointestinal disease; other texts in the *Crash Course* series should be consulted for other systems.

Haematological tests

These, and their results, are described in Fig. 8.27.

Biochemical tests

Liver function tests (LFTs) are one of the most commonly requested biochemical investigations, and not always because a hepatic cause of disease is suspected—for example, they are also useful when assessing liver function before a certain drug is prescribed. They are discussed in detail below; other biochemical tests concerning the gastrointestinal system are summarized in Fig. 8.28.

The functions of the liver are described in Chapter 6 (see Fig. 6.10). Liver 'function' can be assessed by measurement of serum levels of albumin, bilirubin, urea, glucose and prothrombin time.

Included in the term LFTs are the liver enzymes, i.e. aminotransferases (AST and ALT), alkaline phosphatase and γ-glutamyltransferase (see below). Although these actually give no information about liver function, raised serum levels reflect some degree of damage to the liver.

Routine haematology tests

Parameter	Level	Inference
HB	Low	Dietary iron deficiency, malabsorption, or blood loss (achlorhydia, gastrectomy, coeliac disease)
WCC	Low High	Viral infection (e.g. hepatitis) bacterial infection, colonic inflammation, alcoholic hepatitis, steroids
Platelets	Low High	Portal hypertension and hypersplenism Inflammatory disease (e.g. Crohn's) or chronic GI blood loss
MCV	Low High	Iron deficiency Reticulocytosis (recent bleed), macrocytosis (B_{12} deficiency or alcoholic liver)

Prothrombin time

Prothrombin time is a functional test measuring the interaction between a cascade of clotting factors, all of which are made in the liver. Therefore, if any one of these is abnormal or deficient, the prothrobin time will be prolonged, making it a very sensitive test of synthetic liver function.

Prothrombin time is also increased in vitamin K deficiency as this fat-soluble vitamin is required for activation of factors II, VII, IX and X.

Jaundice due to obstruction will impair absorption of vitamin K so prolonged prothrombin time in obstructive jaundice can be corrected by giving vitamin K. However, in the presence of hepatocellular damage, where synthesis of other clotting factors is affected, vitamin K administration will have no effect.

Hepatic enzyme assays

Aminotransferases (transaminases) are enzymes present in hepatocytes which leak into the plasma in liver cell damage.

Alanine aminotransferase (ALT) is present in the cytoplasm of hepatocytes and its level increases in hepatocellular injury. Aspartate aminotransferase (AST) is a mitochondrial enzyme present not only in the liver but also in cardiac muscle, the kidneys and the brain. Because of this it is less specific than ALT, as conditions affecting these other organs, e.g. myocardial infarction, muscle injury and congestive heart failure, will also cause it to rise.

Alkaline phosphatase is an isoenzyme present in the canalicular and sinusoidal membranes of the liver. It is also present in bone (it is produced by osteoblasts), and less importantly in the intestine and placenta.

Routine biochemistry

Parameter	Level	Inference
Urea	Low High	Malabsorption or liver disease Slightly (up to 14 mmol/L): dehydration (nausea, vomiting, Addison's) Moderate (up to 20 mmol/L): profound dehydration, GI bleed (protein load) Severe (more than 20 mmol/L): renal failure, hepatorenal syndrome
Sodium (Na)	Low	Common in diarrhoea, vomiting, alcoholic liver disease, diuretics
Potassium (K)	Low High	Common in diarrhoea, vomiting, alcoholic liver disease, loop diuretics Possible renal failure, diuretics especially spironolactone
Calcium (Ca)	Low High	Correct for albumin, common in coeliac disease Associated with malignant disease, hyperparathyroidism
Magnesium (Mg)	Low	Commonly in malnutrition, malabsorption, alcoholic diseases
Creatinine	High	Renal failure (all causes)
Glucose	High	Hyperglycaemia can cause abdominal pain, dehydration and acidosis Acute and chronic pancreatitis can lead to high glucose in serum

Levels rise following damage to any of these structures, but in practice a commensurate rise in g-glutamyltransferase is usually taken to indicate hepatic origin. Hepatic alkaline phosphatase is raised in infiltration of the liver, cirrhosis and cholestasis (from both intrahepatic and extrahepatic causes). The highest levels are seen in hepatic metastases and primary biliary cirrhosis.

γ-Glutamyltransferase (γ-GT) is an enzyme present in the mitochondria of many tissues, including the liver. If γ-GT is raised but alkaline phosphatase levels are normal, the cause of the damage is probably alcohol. If both γ-GT and alkaline phosphatase are high, the cause may be cholestasis or intrahepatic malignancy. If the alkaline phosphatase is raised, but the γ-GT is normal, then one should suspect bone disease, e.g. Paget's disease, or pregnancy.

When interpreting the results of liver enzyme assays, patterns of abnormality are important in diagnosis (Fig. 8.29):

- Predominantly raised levels of AST and ALT reflect hepatocellular damage
- Predominantly raised alkaline phosphatase and γ-GT indicate cholestasis or intrahepatic abscess and malignancy.

Fig. 8.29 Elevation of liver enzymes, and their significance. (Reproduced with permission from Fox C, Lombard M. Crash Course: Gastroenterology, 3rd edn. Edinburgh: Mosby, 2008.)

Elevation of liver enzymes	
Liver enzymes	Significance
AST (aspartate aminotranferase)	Very high (thousands) in acute hepatitis or necrosis. Moderate (approx. 500) in chronic active inflammatory disease. Mild (>300) in portal tract damage, focal hepatitis. Also present in muscle (raised in myocardial infarction)
ALT (alanine aminotranferase)	As for AST, but more specific to liverIn alcoholic hepatitis usually less than AST by ratio of 2
Alkaline phosphatase	Highest in cholestatic syndromes (portal tract disease or bile duct obstruction). Remember other sources: bones (especially young), placenta (females), intestine (rare)
Gamma-glutamyl transferase	Very labile enzyme, often mildly elevated. Highest levels in portal tract disease and alcoholics

Liver screen

As there are many causes of liver failure it is sometimes useful to carry out a number of other tests especially if the standard LFTs are deranged. These are shown in Fig. 8.30.

Histology and cytology

Histology is the study of tissue samples taken by biopsy or following surgical removal. The sample may be examined using light microscopy or electron microscopy. Histological examination is useful in cases of malignancy, or in diseases where there are structural changes, e.g. Crohn's disease.

Cytology is the study of cell samples taken by means of swabs or fine-needle aspiration. The cells are stained and examined under a microscope to detect the presence of abnormal, e.g. neoplastic, and inflammatory cells.

Microbiology

Medical microbiology is the study of microorganisms and their effects on humans. Bacteria, viruses, fungi and parasites can cause disease. A typical request to the microbiology laboratory would be for microscopy, culture and (antibiotic) sensitivity. In gastrointestinal disease, samples for microbiological investigation include raw stools and swabs.

Many bacteria, fungi and parasites can be identified using light microscopy, but viruses are too small so other methods such as electron microscopy or serological testing must be employed for their detection. Gram staining of microscopic samples is particularly useful, as it classifies bacteria as being either Gram-positive or Gram-negative, allowing provisional identification.

Culture is a slower method of identification. Some bacteria require certain types of culture medium to grow. It is also useful in deciding which antibiotic is most effective against a particular organism.

A simple sensitivity test involves smearing samples on an agar plate, placing antibiotic discs onto the plate and then incubating it. Small patches of agar on which no bacteria have grown can be seen around those antibiotics that are most effective against the bacteria in question. Other, more sophisticated sensitivity tests are available but are not within the scope of this book.

Breath tests

The general principle of a breath test is that if an enzyme which catalyses a reaction causing the production of gases such as hydrogen or CO_2 is present in the gut lumen, then giving the patient the relevant substrate will cause the gas to be detectable in the patient's breath (Fig. 8.31).This is because the gas is absorbed by diffusion and then exhaled via the lungs.

Fig. 8.30 Table showing the liver screen.

Test	Clinical significance
α_1-antitrypsin	Deficiency of α_1-antitrypsin can produce cirrhosis.
α-fetoprotein	This is raised in patients with hepatocellular carcinoma and in pregnant women. Less elevated levels are found in hepatitis, teratoma and chronic liver disease.
Ferritin	In haemochromatosis, the serum ferritin will be raised due to the increased serum iron, as will transferrin saturation levels. It is most commonly raised in diabetes mellitus, alcoholic liver disease or arthritis but levels >1000 ng/ml need to be investigated further.
Caeruloplasmin	This is relevant if Wilson's disease is suspected. Patients will have low levels of the protein, although occasionally there is no apparent abnormality. Note that any cause of advanced liver failure may cause low caeruloplasmin.
24-hour urinary copper	As with caeruloplasmin, this aids in the diagnosis of Wilson's disease. The urinary excretion rate of copper will be raised.
Viral hepatitis serology for hepatitis A, B and C viruses	This is useful to screen for an infective cause. The presence of anti-viral IgM suggests an acute infection, while the presence of IgG suggests immunity due to past infection or vaccination.
Autoantibody screen	Certain diseases are associated with particular autoantibodies, for example autoimmune hepatitis (anti-smooth muscle and anti-nuclear in type I; anti-liver-kidney-microsomal in type II), primary biliary sclerosis (anti-mitochondrial) and primary sclerosing cholangitis (perinuclear anti-neutrophil cytoplasmic antibodies, p-ANCA).
Glucose, lipids and HbA1c.	To screen for metabolic diseases, e.g. diabetes mellitus which may have symptoms common to liver disease. For instance, acute liver failure can cause hypoglycaemia.

An example of this is the hydrogen breath test, which can be performed after giving the patient a lactulose solution to drink. This can detect an overgrowth of bacteria if there are more than 20 parts per million of hydrogen gas in less than 2 hours. Normally, breath hydrogen is undetectable, hence raised levels suggest bacterial hydrolysis. In a similar way, lactase deficiency can be detected by giving a lactose drink.

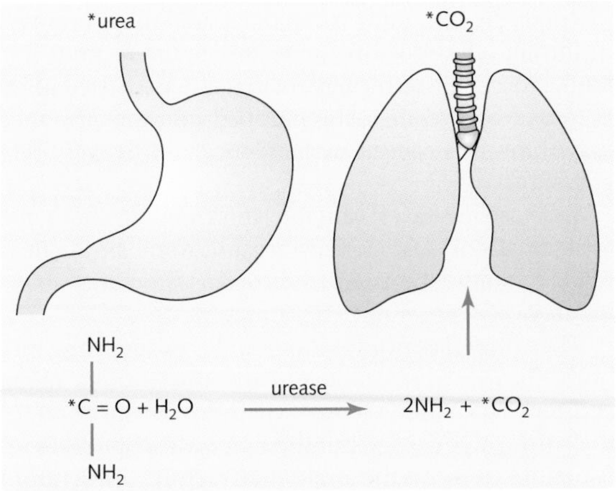

A urea breath test can be performed to confirm the presence of *Helicobacter pylori* in the stomach. This uses 14 C-urea or 13 C-urea isotopes. The *H. pylori* urease enzyme converts the urea to ammonia and radiolabelled CO_2, which is collected in a breath sample. It is a good non-invasive investigation.

Fig. 8.31 The basis of a breath test. The example shown here is the urea breath test for detection of H. pylori, where the bacterial urease splits radiolabelled urea into ammonia and CO_2, the latter of which is detected in the exhaled breath. (Reproduced with permission from Fox C, Lombard M. Crash Course: Gastroenterology, 2nd edn. Edinburgh: Mosby, 2004.)

Oesophageal manometry

Oesophageal manometry measures pressure changes in different parts of the oesophagus and is used to investigate suspected motility disorders.

A fluid-filled continuously perfused catheter is passed through the nose into the oesophagus, in much the same way as a nasogastric tube. Contraction of the oesophagus causes a pressure change that is transmitted up the fluid column and recorded as a trace.

In normal individuals, a pressure wave should pass down the oesophagus to the lower oesophageal sphincter, which then relaxes to allow the oesophageal contents to pass into the stomach. Abnormal traces are seen in motility disorders, e.g. achalasia.

Investigation of gastric function

Refluxed acid may overwhelm the normal protective lining of the oesophagus, leading to ulceration. Suspected reflux may be investigated by measuring the pH in the lower oesophagus over the course of 24 hours with a pH-sensitive probe.

A normal trace shows a pH above 4 for most of the time—if the pH is below 4 for more than 4% of the time significant reflux is said to have occurred.

Disorders of gastric acid secretion may be investigated using the pentagastrin test. The patient fasts overnight and the resting juice in the stomach is aspirated using a nasogastric tube. Pentagastrin, a synthetic analogue of gastrin, is then given (6 mg/kg body weight) to stimulate acid secretion, and gastric contents are again aspirated for 1 hour and analysed.

Generally, a large volume of resting juice suggests gastric stasis, a high acid secretion suggests Zollinger–Ellison syndrome and a failure to stimulate acid secretion with pentagastrin indicates achlorhydria.

Plasma levels of gastrin (a hormone which stimulates gastric acid secretion and growth of the gastric mucosa) may also be measured. The levels of gastrin will be high in the Zollinger–Ellison syndrome as G cells in the pancreas, duodenum or, more rarely, the stomach, secrete large amounts of gastrin in this disorder and cause hyperacidity, leading to ulceration.

ENDOSCOPIC EXAMINATIONS

Endoscopy gives valuable information about the gastrointestinal tract. It allows visualization of the interior of the alimentary tract on a monitor.

Endoscopy can also be used therapeutically for the following:

- Removal of submucosal lesions or polyps (polypectomy, sub-mucosal resection)
- Control of bleeding, e.g. variceal banding or diathermy
- Relief of strictures, e.g. with stents
- Treatment of tumours, e.g. with lasers
- Gallstones in the bile duct (retrieval or sphincterotomy).

Gastroscopy (oesophagogastroduodenoscopy – OGD)

In this procedure, the patient is laid on the left side and the endoscope is passed down the oesophagus. Patients must fast overnight beforehand and the endoscopy is performed as a day-case procedure.

Some patients are given mild sedation (which can cause slight amnesia), but many manage with just an oral local anaesthetic spray.

Gastroscopy is commonly used to investigate upper gastrointestinal disorders. Forceps for taking biopsies can be passed through the biopsy channel of the endoscope.

> **Clinical Note**
>
> Gastroscopy should not be performed in patients with upper gastrointestinal bleeding until the haemorrhage is controlled, and the patient is stabilised as the procedure can increase the severity of the haemorrhage.

Colonoscopy, sigmoidoscopy and proctoscopy

Proctoscopy is commonly performed in out-patients and involves the use of a proctoscope, a rigid tube with a detachable, disposable end that is used for one patient only and then removed and thrown away. Before the proctoscope is used, an obturator is inserted into its lumen to avoid the discomfort of inserting a hollow tube into the patient's anal canal and the end of the instrument is well lubricated.

The patient is then asked to lie on the left side with knees drawn up to the chest; the proctoscope is gently inserted; the obturator is removed; and air is pumped in through the proctoscope to inflate the rectum. It is kinder to explain to the patient that any associated noise is caused by the air being pumped in, otherwise they may think it is caused by flatulence and become very embarrassed!

Proctoscopy gives valuable information about the anal canal and rectum but, because the instrument is rigid, it cannot be used to visualize structures above the flexure.

The fibre sigmoidoscope and colonoscope are both flexible instruments, with the former being shorter. The colonoscope will allow inspection of the entire large bowel, but the sigmoidoscope gives information only on the anal canal, rectum and sigmoid colon.

The procedure in sigmoidoscopy and colonoscopy is similar to proctoscopy. However, bowel preparation, e.g. with sodium picosulphate to clear out the bowel, is required prior to colonoscopy. Patients are given analgesia and may be sedated for the procedure.

Endoscopic ultrasound

Endoscopic ultrasound (EUS) is a relatively new procedure in which an ultrasound image is obtained while performing an endoscopy. It is used to view the ampulla of Vater, as well as the GI tract and the pancreas. The ultrasound transducer is incorporated into the end of the endoscope to produce images alongside the camera image (Fig. 8.32).

Endoscopic retrograde cholangiopancreatography

Endoscopic retrograde cholangiopancreatography (ERCP) involves injection of contrast material into the biliary and pancreatic systems, via endoscopy, followed by radiological screening (Fig. 8.33).

Diathermy instruments and grasping forceps can be passed through the endoscope and used to remove stones in the common bile duct after the sphincter of Oddi has been incised (sphincterotomy). Obstructions in the biliary tree can also be relieved using a stent.

ERCP may introduce infection leading to cholangitis and prophylactic antibiotics are usually given. Pancreatitis may also occur.

Nowadays, EUS or magnetic resonance cholangiopancreatography (MRCP – see below) is used for diagnosis and ERCP is reserved for therapeutic purposes only.

IMAGING OF THE GASTROINTESTINAL SYSTEM

Plain radiography and contrast technique

Substances absorb X-rays to different extents, depending on their atomic number. Those that absorb most appear white, e.g. bone, while those that absorb least, e.g. air, appear black.

Borders are seen only at the interfaces between different densities, e.g. the interface between the wall of the stomach and the gastric air bubble, but may be enhanced by the introduction of contrast media, for example, barium.

When commenting on any X-ray, always follow the same order. Do not come straight out with a diagnosis, evident though it may be!

1. Check that the film has been taken properly and the information recorded on it:
   - Look at the name and the date. Is it the correct patient and the X-ray you want to examine?
   - Is it an AP (anteroposterior) or PA (posteroanterior) film?

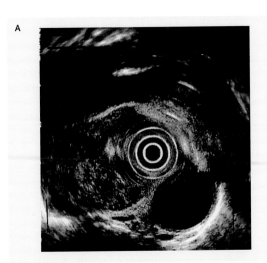

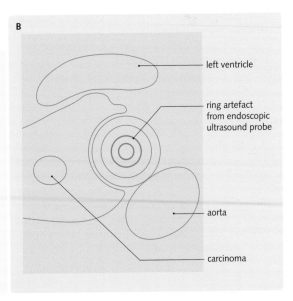

Fig. 8.32 Endoscopic ultrasound image of oesophageal carcinoma (A) and explanatory diagram (B). ([A] Reproduced with permission from Haslett C et al. Davidson's Principles and Practice of Medicine, 19th edn. Edinburgh: Churchill Livingstone, 2002.)

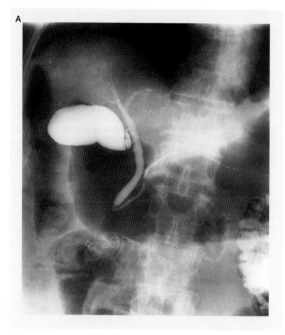

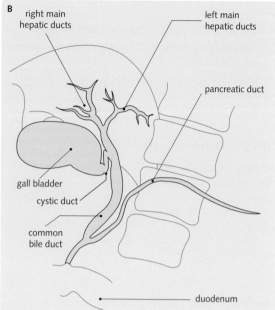

Fig. 8.33 Endoscopic retrograde cholangiopancreatography (ERCP) image showing a normal biliary and pancreatic duct system (A) and explanatory diagram (B). ([A] Reproduced with permission from Haslett C et al. Davidson's Principles and Practice of Medicine, 18th edn. Edinburgh: Churchill Livingstone, 1999.)

- Check the alignment of the spine (or the clavicles on a chest X-ray). Was the patient straight when it was taken? If not, organs may be displaced and look abnormal, even if they are not
2. Check the outlines of all the structures you would expect to see on a normal X-ray. Are they all visible? Can you see anything you would not normally expect? Is any area more (or less) opaque than normal?
3. Describe the gross pathology that might have caused these abnormalities, e.g. stricture in the oesophagus, rose-thorn ulcers in the ileum
4. Suggest the most probable diagnosis and some differential diagnoses.

Abdominal radiographs

Abdominal films may be taken with the patient supine (best for seeing the distribution of gas) or erect (better for spotting air under the diaphragm and for seeing fluid levels).

The intestines are lower down in erect X-rays than in the supine position. Before X-rays became available doctors had seen intestines only in supine bodies at dissections and operations and a number of unfortunate people had completely unnecessary operations to hitch up their guts when erect abdominal X-rays were first taken! Look at the pattern of gas (central in ascites, displaced to the left lower quadrant in splenomegaly). Extraluminal gas in the liver or biliary system suggests

a gas-forming infection or the passing of a stone. In the colonic wall it suggests infective colitis.

Important causes of air under the diaphragm are:

- Perforation of the bowel – this is an emergency and should not be missed
- A section of intestine lying between the liver and the diaphragm
- A gas-forming infection
- A pleuro-peritoneal fistula (tuberculosis, trauma or carcinoma), following surgery or laparoscopy.

Look for opaque areas of calcification, commonly caused by stones (although only 10% of gallstones are radio-opaque), pancreatitis or atherosclerosis.

Fig. 8.34 shows the structures normally visible on plain abdominal X-ray.

Contrast radiographs

These may be single (barium only) or double contrast (e.g. air and barium). Double-contrast films give a better picture of surface mucosa.

Barium may be administered orally and different parts of the gastrointestinal tract can be visualized using this technique depending on the delay before taking the X-ray. A barium enema is often used to visualize the lower gastrointestinal tract (Fig. 8.35). Barium investigations have largely been replaced by contrast CT and endoscopy.

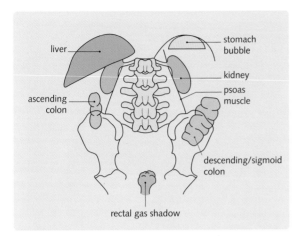

Fig. 8.34 Structures normally visible on plain abdominal X-ray. (Reproduced with permission from Hope RA et al. Oxford Handbook of Clinical Medicine, 3rd edn. Oxford: Oxford University Press, 1993.)

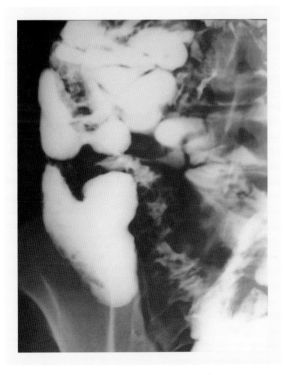

Fig. 8.35 A small bowel barium study in Crohn's disease showing narrowing and distortion of the terminal ileum. (Courtesy of Dr A Grundy, St George's Hospital, London.)

Angiography

Angiography is a form of contrast imaging used to visualize blood vessels. It may show the site of gastrointestinal bleeding (although endoscopy is often the investigation of choice) and the blood supply to specific organs such as the liver (showing architectural abnormalities). It is now rarely used as MR and contrast CT can demonstrate the same detail.

Computerized tomography

Computerized tomography (CT) scanners produce computerized images of the body in a series of slices, based on the amount of X-rays absorbed by different tissues at different angles (Fig. 8.36). They are more effective for imaging soft tissues (including tumours) than radiography, and the level of radiation is generally lower. CT scans may be plain or contrast; contrast is often used to delineate the bowel.

Magnetic resonance imaging

Magnetic resonance imaging (MRI) scanners are large electrical coils that align the nuclei of hydrogen atoms in the body so that they lie parallel to each other (normally they lie in random directions).

The nuclei are then temporarily knocked out of alignment by radio pulses and they emit radio signals as they fall back into alignment. These signals are analysed to produce sliced images of the body, similar to CT scans.

MRI scans are often preferred in pregnancy as they do not use radiation, but they can interfere with pacemakers, hearing aids and other electrical devices.

> **Clinical Note**
>
> In many cases, CT is preferred over MRI, as it is faster, exposes the patient to lower levels of radiation and costs less.

As its name suggests, MRCP (magnetic resonance cholangio-pancreatography) uses a large magnet surrounding the body to detect differences in the electromagnetic characteristics of different body components or fluids. The signals obtained are compiled by computer graphics into very detailed anatomical images which can be used to visualize the common bile duct and pancreatic duct. However, because it is not invasive it cannot be used for therapeutic purposes.

Another related, but also not endoscopic, investigation is percutaneous transhepatic cholangiography, which is an interventional radiological technique. While it can be used for therapeutic interventions, it does not allow the visualization of the ampulla of Vater or pancreatic duct.

Fig. 8.36 Computerized tomography (CT) scan of a renal cyst. The cyst (C) is displacing the pelvicalyceal system (compare with right kidney, K). (L = liver.) (Courtesy of Dr A Grundy, St George's Hospital, London.)

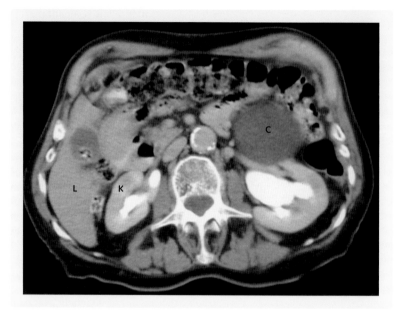

Radioisotope scanning

Radioisotope scanning is used to study the uptake of isotopes by various organs.

Different isotopes are taken up by different organs and structures. 'Hot' lesions are those which take up more isotope than the surrounding tissue, while 'cold' ones take up less.

An example of radioisotope scanning is the use of technetium (^{99m}Tc) colloid to scan the liver and assess gastric emptying. Another is ^{99m}Tc HIDA (hepatic iminodiacetic acid) which is used to scan the biliary tree, as it is taken up by the liver, cleared to the gall bladder and excreted in the bile. Liver lesions greater than 2 cm in diameter show up as cold spots in scanning with ^{99m}Tc colloid.

Ultrasonography

Ultrasonography has been used since the 1970s and is often the investigation of choice for abdominal masses.

Ultrasonographic machines emit very-high-frequency sound waves, which pass readily through fluids, but are reflected back from acoustic interfaces such as soft tissue, bone or gas. The reflected echoes are then analysed to produce images.

Ultrasonographic scans are non-invasive and safe in pregnancy.

Single best answer (SBA) questions

1. A term baby is born with a vitelline duct still present. Her baby check was normal and she was discharged 2 days after birth. She remains well until she attends university at 19 years of age, when she develops colicky abdominal pain. What is the likely cause?
   a. Appendicitis
   b. Meckel's diverticulum
   c. Exomphalos
   d. Gastroschisis
   e. Atresia

2. A 56-year-old man presents to the GP complaining of weight loss of 2 kg over 3 months and lethargy. On further question he reveals that his stools are paler than normal, and his urine dark in colour. He denies being in any pain. On examination his sclerae look yellow. What is the most likely diagnosis?
   a. Gallstones
   b. Acute pancreatitis
   c. Autoimmune hepatitis
   d. Pancreatic cancer
   e. Hepatocellular carcinoma

3. A 78-year-old female is admitted to the surgical assessment unit with severe, sudden onset, abdominal pain for the past 3 days along with bloody diarrhoea for the past 24 hours. She has a past medical history of atrial fibrillation. Bloods are unremarkable apart from an elevated lactate. What is the most likely diagnosis?
   a. Ulcerative colitis
   b. Colorectal carcinoma
   c. Angiodysplasia
   d. Crohn's disease
   e. Ischaemic bowel

4. A 40-year-old gentleman has been suffering from reflux symptoms for 1 year. He drinks approximately 40 units of alcohol a week, and has recently managed to give up smoking. His GP send him for an upper GI endoscopy for further investigation. This looked suspicious for Barrett's Oesophagus so a biopsy was taken. What would you expect the histology to show?
   a. Columnar cells
   b. Squamous cells
   c. Glandular cells
   d. Transitional cells
   e. Connective tissue cells

5. A 52-year-old female attended her local walk-in centre complaining of tiredness. On further questioning she had pruritus. A full panel of blood tests were sent off, and she was informed later in the week that one of the tests had come back positive, for mitochondrial autoantibodies. What is the diagnosis?
   a. Primary biliary cirrhosis
   b. Secondary biliary cirrhosis
   c. Primary sclerosing cholangitis
   d. Autoimmune hepatitis
   e. Wilson's disease

6. A 58-year-old male went to the GP complaining of feeling more tired than usual. He also felt that he had become more 'tanned' throughout the winter months. On examination he had hepatomegaly. What is the diagnosis?
   a. Wilson's disease
   b. Secondary biliary cirrhosis
   c. Iron-deficient anaemia
   d. Vitamin B_{12} deficiency
   e. Haemochromatosis

7. A 10-month old baby was admitted to the children's ward with vomiting. The parents said he seemed generally unwell, crying more than usual and drawing his knees up to his chest. When the nurses changed his nappy they noticed that his stools were loose, and looked redder than normal. What is the diagnosis?
   a. Pyloric stenosis
   b. Gastroenteritis
   c. Intussusception
   d. GORD
   e. Duodenal atresia

8. A 57-year-old alcohol dependant lady presented for the first time to A&E with abdominal pain and a distended abdomen. Examination of the abdomen reveals the presence of spider naevi and shifting dullness evident. She is treated for decompensated alcoholic liver disease. What vitamin should she be given intra-venously?
   a. Vitamin A
   b. Vitamin B_1
   c. Vitamin B_{12}
   d. Vitamin C
   e. Vitamin D

9. A 32-year-old lady with type 1 diabetes went to the see her GP complaining of a 10-day history of pain when swallowing both fluid and liquids. She had recently completed a course of antibiotics for a urinary tract infection. She has been referred for an OGD. What is this most likely to show?
   a. Scleroderma
   b. Oesophageal carcinoma
   c. Achalasia

d. Oesophageal candidiasis
e. Benign oesophageal stricture

10. A 50-year-old male attended A&E with large volume haematemesis. On examination he has gynaecomastia and spider naevi. PR examination revealed black stool. What is the most likely cause of his upper GI bleed
    a. Oesophageal varices
    b. Oesophagitis
    c. Mallory-Weiss tear
    d. Duodenal ulcer
    e. Gastric carcinoma

11. A 21-year-old female presents to the hospital with sudden onset acute abdominal pain. On examination she is tender in the right iliac fossa with guarding. She has tachycardia and is hypotensive. What would be your initial management?
    a. Abdominal X-ray
    b. Pregnancy test
    c. IV fluids
    d. Urine dipstick
    e. Abdominal ultrasound

12. A 46-year-old female presents with to A&E with severe upper abdominal pain. On examination she is tender in the left upper quadrant and her sclera look jaundiced. Her temperature is 38.2°C. Her bloods showed a raised alkaline phosphatise and bilirubin. What is the most likely diagnosis?
    a. Liver abscess
    b. Gallstone ileus
    c. Appendicitis
    d. Viral hepatitis
    e. Cholangitis

13. A patient is brought into hospital after having a witnessed seizure lasting 2 minutes. He is known to have hepatic cirrhosis, and has become confused and disorientated over the past few days. On examination he has a coarse flap with outstretched hands. What is the most likely diagnosis?
    a. Hyponatraemia
    b. Hepatic encephalopathy
    c. Carbon dioxide retention
    d. Epilepsy
    e. Illicit drug use

14. A 21-year-old male, who had been feeling unwell with flu-like symptoms for the past week went to see the GP as his eyes looked yellow. Routine bloods showed a bilirubin of 68 µmol/L, however the rest of his liver function tests were normal. What is the most likely diagnosis
    a. Viral hepatitis
    b. Rotor syndrome
    c. Gilberts syndrome
    d. Dubin–Johnson syndrome
    e. Gallstones

15. A 23-year-old medical student organises her elective in India. Whilst there she develops fever, diarrhoea and abdominal cramps. The symptoms persist for a week, before she visits a doctor for some advice. What is the most likely cause?
    a. Giardiasis
    b. Hepatitis A
    c. Salmonellosis
    d. Yersiniosis
    e. Rotavirus

16. A 68-year-old male was referred for an urgent clinic appointment after a change in bowel habit. Colonoscopy and biopsy confirmed colorectal adenocarcinoma which was resected. Histology showed spread to the muscle layer and bowel wall, without any involvement of lymph nodes. What Dukes staging is this?
    a. Dukes A
    b. Dukes B
    c. Dukes C1
    d. Dukes C2
    e. Dukes D

17. A 51-year-old male had been been diagnosed last year with chronic respiratory disease, which was fairly severe and affected his mobility. This had come as a shock as he had never previously smoked. His liver function tests had previously been mildly deranged. He went to see his GP as he looked more yellow than normal. What is the most likely cause?
    a. Gilbert's syndrome
    b. Mirizzi's syndrome
    c. Haemochromatosis
    d. Alpha-1-antitrypsin deficiency
    e. Alcoholic hepatitis

18. A 67-year-old lady presents with weight loss of 3 kg over 4 months and intermittent abdominal pain. Examination is unremarkable apart from an enlarged supraclavicular lymph node on the left side of the body. What is the most likely diagnosis?
    a. Cholangiocarcinoma
    b. Pancreatic cancer
    c. Sigmoid cancer
    d. Hepatocellular carcinoma
    e. Gastric cancer

19. A 17-year-old female presents to the GP complaining of feeling tired all the time. On further questioning she admits to having heavy periods. Routine blood tests are done which show a Hb of 7.9 g/dL, and a MCV of 72.6. What would the likely management plan be?
    a. Vitamin B_{12} injections
    b. Thiamine tablets
    c. Iron tablets
    d. Vitamin C supplements
    e. Folate supplements

20. A 71-year-old male presents to the GP with weight loss, lethargy and decreased appetite over the past 6 months. The GP organises for bloods to be taken and requests tumour markers. AFP comes back elevated at 58 g/L. What is this suggestive of?

a. Hepatocellular carcinoma
b. Cholangiocarcinoma
c. Ampullary adenoma
d. Colorectal cancer
e. Pancreatic cancer

21. A 21-year-old female presented to A&E complaining of vomiting blood. She had been out the previous night and drank copious amounts of alcohol, and had been vomiting several times throughout the day. Examination was unremarkable, and there was no evidence of black stools. A nurse witnessed a vomit and reported that there were just small amount of red streaks in it. What is the most likely diagnosis?
a. Alcoholic hepatitis
b. Acute gastritis
c. Gastric ulcer
d. Oesophageal varices
e. Mallory–Weiss tear

22. A 23-year-old university student presented with general flu-like symptoms for 2 weeks including a sore throat. On examination she has enlarged cervical lymph nodes. Routine blood tests show, bilirubin 27 μmol/L, ALT 494 IU/L, GGT 62 IU/L, WCC 13.3, lymphocytes 6.0. What is the likely cause of the raised liver enzymes?
a. Gilbert's syndrome
b. Gallstone
c. Viral illness
d. Autoimmune hepatitis
e. Acute pancreatitis

23. A 50-year-old male was being treated on a surgical assessment ward for acute pancreatitis. His initial GLASGOW score was 2. On ward round, 7 days after admission the consultant requested an investigation to look for any evidence of pancreatic necrosis. What is the imaging used normally?
a. MRI abdomen
b. USS abdomen
c. Abdominal X-ray
d. CT abdomen
e. EUS

24. A 70-year-old male presented with central intermittent abdominal pain for the past 3 weeks. On examination he had mild epigastric tenderness without any signs of peritonitis. He is a known heavy smoker and mentioned he had recently had an USS scan done on his neck as an investigation for dizzy spells. What is the most likely cause?
a. Mesenteric ischaemia
b. Chronic pancreatitis
c. Duodenal ulcer
d. Gastric carcinoma
e. Appendicitis

25. A 47-year-old female presents with severe intermittent abdominal pain over the last 2 months. She has had multiple previous admissions with acute pancreatitis.

Her most recent CT scan showed calcified deposits in the pancreas. She denies any alcohol intake for the past 6 months. What is the most likely diagnosis?
a. Acute pancreatitis
b. Chronic pancreatitis
c. Mesenteric ischaemia
d. Pancreatic cancer
e. Gastric ulcer

26. A 5-week-old baby was brought into A&E vomiting. The mother reported a 3-day history of vomiting large amounts following every feed. The baby was born at 39 weeks without any complications and had been putting weight on well post birth. On examination the doctor could palpate a sausage-shaped mass in the right upper quadrant. What is the most likely diagnosis?
a. Pyloric stenosis
b. Neonatal jaundice
c. Duodenal atresia
d. Diaphragmatic hernia
e. Acute gastritis

27. A 24-year-old male was referred for a colonoscopy to investigate his symptoms of weight loss and diarrhoea. The endoscopist thought that they could view skip lesions in the terminal ileum and took several biopsies. What is the histology most likely to show?
a. Ulcerative colitis
b. Coeliac disease
c. Irritable bowel syndrome
d. Crohn's disease
e. Bacterial enterocolitis

28. A 16-year-old female attends the GP surgery to ask for some advice. She suffers from severe travel sickness. The GP prescribes an anti-emetic. Which one is likely to be the most effective?
a. Levomepromazine
b. Ondansetron
c. Metoclopramide
d. Domperidone
e. Cyclizine

29. A 67-year-old male noticed a swelling in the right groin region that appears to 'come and go'. On examination there is a reducible 2 x 2 cm mass that appears to lie inferior to the inferior gastric vessels. What hernia is this most likely to be?
a. Incisional hernia
b. Direct inguinal hernia
c. Indirect inguinal hernia
d. Femoral hernia
e. Umbilical hernia

30. A 32-year-old male presented with abdominal pain and vomiting. He described the pain as a sudden onset, severe pain which radiates through to his back. He had an ultrasound earlier this year which showed gallstones. You suspect acute pancreatitis. What investigation is used to confirm this?
a. Arterial blood gases

b. U&Es
c. Serum amylase
d. Abdominal X-ray
e. CT abdomen

31. A 38-year-old male visits his GP complaining of intermittent abdominal pain. This is epigastric in nature and radiates through to the back. It is more severe before meal times and relieved by eating. A C14 breath test is arranged which comes back positive. What is the most likely diagnosis?
a. Duodenal ulcer
b. GORD
c. Barrett's oesophagus
d. Achalasia
e. Gastric ulcer

32. A 56-year-old woman is having an OGD to investigate her symptoms of dysphagia. The endoscopist can see a lesion in the distal oesophagus and takes a needle biopsy to send for histology. What is the first layer that the needle would go through?
a. Submucosa
b. Circular smooth muscle
c. Serosa
d. Mucosa
e. Longitudinal smooth muscle

33. A 41-year-old woman visits the GP complaining of a sore mouth. On examination her tongue is very tender, and she feels that it has changed colour slightly. She was recently started on vitamin B_{12} injections for pernicious anaemia. What is the likely cause?
a. Candidiasis
b. Herpes simplex virus
c. Glossitis
d. Sialadenitis
e. Carcinoma of the tongue

34. The defence system of the small intestine comprises of T and B lymphocytes. B lymphocytes are responsible for producing antibodies which act in the gut lumen. Which is the main antibody that is produced?
a. IgG
b. IgA
c. IgM
d. IgE
e. IgD

35. A patient had been in hospital for several weeks following a car crash. Whilst in he developed offensive-smelling diarrhoea, passing at least six motions a day. He had a stool sample sent off which confirmed *Clostridium difficile*. Which of the following antibiotics is considered high risk for developing pseudomembanous colitis?
a. Cefotaxime
b. Vancomycin
c. Flucloxacillin
d. Doxycycline
e. Ciprofloxacin

36. A 32-year-old male of Asian origin presents with weight loss, diarrhoea and stools that are difficult to flush away. He had a colonoscopy, and a biopsy later confirmed villous atrophy. He was started on a gluten free diet; however his symptoms failed to improve. What is the most likely diagnosis?
a. Tropical sprue
b. Coeliac disease
c. Chronic pancreatitis
d. Crohn's disease
e. Irritable bowel syndrome

37. A 46-year-old female presented to the GP with a change in bowel habit for the past 2 months. She is having looser stools than normal with blood mixed in with the stools. There is no history of any abdominal pain. What would be your first choice investigation?
a. Abdominal X-ray
b. Faecal occult blood
c. Abdominal CT
d. Ultrasound abdomen
e. Colonoscopy

38. A 58-year-old male, who has a long past medical history of achalasia, presents with symptoms of weight loss and worsening dysphagia. He is referred for an urgent OGD, which shows a lesion in the upper third of the oesophagus suspicious for oesophageal cancer. What is the likely histological type to be shown on biopsy?
a. Adenocarcinoma
b. Lymphoma
c. Small cell carcinoma
d. Squamous cell carcinoma
e. Melanoma

39. A 70-year-old male has pancreatic cancer. He has been recently started on strong opioids to control his pain. He is visited by the palliative care nurses and complains of difficulty in opening his bowels, stating that his stools are much harder than they used to be. What is the most appropriate laxative to put him on?
a. Lactulose
b. Sodium docusate
c. Fybogel
d. Movicol
e. Senna

40. A 68-year-old woman presents to the GP feeling lethargic and more breathless than usual. Routine bloods are taken which show a HB of 8.1 g/dL and a MCV of 107.3. What is the most likely cause of her anaemia?
a. Iron-deficiency anaemia
b. Anaemia of chronic disease
c. Pernicious anaemia
d. Haemolytic anaemia
e. Thalassaemia

Extended matching questions (EMQs)

For each scenario described below, choose the most likely corresponding option from the list given. Each option may be used once, more than once, or not at all.

1. Diarrhoea

A. Ulcerative colitis
B. Colon cancer
C. Gastroenteritis
D. Giardiasis
E. Crohn's disease
F. Coeliac disease
G. Pseudomembranous colitis
H. Thyrotoxicosis
I. Irritable bowel syndrome

1. A 25-year-old male gives a history of diarrhoea for 1 week. He has no associated abdominal pain, vomiting or rectal bleeding. Past medical history reveals he was treated with antibiotics by his GP 2 weeks ago for a skin infection. Standard stool culture is negative.
2. A 72-year-old gentleman visits the GP complaining of weight loss, and opening his bowels more frequently, up to four times a day. He has no abdominal pain or PR bleeding, but on examination he is noted to look pale.
3. A 23-year-old woman has been seen by the GP on two occasions over the last 5 years complaining of loose stool, with intermittent lower abdominal pain, which she describes as cramps. She stopped smoking 3 months ago, and feels that her symptoms are getting worse, and has also noticed some blood mixed in with her stools.
4. A 24-year-old woman gives a 10-year history of intermittent lower abdominal pain and loose stools. She denies any PR bleeding, although suggests that her symptoms often correspond to when she feels under stress at work.
5. A 67-year-old woman visits the GP having had diarrhoea for 3 months. She denies any abdominal pain but admits to loosing 1 stone in weight recently although denies eating any less than usual. She is concerned as her brother has been recently diagnosed with bowel cancer. On examination it is noted that her pulse is irregular.

2. Vomiting

A. Gastric cancer
B. Acute gastritis
C. Small bowel obstruction
D. Peptic ulcer disease
E. Hypercalcaemia
F. Rotavirus infection
G. Autonomic neuropathy
H. Acute pancreatitis
I. *Salmonella* infection

1. An 82-year-old man with metastatic prostate cancer is admitted to hospital with 'general deterioration'. He has been vomiting over the past week, is constipated, more fatigued than normal and has some non-specific abdominal pain. CT scan picks up some renal stones.
2. A 58-year-old woman presents to A&E with vomiting for the past 48 hours. She has associated epigastric pain, which is colicky in nature. Further questioning reveals she has not opened her bowels for 4 days, and past medical history reveals she underwent a laparotomy 10 years ago. Her abdomen is very distended and tender.
3. Passengers on a cruise ship have been quarantined after there has been an outbreak of vomiting on board among staff and passengers. The illness is self-limiting, and after a few days of boarding, and a deep clean the ship is able to continue its journey.
4. A 65-year-old male with type 2 diabetes is admitted to hospital on four separate occasions over the past year with vomiting. Each time, he is discharged after 5–7 days once the episode has settled. OGD was essentially normal. Full examination reveals a painless ulcer on his right foot.
5. A 34-year-old lady attends her local walk-in centre after vomiting several times over the day. She has some associated abdominal pain, and nothing abnormal was found on examination. She mentioned that she had eaten a takeaway last night.

3. Acute abdominal pain

A. Appendicitis
B. Diverticulitis
C. Gastric ulcer
D. Acute pancreatitis
E. Crohn's disease
F. Ectopic pregnancy
G. Bowel Obstruction

H. Cholecystitis

I. Duodenal ulcer

1. A 26-year-old woman presents with a 4-hour history of severe, sudden onset right iliac fossa pain. On examination she looks unwell, her blood pressure is 79/48 and she is very tender, with guarding on palpation of the right iliac fossa

2. A 44-year-old male is brought into A&E with severe upper abdominal pain worsening over the past 24 hours. He has also been vomiting. On examination he is tachcardic, hypotensive, and is abdomen is generally very tender. His wife informs you that a recent scan showed gallstones.

3. A 65-year-old male presented with colicky abdominal pain with associated vomiting for the past 3 days. On examination the abdomen was distended, tympanic and tender. Auscultation revealed tinkling bowel sounds.

4. A 31-year-old female is seen by the GP with a 1-month history of epigastric pain. He describes a dull aching pain that wakes hip up from sleep, but then tends to improve throughout the day.

5. A 73-year-old woman is admitted with left lower quadrant pain, which is colicky in nature. She has a fever and on examination she has mild left iliac fossa tenderness. Her bloods show a raised WCC.

4. Chronic abdominal pain

A. Gastric cancer

B. Chronic pancreatitis

C. Peptic ulcer disease

D. Crohn's disease

E. Irritable bowel syndrome

F. Chronic cholecystitis

G. Mesenteric ischaemia

H. Pancreatic carcinoma

I. Crohn's disease

1. A 51-year-old lady has been having intermittent abdominal pain for several months, mainly in the right upper quadrant. She gets approximately one episode a week, which is associated with nausea. Examination is unremarkable. Bloods show a mild nutrophilia and an elevated CRP.

2. A 58-year-old male has been having intermittent abdominal pain, with each episode lasting between 5–10 days. He describes central pain, which radiates to his back and pale offensive smelling stools which are difficult to flush away. Blood tests show a raised GGT.

3. A 49-year-old male complains of a 6-month history of epigastric pain. His GP has prescribed him a proton pump inhibitor, but he doesn't feel that this has helped his pain. He also mentions he is more fatigued than usual, and feels that he has lost some weight.

4. A 26-year-old female has a 2-year history of intermittent episodes of right-sided abdominal pain accompanied by loose stools. She also describes weight loss and lethargy. Examination is unremarkable. She admits to her GP that she is concerned her symptoms are getting worse.

5. A 71-year-old male has been having upper abdominal pain that radiates through to his back for 6 weeks. There has been no associated vomiting or change in bowel habit. His appetite is less than normal, and his wife is concerned that he has recently lost 2 stone in weight.

5. Dysphagia

A. Oesophageal candidiasis

B. Barrett's oesophagus

C. Achalasia

D. Oesophageal web

E. Oesophageal carcinoma

F. Oesophageal stricture

G. Scleroderma

H. Oesophageal dysmotility

I. Presence of a foreign body

1. A 56-year-old woman presents with difficulty swallowing over the past few months. Further questioning reveals that she feels more tired than usual, but there is no history of recent weight loss. A full blood count shows a low HB, and a low MCV.

2. A 43-year-old male who has a long history of gastro-oesophageal reflux disease presents with difficulty swallowing. The rest of the history and examination were unremarkable. There is no history of weight loss.

3. A 31-year-old female with intermittent history of swallowing difficulties, occurring with both solids and liquids. She also mentions that she has been admitted to A&E earlier on in the year with an episode of central chest pain. She was reassured that nothing was wrong with her heart, and discharged.

4. A 69-year-old male attends his GP with difficulties swallowing. Originally he was having problems with solid food, but now he is struggling with a soft diet too. He has lost 3 stone in weight over the past few months, but attributes this to his change in diet.

5. A women undergoing chemotherapy for breast cancer, presents with a 1-week history of a sore throat with pain on swallowing. She says that food doesn't taste right to her.

6. Jaundice

A. Alpha-1-antitrypsin deficiency

B. Primary biliary cirrhosis

C. Gallstones

D. Pancreatic cancer

E. Alcoholic hepatitis

F. Gilbert's syndrome

G. Sclerosing cholangitis

H. Epstein–Barr virus

I. Hepatitis A

1. A university student was admitted to hospital after a friend noticed that he looked jaundiced. He otherwise felt well, apart from some coryzal symptoms. On examination he was obviously jaundiced, had a temperature of 38° C, and had some palpable cervical lymph nodes and tender hepatomegaly. The LFTs are elevated and atypical lymphocytes appear on the blood film.

2. A 67-year-old male has noticed that he's gotten progressively more yellow over the past month. He denies any abdominal pain, but feels he may have lost weight over the past few weeks. Examination was unremarkable, with no signs of hepatomegaly. Abdominal ultrasound showed a dilated biliary tree.

3. A 35-year-old female presented to his GP with jaundice, which had been getting worse over the last 2 weeks. He otherwise felt well apart from some intermittent right upper quandrant pain. He has a past medical history of ulcerative colitis, for which he takes mesalazine. Bilirubin was 63, and alkaline phosphatise was also elevated. The other liver enzymes are normal.

4. A 42-year-old man is admitted with jaundice and confusion. He is unable to give a history, is clearly jaundiced, and has a coarse tremor in his hands on examination. His initial full blood count shows a HB of 8.2, and a MCV of 104.3.

5. A 26-year-old lady presents with right upper quadrant pain and jaundice. On further questioning she reveals that she has pale stools and dark urine. On examination she is tender in the right upper quadrant.

SBA answers

1. **b.** Meckel's diverticulum
   Meckel's diverticulum is the remnant of the vitelline duct present in embryonic life. It connects the developing embryo with the yolk sac. It is often asymptomatic, however acute inflammation of the diverticulum may occur, mimicking acute appendicitis. The mucosa at the mouth of the diverticulum may become inflamed and lead to intussusceptions and obstruction, or the diverticulum may perforate and cause peritonitis.

2. **d.** Pancreatic cancer
   The most likely diagnosis here is carcinoma of the head of the pancreas. The tumour obstructs the common bile duct causing jaundice and dark urine because of conjugated hyperbilirubinaemia. The faeces are pale due to a lack of stercobilinogen. Painless jaundice is typically the presenting feature of carcinoma of the head of the pancreas, along with weight loss.

3. **e.** Ischaemic bowel
   Ischaemic bowel is difficult to diagnose and commonly missed. It usually presents as abdominal pain out of proportion to clinical findings and investigations, and is often a diagnosis of exclusion; however the presence of metabolic acidosis helps. It rarely occurs in patients less than 60 years old. CT angiogram is the investigation of choice.

4. **a.** Columnar cells
   Barrett's oesophagus is when prolonged injury results in the normal squamous epithelium of the lower oesophagus being replaced by columnar epithelium. This metaplastic change may be followed by dysplastic change, which predisposes to malignant transformation. The majority of patients present with a long history of reflux.

5. **a.** Primary biliary cirrhosis
   Primary biliary cirrhosis (PBC) is an autoimmune disorder and predominantly affects women, especially those 40–50 years of age, more than men. All patients with PBC have antimitochondrial autoantibodies and this, together with raised serum alkaline phosphatase, is diagnostic for the condition. Patients often present with pruritus and fatigue, and jaundice can be present at a later stage: some patients have xanthelasma.

6. **e.** Haemochromatosis
   Primary haemochromatosis is an autosomal recessive disorder characterized by the absorption of too much iron, which then accumulates (as haemosiderin) in the liver, pancreas, heart, pituitary and joints. The commonest presentation is an incidental finding of abnormal liver enzymes or raised ferritin level. Symptoms are rare in women of child-bearing age as menstrual losses and pregnancy compensate for the excess iron absorption. Symptomatic presentation in males is usually in the fourth or fifth decade and can be obscure such as loss of libido and hypogonadism, secondary to dysfunction of the pituitary gland or can include diabetes mellitus or arthritis.

7. **c.** Intussusception
   Intussusception occurs when one segment of bowel slides inside the adjacent segment, like a telescope. The most common site is at the ileocaecal valve. Patients typically present aged 5–12 months of age, with periods of screaming, vomiting, blood in the faeces ('redcurrant jelly') and drawing up of the legs. The child is pale and a sausage-shaped mass may be felt on palpation of the abdomen.

8. **b.** Vitamin B_1
   Vitamin B_1 is also known as thiamine. Thiamine deficiency is very common in people who drink excess alcohol due to several factors. These patients generally have a poor oral diet, and thiamine is also a coenzyme in alcohol metabolism. It is essential that it is given quickly in patients who have decompensated liver failure as thiamine deficiency can lead to Wernicke's encephalopathy. It is always given intravenously in the acute presentation as it is poorly absorbed orally in people who are alcohol-dependent.

9. **d.** Oesophageal candidasis
   Patients with diabetes are more prone to getting candidiasis, as high sugar levels lead to better conditions for the yeast to grow. It is also only a short 10-day history which also favours candidiasis over some of the more chronic conditions listed.

10. **a.** Oesophageal varices

The examination findings here show evidence of liver disease. This helps point to the diagnosis of oesophageal varices as the cause of the upper gastrointestinal bleed. In patients with cirrhosis of the liver and portal hypertension the raised pressure in the portal system causes the site of a connection between the systemic and portal venous systems to open up and enlarge. The enlarged veins protrude into the lumen of the lower oesophagus and may burst, resulting in haematemesis. A man with this history could also be prone to a Mallory–Weiss tear without varices but usually there would be a history of retching or vomiting before blood appears. The diagnoses rarely cause large volume haematemesis.

11. **c.** IV fluids

There is clinical evidence of shock with the patient being tachycardic and hypotensive, so the initial management should be resuscitation with IV fluids. All of the other investigations are relevant, and should be done once the patient is haemodynamically stable.

12. **e.** Cholangitis

The triad of symptoms which includes fever, abdominal pain and jaundice are typical in cholangitis. Cholangitis occurs when gallstones become impacted in the bile duct; the bile which is unable to escape becomes concentrated and infected, resulting in acute cholecystitis. This causes a rise in the LFTs, particularly bilirubin and alkaline phosphatase. The other diseases do not cause jaundice with pain.

13. **b.** Hepatic encephalopathy

Hepatic encephalopathy is a neurological disorder caused by metabolic failure of the hepatocytes and the shunting of blood around the liver (due to cirrhosis or after portocaval anastomosis). It may occur in both chronic and acute liver failure, and results in the exposure of the brain to abnormal metabolites, causing oedema and astrocyte changes. Symptoms include disturbances in consciousness (ranging from confusion to coma and death), asterixis (coarse flap of outstretched hand) and fluctuating neurological signs including seizures, muscular rigidity and hyperreflexia.

14. **c.** Gilbert's syndrome

The isolated rise in the bilirubin within the liver function tests is suggestive of Gilbert's syndrome. This is a congenital disorder caused by patients having a reduced amount of the enzyme UDP-glucuronyl transferase (UGT-1), which conjugates bilirubin with glucuronic acid. There is only a slight increase in serum bilirubin (unconjugated), often after prolonged starvation or intercurrent illness. The syndrome is asymptomatic, although some patients complain of fatigue.

15. **a.** Giardiasis

Giardiasis, prevalent in the tropics, is an important cause of traveller's diarrhoea. It is caused by the flagellate protozoan *Giardia lamblia*, which lives in the duodenum and jejunum and is transmitted by the faecal–oral route. Patients may be asymptomatic, or alternatively, symptoms of diarrhoea, malabsorption and abdominal pain or bloating may develop within 1 or 2 {ts}weeks of ingesting cysts. Diagnosis is by stool microscopy, and treatment is with metronidazole. Hepatitis A can also be picked up when travelling abroad, however this is usually asymptomatic, or presents as fever, jaundice and malaise.

16. **b.** Dukes B

Dukes' classification is most widely used to stage, and predict the prognosis of colorectal carcinoma. Dukes' stages are:

Stage A: invaded submucosa and muscle layer of the bowel, but confined to the wall.

Stage B: breached the muscle layer and bowel wall, but no involvement of lymph nodes.

Stage C1: spread to immediately draining pericolic lymph nodes.

Stage C2: spread to higher mesenteric lymph nodes.

Stage D: distant visceral metastases.

17. **d.** Alpha-1-antitrypsin deficiency

The history here of both COPD and derranged liver function test is suggestive of α_1-antitrypsin deficiency. α_1-Antitrypsin is a serum protein that is produced in the liver and has antiprotease effects. One in ten northern Europeans carries a deficiency gene, which is autosomal recessive in inheritance. Symptoms include basal emphysema in about 75% of homozygotes and liver cirrhosis in approximately 10%. Heterozygotes have an increased risk of developing emphysema if they smoke. None of the other diagnoses given have a link with respiratory disease.

18. **e.** Gastric cancer

An enlarged supraclavicular lymph node of the left side of the body is also known as Virchow's node. This is highly suggestive of carcinoma of the stomach. Patients with a palpable Virchow's node should be referred for an OGD for further investigation.

19. c. Iron tablets

The low haemoglobin and low MCV suggests microcytic anaemia. In females of menstrual age the most common cause of this is iron-deficiency anaemia caused by menorrhagia, sometimes on a background of an iron-deficient diet. Patients should have further bloods sent off for iron studies to confirm the diagnosis, and then be started on iron tablets such as ferrous sulphate if appropriate. If patients had either vitamin B_{12} or folate deficiency, then the MCV should be high.

20. a. Hepatocellular carcinoma

A raised AFP is associated with hepatocellular carcinoma. In younger males a raised AFP, along with a raised β-HCG is also indicative of germ cell tumours. However, with hepatocellular carcinoma often the rest of the LFTS are deranged as well.

21. e. Mallory–Weiss tear

A Mallory–Weiss tear is a tear at the gastro-oesophageal junction. It is caused by prolonged retching or coughing and a sudden increase in intra-abdominal pressure. It is most common in alcoholics and presents as haematemesis. All of the other answers can cause an upper gastrointestinal bleed, however the history given of prolonged vomiting preceding haematemesis is suggestive of a Mallory–Weiss tear.

22. c. Viral illness

The raised WCC and raised lymphocyte count is suggestive of an acute viral illness, whilst the rise in the LFTs, in particular the transaminases, suggests a hepatitis type of picture. There are several causes of a viral hepatitis which include Epstein–Barr virus, hepatitis A, drugs such as antibiotics and alcohol. Further investigations to determine the exact cause would be required. Generally the treatment would be supportive.

23. d. CT abdomen

When acute pancreatitis is diagnosed, the focus should be on the acute management. Once the patient has recovered from the initial attack, they require further imaging to assess if there has been any damage to the pancreas. In particular, the consultant is looking for any evidence of pancreatic necrosis. CT scan is the most appropriate investigation in order to view the pancreas properly and any soft tissue damage. CT is normally done prior to an MRI due to the lower cost and the lower levels of radiation to the patient.

24. a. Mesenteric ischaemia

The key to diagnosis here is in the history. The neck USS is likely to be a carotid Doppler scan, suggesting there may be a history of ischaemia. Smoking is also considered a risk factor for this. Mesenteric ischaemia generally only affects people over 50 years of age and is associated with conditions causing arterial emboli and thrombosis. It presents as a colicky poorly localized pain with minimal tenderness in the early stages, leading eventually to signs and symptoms of peritonitis.

25. b. Chronic pancreatitis

Chronic pancreatitis is an on-going inflammation of the pancreas accompanied by irreversible architectural changes. Alcohol consumption causes more than 85% of cases, and is the most common cause of pancreatitis in developed countries. High-fat and -protein diets amplify the damage done by alcohol. Other causes include: idiopathic chronic pancreatitis; trauma and scar formation, leading to the obstruction of the main pancreatic duct; previous episodes of acute pancreatitis predispose to others although they may often be subclinical; cystic fibrosis resulting in protein plugs in the duct system; hereditary forms of pancreatitis. Patients normally present with a history of prolonged ill-health with chronic epigastric pain, usually radiating through to the back.

26. a. Pyloric stenosis

Pyloric stenosis, or narrowing, occurs in about 1 in 150 male infants and 1 in 750 female infants. Stenosis is caused by hypertrophy of the circular muscles of the pylorus, obstructing the pyloric canal and the flow of contents from the stomach into the duodenum. Typically, it presents 4–6 weeks after birth with projectile vomiting within half an hour of a feed. Note that there is no bile in the vomit because the obstruction is proximal to the ampulla of Vater. Peristaltic waves are visible in the child, a sausage-shaped mass (the enlarged pylorus) can be felt in the right upper quadrant and the hypertrophied pyloric muscle can be observed using ultrasonography. Treatment is surgical.

27. d. Crohn's disease

In a young adult, the history of diarrhoea and weight loss should be investigated by a colonoscopy to look for inflammatory bowel disease. The presence of skip lesions in the colon indicates that Crohn's is the most likely diagnosis. Crohn's disease may affect any part of the gastrointestinal tract from the mouth to the anus. Endoscopy usually shows skip lesions and deep ulcers and fissures in the mucosa. Ulcerative colitis usually starts in the rectum and it may extend proximally, although never beyond the colon. Unlike Crohn's, which commonly shows skip lesions, ulcerative colitis is continuous. Areas of normal gut are not found between lesions.

28. **e.** Cyclizine

Cyclizine is an antiemetic from the H1-receptor antagonist class. These are effective against motion sickness, as these receptors are found in the vestibular nuclei, and against vomiting caused by substances acting in the stomach

29. **b.** Direct inguinal hernia

A hernia is the protrusion of any organ or tissue through its coverings and outside its normal body cavity. If reducible, hernias can be pushed back into the compartment from which they came from. Inguinal hernias are the most common site and may be direct (protruding through the posterior wall of the inguinal canal), or indirect (passing through the inguinal canal). Indirect hernias are much more common, and lie lateral to the inferior epigastric vessels. Direct inguinal hernias are less common and they lie medial to the inferior epigastric vessels.

30. **c.** Serum amylase

Diagnosis of acute pancreatitis is by measurement of serum amylase. It is normally greatly elevated (five times or more) in acute pancreatitis. The rest of the investigations are relevant once acute pancreatitis has been diagnosed. The U&Es and arterial blood gases should be done in order to ascertain the severity of the disease, by using the Glasgow criteria. Abdominal X-ray may show an absent psoas shadow and an air-filled dilatation of the proximal jejunum. CT is typically done after the acute event to assess the degree of damage to the pancreas.

31. **a.** Duodenal ulcer

The positive C14 breath test is indicative of the presence of *H. pylori*, which is closely associated with peptic ulcer disease. The history given means the diagnosis is most likely to be a duodenal ulcer. With duodenal ulcers, classically the epigastric pain is said to be relieved by food or antacids, and exacerbated by hunger. The epigastric pain with gastric ulcers is characteristically associated with food.

32. **d.** Mucosa

The gastrointestinal tract maintains the same basic structure throughout its length. From the innermost to the outermost, the layers which comprise the basic structure are the mucosa (composed of the epithelial layer, lamina propria and muscularis mucosae), submucosa, two smooth layers (the inner is circular, and the outer longitudinal) and finally the serosa.

33. **c.** Glossitis

Glossitis is inflammation of the tongue. It may occur in anaemia and certain other deficiency states, most notably vitamin B_{12} deficiency. The most common symptoms are difficulty with chewing and swallowing foods, tender tongue, smooth tongue swelling, and a change in colour (is paler if caused by pernicious anaemia).

34. **b.** IgA

The defences of the small intestine are in the most part due to T and B lymphocytes. The main type of antibody produced by intestinal B cells is IgA, the major immunoglobulin of external secretions. IgA prevents microorganisms from entering the gut lumen as it binds and neutralizes them directly without the need for other effector systems. A much smaller amount of IgM is also secreted by the intestinal B cells.

35. **a.** Cefotaxime

Pseudomembranous colitis is caused by an overgrowth of *Clostridium difficile*, a bacillus which is carried by 2% of the population, asymptomatically. It usually occurs post antibiotic therapy which suppresses the normal colonic flora allowing *C. difficile* to proliferate. Pseudomembranous colitis is associated mainly with broad-spectrum antibiotics; however cephalosporins are considered the highest-risk group. Cefotaxime is a third-generation cephalosporin antibiotic.

36. **a.** Tropical sprue

The symptoms of weight loss, diarrhoea and steatorrhea are classic symptoms for malabsorption. The colonoscopy findings of villous atrophy is suggestive initially of coeliac disease, however you would expect the patient's symptoms to improve with a gluten-free diet. Tropical sprue is a chronic, progressive malabsorption in patients from the tropics (mainly the West Indies and Asia) associated with abnormalities of small intestinal structure and function. It is thought to have an infective cause. Like coeliac disease, there is villous atrophy, although obviously a gluten-free diet is of no help. Treatment is with broad-spectrum antibiotics.

37. **e.** Colonoscopy

This history of a change in bowel habit for greater than 6 weeks with PR bleeding is one of the criteria of the NICE guidelines for an urgent 2-week referral for patients of any age. This should include an urgent colonoscopy and review by a colorectal surgeon.

38. **d.** Squamous cell carcinoma

Achalasia is a known risk factor for the development of squamous cell carcinoma of the oesophagus. This is thought to be caused by chronic inflammation and stasis within the oesophagus. Other risk factors for the development of squamous cell carcinoma are smoking, alcohol, tylosis and Plummer–Vinson Syndrome.

39. **b.** Sodium docusate

This patient's constipation has been caused by the strong opioids he is taking. His main problem is hard stools, so the first-line laxative should be a faecal softener. Sodium docusate is the only faecal softener in the answers given. If he is still having problems with constipation, then it would be appropriate to add in a different class of laxative.

40. **c.** Pernicious anaemia

The low haemoglobin and high MCV is indicative of macrocytic anaemia. Pernicious anaemia is the only answer given here that is a cause of macrocytic anaemia. Iron-deficient anaemia and thalassaemia are both causes of microcytic anaemia, whilst anaemia of chronic disease and haemolytic anaemia are causes of normocyctic anaemia.

EMQ answers

1 Diarrhoea

1. G. Pseudomembranous colitis is caused by the *Clostridium difficile* toxin. This is often associated with recent antibiotic use, including cephalosporins and penicillins. A separate *C. difficile*-specific stool sample has to be sent off to detect it.

2. B. Colon cancer needs to be considered in anyone over the age of 55 who presents with a change in bowel habit, weight loss and anaemia.

3. A. The history of diarrhoea with blood in her stools, suggests that the patient could have inflammatory bowel disease. With ulcerative colitis, smoking has a protective effect and some patients have their first acute attack of colitis once they have given up smoking.

4. I. This lady has a similar history to the lady in the question above, however there has been no PR bleeding or weight loss. Given the long duration of her symptoms the most likely diagnosis is irritable bowel syndrome.

5. H. This lady's history of weight loss with a good appetite, and an irregular pulse on examination point to thyrotoxicosis as the cause of her diarrhoea.

2 Vomiting

1. E. Hypercalcaemia may occur in patients with a history of cancer. It can cause a variety of symptoms, which can sometimes be grouped into 'moans, bones, groans and stones'.

2. C. History and examination is suggestive of small bowel obstruction, which is likely to be caused by adhesions from her previous surgery.

3. F. Rotovirus is a common cause of outbreaks of vomiting when there are several people in the same place, such as cruises, hospitals and schools.

4. G. Autonomic neuropathy can cause gastric dysmotility. Symptoms include vomiting and a sensation of early satiety, which occurs as a result of gastric emptying.

5. B. This short history of vomiting following a takeaway points to acute gastritis.

3 Acute abdominal pain

1. F. The very short history here favours ectopic pregnancy, and she also has evidence of significant intravascular loss. The differential here is appendicitis, however the onset is usually over a longer period of time, and the pain may initially start centrally.

2. D. Gallstones are one of the commonest causes of acute pancreatitis. The history of abdominal pain and vomiting support this. She has evidence of shock, which is likely to be the result of a metabolic acidosis.

3. G. The tinkling bowel sounds are diagnostic of obstruction. The vomiting suggests that the obstruction is high up in the gastrointestinal tract.

4. I. This pain is typical of duodenal ulcers where the pain is often eased by food, and gets worse throughout the night. In contrast, with gastric ulcers the pain tends to be precipitated by food.

5. B. The location of the pain and the raised WCC is suggestive of diverticulitis. This should be confirmed by CT scan.

4 Chronic abdominal pain

1. F. There is evidence of inflammation, and the site of pain suggests that it is of biliary origin. An abdominal ultrasound would be able to confirm this.

2. B. The raised GGT suggests alcohol excess. Exacerbations of chronic pancreatitis are often related to alcohol use. Pancreatic exocrine hyposecretion leads to steatorrhoea.

3. A. Patients should be investigated for gastric cancer if they have any of the following ALARMS symptoms (Anaemia, Loss of weight, Anorexia, Refractory to medications, Melaena, Swallowing problems).

4. D. Crohn's disease can present with all of the listed symptoms. Not all colitis initially presents with PR bleeding, and many patients just have constitutional symptoms.

5. H. Pancreatic carcinoma is often associated with severe abdominal pain radiating to the back along with significant weight loss.

5 Dysphagia

1. **D.** Oesophageal web is associated with Plummer–Vinson syndrome, which is associated with dysphagia and iron-deficient anaemia, which is suggested from the blood results.
2. **F.** Strictures are a complication of longstanding reflux disease. This is due to gastric acid causing damage to the mucosa. Surgical intervention is required.
3. **C.** This is a typical history of achalasia. The chest pain was caused by oesophageal spasms.
4. **E.** Oesophageal carcinoma needs to be excluded in patients with progressive dysphagia and significant weight loss.
5. **A.** This patient is immunosuppressed whilst having chemotherapy, which puts patients at risk for mucosal candidiasis.

6 Jaundice

1. **H.** The history and examination findings are consistent with infective mononucleosis. Atypical lymphocytes are common. Treatment is mainly supportive.
2. **D.** Painless jaundice is suggestive of carcinoma of the head of the pancreas. This would account for the ultrasound findings.
3. **G.** There is a crossover between ulcerative colitis and sclerosing cholangitis in 10% of patients. It is actually more common in males.
4. **E.** Severe, acute alcoholic hepatitis can cause hepatic encephalopathy. His macrocytic anaemia gives a clue that he drinks excess alcohol.
5. **C.** This patient has symptoms of cholestasis. The presence of right upper quadrant pain makes gallstone the most likely diagnosis.

Glossary

achalasia A condition in which the lower oesophageal sphincter goes into spasm and there is loss of coordinated peristalsis in the lower oesophagus

achlorhydria Absence of gastric hydrochloric acid

acinus A general definition is a sac or cavity surrounded by secretory cells of a gland. See individual chapters for more specialized definitions

ascites accumulation of fluid in the peritoneal cavity

asterixis A flapping tremor seen in liver disease or carbon dioxide retention when the hands are outstretched

atresia Congenital absence of a duct or opening

borborygmi Bowel sounds

cachexia Abnormally low weight with a wasted appearance and weakness, usually seen in chronic disease, e.g. malignancy

cholangiocarcinoma Carcinoma of the bile ducts

cholangitis Inflammation of the bile ducts

cholelithiasis Gallstone disease

cirrhosis A condition in which the liver undergoes nodular fibrosis in response to injury and/or cell death. A number of complications may ensue, including liver failure and portal hypertension

dysentery An infection of the gut causing severe bloody, mucoid diarrhoea

endoscopy Any investigation using an instrument (an endoscope) to view the inside of a body cavity, e.g. the gut. Examples include gastroscopy, proctoscopy and colonoscopy

ERCP Endoscopic retrograde cholangiopancreatography, a radiological diagnostic or therapeutic technique in which the pancreatic duct and bile ducts are visualized by passing a catheter through a duodenoscope into the ampulla of Vater and injecting a radio-opaque dye into the biliary tract. See also MRCP

faecaliths Small, hard masses of faeces which may cause obstruction, e.g. of the appendix

fistula An abnormal connection between two epithelium-lined surfaces, e.g. the gut and the bladder

glossitis Inflammation of the tongue

haustra The pouches on the external surface of the colon

melaena Faeces which are black and tarry due to the presence of partly digested blood originating from higher up the alimentary tract

mesentery A double layer of peritoneum which attaches an organ, or part of an organ, to the posterior abdominal wall and confers motility. Not all abdominal organs have mesenteries

MRCP Magnetic resonance cholangiopancreatography, a radiological diagnostic technique using magnetic resonance imaging to visualize the pancreatic duct and bile ducts. Unlike ERCP, it is not invasive and cannot be used for therapeutic purposes. See also ERCP

omentum A double layer of peritoneum attaching the stomach to other abdominal organs, e.g. the liver and large intestine. There are two omenta, the greater omentum and the lesser omentum

plicae circulares Circular folds in the small intestine which extend across its entire width and are visible on radiographs. Also known as valvulae conniventes or Kerckring's valves

porta hepatis The opening on the visceral surface of the liver through which its associated nerves and vessels (hepatic artery, portal vein, hepatic ducts and lymphatics) pass

portosystemic anastomosis A connection between the hepatic portal and systemic venous systems. They are not significant except in portal hypertension, in which they may distend and possibly bleed

pseudocyst A fluid-filled sac which is not covered by epithelium, e.g. a pancreatic pseudocyst (cf. a true cyst, which has an epithelial lining)

salivon The basic unit of a salivary gland

stenosis An abnormal narrowing of a tube or opening

stomatitis Ulceration of the oral mucosal surface

tenesmus The sensation of incomplete evacuation of the bowels, especially after defecation

volvulus Twisting of part of the intestine, which may lead to infarction or obstruction

Index

Note: Page numbers followed by *b* indicate boxes, *f* indicate figures and *ge* indicate glossary terms.